CRC Handbook
of
PAF and
PAF Antagonists

Editor

Pierre Braquet

Directeur General/Directeur de la Recherche
Institut Henri Beaufour
Le Plessis Robinson, France

CRC Press
Boca Raton   Ann Arbor   Boston

Library of Congress Cataloging-in-Publication Data

CRC handbook of PAF and PAF antagonists / editor, Pierre Braquet.

   p.   cm.

   Includes bibliographical references.

   Includes index

   ISBN (invalid) 0-8493-3524-3

   1. Platelet activation factor. 2. Platelet activating factor-
-Antagonists--Structure-activity relationships. I. Braquet, P.
(Pierre)

   [DNLM: 1. Platelet Activating Factor--antagonist & inhibitors.
2. Platelet Activating Factor--physiology. 3. Platelet Activation-
-physiology. QU 93 C911]

QP752.P62C73 1991

612.1′15--dc20

DNLM/DLC

for Library of Congress

90-15177
CIP

Direct all inquiries to CRC Press, Inc., 2000 Corporate Blvd., N.W., Boca Raton, Florida 33431.

© 1991 by CRC Press, Inc.

International Standard Book Number 0-8493-3524-3

Library of Congress Card Number 90-15177
Printed in the United States

PREFACE

PAF-acether is a phospholipid mediator of allergy and inflammation whose structure is 1-O-alkyl-2(R)-acetyl-glyceryl-3-phosphocholine. It originates from membrane ether lipid *via* the successive involvement of phospholipase A_2 (that generates the inactive precursor, lyso-PAF) and acetyltransferase, the latter enzyme being activated by a phosphorylation process. PAF-acether is inactivated by membrane and plasma acetylhydrolyse. PAF-acether is generated by various cell types such as polymorphonuclear (PMN) basophils, neutrophils, and eosinophils, monocytes/macrophages, platelets, endothelial cells, mast cells, and organs including kidney and heart.

In vitro, PAF-acether triggers platelet and PMN aggregation and degranulation, induces the generation of arachidonic acid metabolites from various cell types, and inhibits lymphocyte proliferation and interleukin 2 production. *In vivo*, PAF-acether causes bronchoconstriction, bronchial hyperreactivity to various agonists, hypotension, thrombocytopenia and leukopenia, increase in vascular permeability, gastrointestinal damages and acute renal failure. PAF-acether acts *via* specific binding sites present on platelet, neutrophil, and tissue membranes. Recently, several PAF-acether antagonists have been described including structure-related and -unrelated substances. Some of them, such as BN 52021 and BN 52063, are already in clinical trials as antiasthma drugs and extensive studies with these and newly developed compounds will help to determine the actual role of the mediator in health and diseases.

CONTRIBUTORS

Evelyne Audry
Laboratoire de Chimie Analytique
Faculté de Pharmacie
Bordeaux, France

Pierre Braquet
Directeur Général/Directeur de la Recherche
Institut Henri Beaufour
Le Plessis Robinson, France

Colette Broquet
Director, Department of Chemistry
Institut Henri Beaufour
Les Ulis, France

Jean-Claude Colleter
Laboratoire de Chimie Analytique
Faculté de Pharmacie
Bordeaux, France

F. Croizet
Laboratoire de Chimie Analytique
Faculté de Pharmacie
Bordeaux, France

Philippe Dallet
Laboratoire de Chimie Analytique
Faculté de Pharmacie
Bordeaux, France

J. P. Dubost
Professeur
Laboratoire de Chimie Analytique
Faculté de Pharmacie
Bordeaux, France

André Esanu
Institut Henri Beaufour
Le Plessis Robinson, France

Annie Etienne
Director, Department of Pharmacology
Institut Henri Beaufour
Les Ulis, France

Otto R. Gottlieb
Professor
Instituto de Química
Universidade de São Paulo
São Paulo, Brazil

Gunnar Grue-Sørensen
Chemical Research Department
Leo Pharmaceutical Products
Ballerup, Denmark

Masashi Hashimoto
Director of Exploratory Research Lab
Fujisawa Pharmaceutical Co.
Tsukuba, Ibaraki, Japan

Keiji Hemmi
Head of Chemistry
Exploratory Research Lab
Fujisawa Pharmaceutical Co.
Tsukuba, Ibaraki, Japan

Hubert O. Heuer
Head of Laboratory
Department of Pharmacology
Boehringer Ingelheim KG
Ingelheim/Rhein, Germany

David Hosford
Director of Communications
Institut Henri Beaufour
Le Plessis Robinson, France

William J. Houlihan
Director, Chemical Research
Sandoz Pharmaceuticals
East Hanover, New Jersey

Matyas Koltai
Institut Henri Beaufour
Le Plessis Robinson, France

Marie-Hélène Langlois
Laboratoire de Chimie Analytique
Faculté de Pharmacie
Bordeaux, France

Daniel Lavé
Département de Chimie
Centre de Recherches de Vitry
Rhône-Poulenc Santé
Vitry sur Seine, France

Jean-Michel Mencia-Huerta
Director, Department of Immunology
Institut Henri Beaufour
Les Ulis, France

Christian Kaergaard Nielsen
Department of Pharmacology
Leo Pharmaccutical Products
Ballerup, Denmark

Margaret O'Donnell
Department of Pharmacology
  and Chemotherapy
Hoffmann La Roche
Nutley, New Jersey

Masanori Okamoto
Head, Allergy and Inflammation Research
Exploratory Research Lab
Fujisawa Pharmaceutical Co.
Tsukuba, Ibaraki, Japan

Bernadette Pignol
Head of Laboratory
Department of Immunology
Institut Henri Beaufour
Les Ulis, France

Paulete Romoff
Instituto de Química
Universidade de São Paulo
São Paulo, Brazil

Ichiro Shima
Researcher of Chemistry
Exploratory Research Lab
Fujusawa Pharmaceutical Co.
Tsukuba, Ibaraki, Japan

Norihiko Shimazaki
Researcher of Chemistry
Exploratory Research Lab
Fujisawa Pharmaceutical Co.
Tsukuba, Ibaraki, Japan

Muneo Takatani
Research Scientist
Chemistry Research Laboratories
Takeda Chemical Industries, Ltd.
Osaka, Japan

Jefferson W. Tilley
Research Leader
Chemistry Research Department
Hoffmann La Roche
Nutley, New Jersey

Caroline Touvay
Head of Laboratory
Department of Immunology
Institut Henri Beaufour
Les Ulis, France

Susumu Tsushima
Research Head
Chemistry Research Laboratories
Takeda Chemical Industries, Ltd.
Osaka, Japan

Keizo Yoshida
Head of Pharmacology
New Drug Research Lab
Fujisawa Pharmaceutical Co.
Osaka, Japan

Massayoshi Yoshida
Instituto de Química
Universidade de São Paulo
São Paulo, Brazil

TABLE OF CONTENTS

PART I: NATURAL PAF ANTAGONISTS

PART II: SYNTHETIC PAF ANTAGONISTS

PART III: MOLECULAR MODELING

Part I
Natural PAF Antagonists

Chapter 1

RECENT PROGRESS IN PAF ANTAGONIST RESEARCH

Matyas Koltai, David Hosford, André Esanu, and Pierre Braquet

INTRODUCTION

From the discovery of platelet activating factor (PAF, 1-O-alkyl-2-(R)acetyl-*sn*-glyceryl-3-phosphocholine) in the early 1970s, increasing attention has been paid to its antagonists, including natural and synthetic compounds (see for review References 1 and 2) which have been proposed as potential therapeutic agents for the treatment of immunological[3] and inflammatory disorders.[4] The chemical structure of natural PAF antagonists in relation to their biological activity has been recently reviewed.[5]

The application of selective PAF receptor antagonists in experimental research has greatly facilitated extensive accumulation of knowledge on the pathophysiological significance of PAF.[1] Besides the great variety of pathological alterations attributed to the phospholipid mediator, PAF has recently been implicated as a signal molecule in quite a few important physiological feedback mechanisms as well.

This review intends to summarize recent progress in the research of various PAF antagonists achieved in the last 2 or 3 years since the publication of the latest extensive reviews.[1-4] This period may be characterized by the abundance of data concerning the involvement of PAF in the function of various organs and the presence of PAF receptors in cell membranes. Therefore, the considerable part of the review is devoted to the description of PAF effects in various pathophysiological states. The number of natural and synthetic PAF receptor antagonists is also remarkable. On the other hand, none of them have developed as clinically used therapeutic agents, although experimental data are in favor of their clinical application.

The basic molecular mode of action of PAF and its antagonists has been recently summarized,[1,2] indicating that the phospholipid mediator exerts multiple effects, such as inhibition of adenylate cyclase with a concomitant decrease in cellular cyclic adenosine monophosphate (cAMP) level, promotion of arachidonic acid (AA) release, phosphoinositide turnover, increased activity of protein kinase C (PKC) leading to enhanced activity of the Na^+/H^+ antiport, induction of $^{45}Ca^{2+}$ and $^{86}Rb^+$ fluxes, transient depolarization, and an increase in the level of cytoskeletal actin in various cellular systems. These effects can be antagonized by specific PAF receptor antagonists. The capability of the antagonists of interfering with these biologically and pathophysiologically important processes has been confirmed by recent experiments and implicated in a great variety of *in vitro* and *in vivo* biological models. The most important recent progress in the field of PAF research is the recognition of PAF/cytokine interaction as one of the basic cellular mechanisms in the action of the phospholipid mediator. The development of this concept and its application in different pathological conditions are also overviewed. This review is not devoted to summarizing the chemistry of different PAF antagonists and structure activity relationships. In respect of the chemistry, biology, and pharmacology of natural compounds, the reader is referred to a recent review.[5] Concerning the chemical structures of the natural and synthetic PAF antagonists mentioned in the text as well as their classification, the reader is referred to the Appendix. The numbers in bold parentheses refer to the chemical structure of the compounds listed in the Appendix.

PAF AND PAF ANTAGONISTS IN PLATELET FUNCTION AND THROMBOSIS

Platelets have been in the focus of interest in PAF research. The interaction between PAF antagonists and platelets is extensively studied and reviewed.[1,2] New progress in this field is outlined below.

PAF AND ITS RECEPTORS IN PLATELET FUNCTION ASSESSED BY PAF ANTAGONISTS

Although PAF has been known to be generated by a wide variety of cells and tissues, its involvement in various platelet functions is still the subject of intensive research.

In canine platelet membranes, ^{3}H-PAF labels a single population of binding sites in a saturable and reversible manner. The affinity of this binding and the density of binding sites were found to be high.[6] ^{3}H-PAF binding was entirely reversed by unlabeled PAF and exhibited stereoselective discrimination. Furthermore, the displacing potency of the (+)-enantiomer of the PAF antagonist 52770 RP (**9b**) was 45 times higher than that of the (−)-enantiomer. ^{3}H-PAF binding displayed a remarkable specificity in that it was not affected by a variety of classical pharmacological agents; however, it was displayed by several PAF receptor antagonists, such as 5922 RP, CV-6209 (**2**), Ro 19-3704 (**3c**), 52770 RP, brotizolam (**11**), WEB 2086 (**12**), SRI 63-441 (**6a**), L-652,731 (**17**), alprazolam (**10a**), triazolam (**10b**), and BN 52021 (**15**). An analysis of comparing binding affinity and biological activity assessed on washed canine platelets revealed the existence of a highly specific correlation. A photoreactive, radioiodinated derivative of PAF, i.e., 1-O-(4-azido-2-hydroxy-3-iodobenzamido)undecyl-2-O-acetyl-*sn*-glycero-3 phosphocholine (^{125}I-AAGP) was synthesized and used as photoaffinity probe to study the PAF binding sites in rabbit platelet membranes.[7] The nonradioactive analog, IAAGP, induced platelet aggregation. ^{125}I-AAGP was specifically bound to rabbit platelet membranes which then showed several ^{125}I-labeled components by sodium dodecyl sulfate-polyacrylamide gel electrophoresis. A protein species with apparent molecular weight of 52,000 was consistently observed and inhibited specifically by unlabeled PAF at nanomolar concentrations. The labeling was specific since PAF antagonists SRI 63,675 and L-652,731 blocked the appearance of this band. These results suggest that the binding sites of PAF receptor in rabbit platelets reside in the polypeptide of M_r = 52,000. Another study was devoted to establishing whether binding of PAF to its receptor was integral to the stimulation of phosphoinositide-specific phospholipase C (PLC) in rabbit platelets.[8] Saturation binding curves for ^{3}H-PAF were obtained (K_D = 28.72 nM). In comparison, PAF-stimulated PLC activity, as monitored by [3H]-inositol triphosphate production, increased at lower concentrations (EC_{50} = 1.5 nM. Unlabeled PAF inhibited [3H]-PAF binding competitively and demonstrated two binding sites (high and low affinity sites). The inhibitory effects of four PAF antagonists, CV-3988 (**1**), CV-6209, SRI 63-441, and SRI 63-675 on the binding of [3H]-PAF were almost complete, whereas their ability to inhibit PAF-stimulated PLC activity varied. The most potent at inhibiting [3H]-PAF binding was CV-6209, while for inhibition of PLC activity, SRI 63-441 and SRI 63-675 were the most effective.

In a recent study by Dive et al.,[9] three-dimensional electrostatic maps were calculated for six potent antagonists of PAF selected for their apparent structural heterogeneity. The molecules were ginkgolides BN 52020, BN 52021, and BN 52022, the semi-rigid kadsurenone (**16**), a flexible synthetic di*nor* type C furanoid lignan L-652,731 and the triazolothienobenzodiazepine WEB 2086. Calculation of the electrostatic potential generated around all of the above molecules showed the existence of two wells of negative potential or "earmuffs". The molecules also presented a moderate hydrophobic fragment which constitutes a third point of interaction with high affinity binding sites in rabbit and human platelets. These findings suggest that this high affinity acceptor site may be a "polarized cylinder".

To clarify the nature of the interaction of octylonium bromide with PAF receptors, saturation studies of [^{3}H]-PAF binding were made.[10] For comparison, L-652,731 was used. The binding behavior of octylium bromide and L-652,731 indicated that both compounds inhibit competitively the binding of [^{3}H]-PAF to its receptors.

INVOLVEMENT OF PAF IN PLATELET AGGREGATION

The effect of various PAF antagonists on PAF- and adrenalin-induced platelet aggregation was studied.[11] Two non-lipid antagonists, BN 52021 and WEB 2086, at concentrations which completely blocked PAF-induced platelet aggregation, failed to interfere with aggregation by adrenalin. In contrast, Ro 19-3704, a structurally related antagonist of PAF, inhibited concentration-dependently the aggregation induced by adrenalin or by the simultaneous addition of submaximal concentrations of adrenalin and PAF. Reversal of aggregation was obtained when Ro 19-3704 was added to the platelet suspension after adrenalin. Ro 19-3704 was selective for PAF and adrenalin, since it failed to interfere with platelet aggregation induced by AA or adenosine diphosphate (ADP). CV-3988 (1), an antagonist of PAF structurally similar to Ro 19-3704, showed similar activity, while a morpholine analog of PAF having no PAF-like activity failed to interfere with the aggregation induced by adrenalin. Experiments on plasma membrane preparations showed that Ro 19-3704 inhibited ^{3}H-yohimbine binding, in contrast to BN 52021 and the morpholine analog of PAF. This interaction with specific α_2-adrenoceptors seems to be involved as an early step in the mechanism of adrenalin-induced platelet activation.

PAF ANTAGONISTS IN PLATELET AGGREGATION

As important and specific pharmacological tools, PAF antagonists have been widely used for the determination of basic pathophysiological phenomena involved in platelet activation, like identification of specific receptor binding sites,[7] importance of enzymes, e.g., PLC,[8] or significance of specifically triggered pathways in the effect of various autacoids.[11] PAF-induced mobilization of cytosolic free calcium from human platelets and neutrophils as measured by the selective fluorescent indicators of fura-2 and quin 2 was used to assess the effect of specific PAF receptor antagonists, such as L-652,731, kadsurenone, triazolam and alprazolam and the effects were compared to that of diltiazem.[12] In decreasing order of potency was L-652,731, kadsurenone, triazolam, diltiazem and alprazolam in platelets and the antagonists were found to be 7 to 20 times less active in polymorphonuclear leukocytes (PMNL). The results indicate that calcium mobilization can provide a rapid, sensitive and quantitative method for the evaluation of the effects of either agonists or antagonists. Shukla et al.[13] have studied PAF-stimulated protein phosphorylation in ^{32}P-labeled rabbit platelets. Both PAF and thrombin caused a rapid increase followed by a decrease in phosphorylation of several proteins with apparent molecular weights of 20,000, 35,000, 40,000, 65,000, and 150,000. Four separate PAF antagonists drastically reduced PAF response, but did not influence that induced by thrombin. The order of potency was SRI 63-675>SRI 63-441 = CV-6209>CV-3988. There was a homologous desensitization of protein phosphorylation when repeated exposures to PAF were applied, but not when PAF stimulation was followed by thrombin. On the other hand, a lack of protein phosphorylation by PAF or thrombin was observed in platelets pre-exposed to thrombin, demonstrating a heterologous desensitization. These results indicate that phosphorylation of proteins by PAF is a PAF receptor coupled event and that this process is desensitized in platelets pre-exposed to PAF. The fact that both the activation of phosphoinositide-specific PLC and the phosphorylation of proteins are desensitized in PAF-pretreated platelets suggests that a close "regulatory" intercommunication exists between these processes.

Beyond these theoretical aspects, some practical reasons, such as the determination of relative potency, selectivity, and the exact pharmacological profile of various PAF antagonists have become of interest to facilitate the eventual clinical application of these drugs.

O'Donnel and Barnett[14] have studied nine different PAF antagonists to determine their relative potency and equilibrium dissociation constants on rabbit platelets as assessed by the aggregatory response induced by PAF. Log concentration-response curves to PAF were found to be shifted to the right, and the slopes of the Schild plots suggested that the drugs were competitive inhibitors of PAF. The order of magnitude of pA_2 values were as follows: WEB 2086>SRI 63-119 **(3a)**>L-652,731>BN 52021>SRI 63-072 **(5)**>CV-3988 >48740 RP **(9a)**>ketotifen>thiazinamium, indicating that WEB 2086 is the most effective drug among the agents studied. For the first time, these experiments have provided some functional response data for PAF antagonists which are appropriate forms for use in classifying putative PAF receptors and comparative potencies. From these results and toxicity data, the possible therapeutic value of either drug can be specified. In a similar careful pharmacological analysis, the IC_{50} values of different PAF antagonists were compared with a PAF-induced [^{3}H]serotonin release assay.[15] The results obtained showed that the order of magnitude of potency for BN 50739 **(14)**, a new, selective hetrazepine-type PAF antagonist, was higher than WEB 2086, therefore suggesting that it is the most potent agent discovered up to now. The high efficacy of BN 50739 was also confirmed by its protective effect against PAF-induced hypotension in anesthetized rats. Alternatively, BN 50739 was studied in PAF-induced rabbit platelet aggregation *in vivo* and *ex vivo*,[16] and similar results were obtained.

PAF ANTAGONISTS IN THROMBOSIS AND HEMOSTASIS

In comparison to platelet activation, the relationship of PAF to thrombogenesis and other parameters of hemostasis was the subject of relatively few publications.

Weichert and Breddin[17] have reported that N 48740 RP, a pyrrolo(1,2-c)thiazole derivative known to inhibit the effects of PAF, produced a dose-dependent antithrombotic effect in a thrombosis model, in which thrombi produced in small rat mesenteric vessels were assessed by a phase contrast Leitz Orthoplan microscope. Thrombus formation was produced with a Coherent CR-2 supergraphite ion laser (argon laser) in vessels of 25 to 35 μm diameter. This highly developed technique allowed them to study the very initial steps of thrombus formation. As recognized previously, in an *in vitro* system nanomolar concentrations of PAF are able to release of tissue-type plasminogen activator from vascular endothelial cells through a calcium-dependent mechanism which involves phospholipase A_2 (PLA_2) activation and release of arachidonate metabolites. Moreover, when administered intravenously PAF increased fibrinolytic activity in the rat blood. In a recent study, the effect of BN 52021 on PAF-induced changes in fibrinolytic activity was studied in two pharmacological models, *in vivo* in rats and in the isolated perfused pig ear preparation.[18] PAF but not lyso-PAF resulted in a rapid, transient increase in blood fibrinolytic activity in rats. This effect was dose-dependently diminished by BN 52021. The dependence of fibrinolysis on plasminogen activator was measured in fibrin plates prepared with use of both plasminogen-rich and plasminogen-free fibrinogen. BN 52021 was capable of inhibiting tissue plasminogen activator release induced by PAF in both preparations used. This study emphasizes the significance of PAF in blood homeostasis.

EFFECT OF PAF ANTAGONISTS ON POLYMORPHONUCLEAR LEUKOCYTES

PAF RECEPTORS IN POLYMORPHONUCLEAR LEUKOCYTES

PAF acts at specific receptor sites in various cells.[19] By using three specific PAF receptor antagonists, WEB 2086 **(12)**, L-652,631 **(17)**, and BN 52021 **(15)**, in assay systems of PAF-induced aggregation of guinea pigs and rabbits platelets and PMNL as well as PAF-induced PGI_2 generation in guinea pig resident peritoneal macrophages, the presence of PAF receptors was demonstrated.[20] The rank order of potency calculated by the pA_2 values for rabbit platelets and PMNL was WEB 2086 = L-652,731>BN 52021 and was the same for the two cell types. On guinea pig resident macrophages WEB 2086 was tenfold less potent for receptor mediating increased generation of 6-keto-PGF$_{1\alpha}$ than those mediating platelet aggregation. Basal PGI$_2$ production was inhibited by PAF antagonists, but the calcium ionophore A23187-induced generation was unaffected. These results confirm the presence of PAF receptors in PMNL and raise the possibility that there may be a PAF receptor-subtype mediating PGI$_2$ generation.

The antagonism of PAF effects by WEB 2086 assessed by PAF-induced β-glucuronidase release and the receptor binding of [^{3}H]WEB 2086 was investigated in isolated human PMNL.[21] Close concordance between affinity constants for WEB 2086 from functional and radioligand-binding studies suggests that WEB 2086 interacts with the neutrophil PAF receptors and that [^{3}H]WEB may be a useful ligand in investigation of these receptors. Evidence for the existence and ionic modulation of PAF receptors mediating degranulatory responses in human PMNL was recently demonstrated.[22] PAF-induced elastase release from azurophilic granules was completely inhibited by RP 59227 (**9b**), a potent, *d*-enantiomeric PAF antagonist. PAF-induced elastase extrusion was enhanced by physiological concentrations of CaCl$_2$ and MgCl$_2$. These ions were capable of enhancing the number of [^{3}H]PAF binding sites in whole or lysed PMNL without affecting the affinity of the ligand. This suggests an intervention at the level of the signal transduction system leading to degranulation, and provides evidence that calcium and magnesium concentrations in biological fluids modulate PAF receptor density and the associated responses.

MOLECULAR MECHANISM OF PAF RELEASE FROM PMNL

The role of calcium in formation and action of PAF has been extensively studied. PAF has been demonstrated to be able to enhance the release of newly synthesized PAF as measured by [^{3}H]acetate incorporation into PAF in human neutrophils.[23] The response was dose-dependent, rapid, transient and inhibitable by BN 52021. The non-metabolizable bioactive PAF analog (C-PAF), but not lyso-PAF, enhanced the release of newly synthesized PAF. Formyl-methyonyl-leucyl-phenylalanine (fMLP) also stimulated this *de novo* PAF generation. The stimulated PAF release was potentiated by granulocyte-monocyte colony stimulating factor (GM-CSF). The intracellular calcium chelator BAPTA inhibited the rise of intracellular calcium and the release of PAF but not the Na$^+$/H$^+$ antiport activity. PAF release, but not the rise in the intracellular free calcium concentration, was inhibited in pertussis toxin-treated neutrophils stimulated with PAF. The release of PAF in pertussis toxin-treated cells was also inhibited in cells stimulated with fMLP or opsonized zymosan. These results suggest that functional pertussis toxin-sensitive guanine nucleotide regulatory protein and/or one or more of the changes produced by PLC activation are necessary for PAF release produced by physiological stimuli. It appears that PAF release requires a coordinated action of receptor-coupled G-proteins, calcium, and other parameters. Addition of opsonized particles to human neutrophils in suspension leads to a biphasic elevation in the cytosolic free calcium concentration. The rise in intracellular calcium during the second phase is pronounced, in contrast to the rise during the first phase, which is relatively small. The second and large rise in intracellular calcium is brought about by messenger(s) released from cells after addition of opsonized particles. This second rise was not observed in the presence of WEB 2086, indicating that PAF can act as an intracellular messenger affecting calcium homeostasis in human PMNL. The use of the sensitive photoprotein aequorin as a calcium indicator in human PMNL not pretreated with cytochalasin B and stimulated with PAF was used to cast more light on the relative importance of intracellular and extracellular calcium in PMNL function.[25] PAF elicited a concentration-dependent calcium mobilization from PMNL which was abolished by EGTA, suggesting that almost all calcium mobilized by PAF derived from the external medium. Aggregation, enzyme release and leukotriene B$_4$ (LTB$_4$) synthesis, but only a weak stimulus for superoxide anion production, which paralleled calcium mobilization, were triggered by PAF, suggesting an important role for the lipid mediator in neutrophil activation. The effects of PAF were tested in an experimental *in vitro* model suitable for studying the modulatory activity of PMNL on platelet function.[25,26] Platelets were loaded with the calcium sensitive photoprotein aequorin and stimulated by PAF in the presence of autologous PMNL in the platelet ionized calcium aggregometer. Aggregation and luminescence peaks related to cytoplasmic calcium movements were simultaneously recorded in response to PAF.[27] Separate platelet and PMNL suspensions were poorly aggregated, while mixed cellular suspensions showed an amplified aggregatory response. PAF induced a concentration-dependent increase of calcium mobilization in aequorin-loaded platelets. The presence of PAF further increased the calcium release. Platelet thromboxane B_2 (TXB_2) production was also increased in the presence of PMNL. BN 52021 inhibited PAF-induced calcium mobilization, aggregation and TXB_4 production in a dose-dependent manner. In PAF-stimulated mixed cellular suspensions, BN 52021 not only prevented the effect of PAF but possibly blocked the generation and the subsequent release from PMNL of several important mediators that are involved in the PMNL-dependent amplification of platelet activation.

PAF AND PRODUCTION OF EDRF BY NEUTROPHILS

Vascular endothelial cells and neutrophils synthesize and release potent vasodilatory factors, i.e., endothelium-derived relaxing factor (EDRF) and neutrophil-derived relaxing factor (NDRF). One EDRF has been identified as nitric oxide (NO) derived from arginine. Since endothelial cells can be damaged in the presence of activated PMNL, it was recently studied whether PAF could exacerbate neutrophil-induced injury to endothelium-dependent relaxation.[28] Rat aortic rings were precontracted with $PGF_{2\alpha}$ and before addition of unstimulated canine neutrophils or cells stimulated with fMLP in the presence of cytochalasin B, acetylcholine produced maximum relaxation which was moderately decreased by both types of cells. Preincubation of stimulated cells with PAF unmasked injury of endothelium-dependent relaxation to acetylcholine but not to nitroglycerin. Facilitation of this impaired response to acetylcholine by PAF-primed neutrophils was blocked by either the PAF antagonists CV-3988 (1) or catalase. Thus, PAF primes PMNL, resulting in an enhanced impairment of EDRF production by a PAF-mediated process which involves oxygen derived free radicals.

INTERACTION BETWEEN CYTOKINES AND PAF ON NEUTROPHIL FUNCTION

Human blood PMNL and monocytes are known to generate reactive oxygen free radicals under appropriate conditions. Various cytokines, such as tumor necrosis factor (TNF) and γ-interferon have been shown to induce release of oxygen free radicals and PAF. The question whether PAF contributed to the respiratory burst generation induced by these two cytokines was recently investigated.[29] Human recombinant TNF and γ-interferon induced the release of superoxide anion from both PMNL and monocytes in a dose- and time-dependent manner. The free radical generation was greater in PMNL than in monocytes. Concomitant addition of these two cytokines induced superoxide anion generation less than predicted. Preincubation of PMNL and monocytes with BN 52021 and WEB 2086 markedly inhibited superoxide generation induced by TNF and γ-interferon, indicating the involvement of PAF in the phenomenon. The possible involvement of G proteins in the priming by TNFα of PAF-induced superoxide production in human PMNL was studied by Braquet et al.[30] PAF alone failed to evoke any superoxide anion production; however, preincubation with PAF significantly enhanced TNF-induced superoxide generation relative to that induced by the cytokine alone. Two structurally unrelated PAF antagonists, BN 52021 and BN 52111 (7) completely abolished this effect. Furthermore, these agents also induced a marked decrease in superoxide anion production elicited solely by TNF, indicating that this effect of TNF is partially mediated by a mechanism involving endogenous PAF. Pretreatment of PMNL with pertussis or cholera toxin reduced the amplification of superoxide production induced by PAF in TNF-stimulated PMNL. Thus, it seems that these inducers of G proteins are involved in the biochemical mechanism of the amplification process.

Incubation of human neutrophils with PAF stimulated the release of LTB_4 and its o-oxidation products.[31] Pretreatment of PMNL with GM-CSF enhanced, while BN 52021 dose-dependently inhibited this response, confirming that the synthesis of LTs was induced by an interaction between PAF and its cell surface receptor.

INVOLVEMENT OF PAF IN PMNL CHEMOTAXIS AND BACTERIAL KILLING

Inflammatory cells are thought to contribute actively to the pathogenesis of asthma since they infiltrate into the lung tissue. These cells are mobilized by lipid-like and protein-like chemotactic factors. In a recent study, PAF was found to induce a dose-dependent chemotaxis of human PMNL isolated from both healthy subjects and allergic asthmatics.[32] BN 52020, BN 52021 and BN 52022 inhibited PAF-induced neutrophil chemotaxis in both groups in a dose-dependent fashion, but failed to inhibit fMLP- and LTB_4-induced chemotactic responses. The migration of human PMNL was inhibited by PAF and agents inducing PAF production, such as PLA_2 from human monocytes and bee venom, or opsonized zymosan, as measured by capillary tube assay.[33] All these responses were inhibited by the specific PAF receptor antagonist BN 52021, indicating an important role for PAF in PMNL migration.

The *Candida albicans* killing activity of circulating PMNL was enhanced in healthy volunteers subjected to whole-body ultraviolet irradiation[34] and was inhibited by indomethacin treatment. The sera of irradiated patients enhanced the killing activity of granulocytes obtained from untreated individuals. This transfer system was blocked by BN 52021. When guinea pig bone marrow cells were incubated in the presence of PAF, the killing of *Candida parapsilosis* was augmented, and this activity was inhibited by PAF antagonists, CV-6209 (**2**) or FR900452 (**19**).[35] Phagocytosis was shown to be strictly dependent on the availability of CR_1 receptors on the red blood cells and phagocytes.[36] BN 52021 inhibited PAF-induced increase of CR_1-mediated erythrophagocytosis.

PAF ANTAGONISTS ON MACROPHAGES-MONOCYTES

PAF RECEPTORS ON MACROPHAGES

PAF binding by eight murine and human cell lines was analyzed, and only the murine $P388D_1$ macrophage line exhibited specific, high affinity PAF binding sites.[37] Minimal PAF metabolism was observed at the time when binding saturation was achieved. PAF binding reached saturation within 10 min at room temperature and was irreversible. Scatchard analysis of PAF binding revealed a single class of PAF receptors which had a dissociation constant of 0.08 nM. PAF binding was stereospecific, required an *sn*-2 acetyl substituent, and was inhibited by structurally diverse PAF antagonists, including kadsurenone, BN 52021 (**15**), triazolam (**10b**) and CV-3988 (**1**). PAF binding to these receptors resulted in an increase in intracellular free calcium levels in a dose-related manner. These studies demonstrate that macrophages have functional PAF receptors whose affinity and structural specificities are similar to PAF receptors located in other cells. These results were confirmed by Steward and Dusting[20] in guinea pig resident peritoneal macrophages.

The effects of alprazolam, BN 52021, kadsurenone (**16**), L-652,731 (**17**) and SRI 63-119 (**3a**) were studied on PAF-induced chemoluminescence of guinea-pig, *C. parvum*-activated peritoneal macrophages *in vitro*.[38] All antagonists produced a shift to the right in the dose-response curve to PAF. Schild plots for BN 52021, L-652,731, kadsurenone and SRI 63-119 were linear, but only for BN 52021 and kadsurenone did the mean slope not differ significantly from unity. The order of potency was L-652,731 > kadsurenone = BN 52021 > alprazolam (**10a**) > SRI 63-119. The affinity of BN 52021 and kadsurenone for macrophage PAF receptors remained relatively constant irrespective of the activation state of the cells; therefore, this process does not seem to have a role in the expression of macrophage PAF binding sites.

THE ROLE OF PAF IN THE FUNCTIONAL STATE OF MACROPHAGES

As described by Elstad et al.[39] upon stimulation, synthesis and release of PAF can be detected in human mononuclear phagocytes. After adherence for 24 or 48 h mouse peritoneal macrophages, upon a zymosan challenge, synthesized less PAF than that produced by a short term adherence, indicating that adherence inhibited PAF generation. At the same time, adhered cells further synthesized LTC_4. Indomethacin, nordihydroguaieretic acid (NDGA), and BW755C did not alter PAF production; therefore, the inhibitory effect of AA metabolites could be excluded. The enzymatic steps which govern PAF synthesis was also studied. The anabolic process was not shown to be impaired, since the amounts of alkylacylglycero-phosphocholine and lyso-PAF were similar after a short or long adherence of the cells. Addition of synthetic lyso-PAF or acetyl-CoA to intact cells did not increase PAF production in zymosan-stimulated 24 and 48-h-adherent macrophages. The basal level of acetyltransferase was comparable in adherent macrophages at all time intervals studied, and was increased by zymosan challenge.

PAF was demonstrated to modify human peritoneal macrophage cAMP levels in a concentration-dependent manner, showing peak accumulation at $10^{-8}\ M$, then a decline at higher concentrations.[40] Human peripheral blood mononuclear leukocytes were labeled with [^{3}H]inositol to study whether PAF could stimulate phosphoinositol hydrolysis.[41] PAF induced phosphatidylinositol hydrolysis and inositol-1,4,5- triphosphate (IP_3) formation in a dose-related manner. The response was rapid and transient and paralleled the time course of PAF-induced calcium mobilization in the same cells; however, the doses of PAF for inducing IP_3 formation were much higher than those for calcium mobilization. Furthermore, PAF-induced IP_3 formation was inhibited by L-659,989 (**18**), but was not altered by pertussis toxin or cholera toxin. These data suggest that PAF receptors in human peripheral blood mononuclears may be coupled through a pertussis toxin-insensitive guanine nucleotide binding protein to a phosphoinositide-specific PLC. Human U937 cells of committed monocytic origin were used to study the PAF-induced increase of the intracellular calcium concentration using the fluorescence probe fure-2.[42] The naturally occurring stereoisomer (R)PAF and the stable, less hydrolyzable racemic analog PR1501 produced dose-related and rapid elevation of intracellular calcium concentrations. The unnatural stereoisomer (S) and the natural stereoisomer lyso-(R)PAF had no effect. LTB_4 also increased intracellular calcium but the responses were smaller and of shorter duration than those induced by PAF. The order of potency of the PAF antagonists studied was WEB 2086 (**12**) > Ro 19-3704 (**3c**) > L-652,731 > BN 52021 > CV-3988 in respect of the inhibition of suboptimal PAF-induced increase in intracellular calcium levels. In another study on U-937 cells,[43] CV-3988 but not calcium channel blockers inhibited the effect of PAF on phosphatidylinositide metabolism and intracellular calcium mobilization.

INVOLVEMENT OF PAF AND EICOSANOIDS IN MACROPHAGE FUNCTION

Adherent guinea pig alveolar macrophages were stimulated by fMLP *in vitro* and the consecutive release of PAF and various eicosanoids were measured to assess the role of cellular eicosanoid secretion in the release of PAF.[44] Indomethacin suppressed TXB_2 generation, BW A137C, a selective lipoxygenase inhibitor, abolished LTB_4 secretion, while none of these drugs influenced PAF release, indicating that fMLP-induced PAF release is independent of eicosanoid generation. Alternatively, eicosanoid generation appeared to be dependent on intracellular PAF concentration in guinea pig resident peritoneal macrophages.[45] Adherent macrophages contained cell-associated PAF whose level was increased by fMLP, endotoxin and ionophore A23187; however, only endotoxin and A23187 caused release of detectable amounts of PAF into the extracellular medium. Exogenous PAF and each of the above stimuli increased PGI_2 generation in resident macrophages. WEB 2086 (**12**) and CV-6209 (**2**) reduced both basal and stimulated PGI_2 generation; in addition, WEB 2086 inhibited fMLP- and PAF-induced superoxide anion generation as well. Responses to A23187 were not inhibited by either antagonist. Nanomolar concentrations of PAF were described as stimulators of LT synthesis in human monocytes.[46] LTB_4 and peptido-LT production was time- and concentration-dependent, and associated with a receptor-mediated mechanism, since BN 52021 and WEB 2086 prevented the response.

The formation of eicosanoids may be a primary route through which PAF exerts its effects during endotoxemia. Morris and Moore[47] have studied whether PAF could stimulate equine macrophage release of TXB_2 and PGI_2. Peritoneal macrophages were cultured from clinically normal horses and exposed to various concentrations of PAF, endotoxin and SRI 63-441 (**6a**). The media concentrations of TXB_2 were significantly increased above baseline after treatment of macrophages with PAF and endotoxin. TXA_2 release by endotoxin was not prevented by prior treatment of macrophages with SRI 63-441, and even the PAF receptor antagonist enhanced macrophage TXA_2 and PGI_2 synthesis, suggesting that PAF may cause increased TXA_2 release during endotoxemia which may not be preventable by SRI 63-441. These results should be confirmed by other PAF antagonists.

PAF INTERACTS WITH CYTOKINES IN MACROPHAGES

When rat alveolar macrophages were cultured with PAF alone, no change in TNF production was observed;[48] however, the concomitant addition of PAF and muramyl dipeptide to cell cultures markedly enhanced TNF production. Stimulation of TNF production by PAF was blocked by structurally different specific PAF receptor antagonists, BN 52021, CV-3988 and WEB 2086. (S)PAF and lyso-PAF failed to induce significant enhancement in TNF production. In parallel, addition of PAF to alveolar macrophages triggered LTB_4 release in a concentration-dependent manner. Inhibition of 5-lipoxygenase by NDGA or AA-861 blocked both TNF and LTB_4 production induced by PAF, while exogenous LTB_4 partially reversed the blockade, indicating the involvement of endogenous 5-lipoxygenase activity in PAF-induced TNF production. The production of TNFα by human platelet-free monocytes, isolated by conterflow elutriation, was analyzed following stimulation with endotoxin in the absence or presence of graded concentration ranges of PAF.[49] Two concentration ranges showed significant increase in TNF production. A major enhancement was observed at 10^{-8} to 10^{-6} M which was blocked by BN 52021, while a second enhancement was seen at 10^{-15} to 10^{-14} M PAF which was insensitive to BN 52021. These results suggest that PAF can directly modulate cytokine production by human monocytes through interacting with two types of receptors of different affinity and structure. This interesting contribution should be further studied by other specific PAF receptor antagonists.

The effects of PAF in the induction and priming for TNF secretion in peripheral blood monocytes have recently been studied.[50,51] Unlike γ-interferon and endotoxin, the addition of PAF to freshly isolated monocytes triggered rapid, concentration-dependent TNF secretion in the absence of induction of macrophage-mediated cytotoxicity. While biologically active and cytotoxic TNF was detected early after PAF addition, the cytotoxic activity declined thereafter though the antigenic activity remained constant. Monocytes primed with PAF responded by secreting TNF to both pokeweed mitogen and concanavalin A, representing unspecific stimuli, but responded poorly to specific stimulation by PAF, endotoxin and γ-interferon. These findings suggest that PAF may mediate part of its biological activity via the macrophage and further, monocyte secretion of PAF can in turn regulate monocyte function, thereby contributing to the inflammatory response. Using rat spleen macrophages stimulated by endotoxin, the priming effects of PAF on interleukin-1 (IL-1) release were studied.[52] Preincubation of macrophages for 10 min with 10^{-15} M PAF prior to stimulation with endotoxin for 24 h markedly increased the IL-1 activity present in the supernatants whereas no direct effect of PAF was noted. When L-651,392, a lipoxygenase inhibitor or mannitol, a free radical scavenger was added during the preincubation period with PAF, the increase in IL-1 secretion was reversed. Pertussis toxin decreased endotoxin-induced IL-1 activity. Association of pertussis toxin with PAF suppressed the enhancing effect of PAF on the IL-1 activity present in the supernatants from endotoxin-stimulated macrophages. It appears therefore that the enhancing effect of PAF on IL-1 release may be due to the production of lipoxygenase metabolites, leading to superoxide anion production and alterations of cAMP levels.

PAF AND ITS ANTAGONISTS IN THE LYMPHOID SYSTEM

More recently, PAF research has been extended to the lymphoid system. The binding and metabolism of PAF were characterized in Raji, a human Burkitt's lymphoma-derived cell line.[53] These cells metabolized PAF rapidly by deacylation-reacylation through specific binding sites assessed by calcium mobilization. CV-3988 and BN 52021 inhibited the effect of PAF, providing evidence for a functional PAF receptor expressed in lymphocytes.

PAF AND PAF ANTAGONISTS ON EOSINOPHIL CELLS

The presence of eosinophilic infiltrate in the conducting airways of asthmatics has been known for a long time. Eosinophil numbers in peripheral blood can be used as an index of disease severity in bronchial asthma, and the occurrence of eosinophils in bronchoalveolar lavage fluid precedes late-onset responses to allergen in asthmatic patients.

The presence of PAF receptors on eosinophil cells demonstrated with a new ligand [³H]WEB 2086 (**12**) was described by Ukena et al.[54] Using assay systems for intracellular calcium mobilization and superoxide anion generation induced by PAF in eosinophil leukocytes suggested the existence of two subtypes of PAF receptors based on the difference in pA_2 values of WEB 2086.[55]

PAF has been reported to induce a selective accumulation of eosinophils in the airways of guinea pigs[56] and primates.[57] Intraperitoneal injection of PAF in guinea pigs caused a dose-related increase in the number of eosinophils recovered from bronchoalveolar lavage fluid within 24 h.[58] PAF administration was maintained by subcutaneous minipump. Eosinophil accumulation induced by PAF was inhibited in animals treated with dexamethasone, aminophylline, disodium cromoglycate (DSCG), tranilast or ketotifen but not in animals treated with oxatomine, azelastine, amlexanox, ibudilast or AA-861. These results suggest that inhibition of pulmonary eosinophilia may be a necessary property of prophylactic anti-asthma drugs and provide indirect evidence favoring a role for PAF in inducing eosinophilia of asthmatic patients. The significance of eosinophil recruitment into guinea pig lungs after intravenous administration of PAF and allergen has been emphasized.[59] The significance of an interaction between platelets and eosinophils in bronchial hyperreactivity in response to PAF and antigen has been hypothesized.[60] Exposure of guinea pigs to aerosolized PAF induced a dose-dependent increased and predominantly delayed incidence of eosinophils in bronchoalveolar lavage fluid.[61] The response was inhibited by SDZ 64-412 (**6**), a selective PAF antagonist, furthermore by pretreatment with antiasthmatic drugs, such as aminophylline, DSCG, ketotifen, dexamethasone and AH 21-132, but remained unaffected by prior treatment with indomethacin, salbutamol and mepyramine, or by depletion of circulating platelets or neutrophils by intravenous injection of specific antisera.

It has been previously reported that pulmonary eosinophils in eosinophilic pneumonia showed hypodensity and hypersegmentation.[62] It was hypothesized that eosinophil chemotactic factor and certain lymphokines may be involved in the induction of these characteristic features. Chemoattractants, such as eosinophil chemotactic factor A, histamine and PAF could induce both nuclear hypersegmentation and hypodensity in eosinophils. Lymphokines, such as γ-interferon, IL-3 plus GM-CSF and phytohemagglutinin-treated lymphocyte culture medium were able to induce hypersegmented nuclei but IL-2 was without effect. More than

90% of eosinophil cells isolated from normal nonatopic healthy volunteers were defined to be normodense during discontinuous Percoll gradient centrifugation.[63] Isolation of eosinophils from patients with atopic asthma revealed a cell population with 65 to 70% occurrence of hypodense cells that was independent of the total eosinophil cell count. *In vitro* activation of normodense cells by A23187, opsonized zymosan and PAF increased superoxide anion production and induced quantities of hypodense eosinophils in the range found in asthmatic patients. During stimulation, no peroxidase or arylsulfatase B secretion could be measured, even though hypodense eosinophils were produced. The enzymatic activity of eosinophilic peroxidase in normodense cells did not change in the normodense fraction but was increased in the induced hypodense cells after stimulation. Yukawa et al.[64] examined a selective induction of hypodense eosinophils by PAF in guinea pigs. Lyso-PAF had no effect on cell density, while WEB 2086 inhibited the PAF-induced density shift. These results indicate that a single mediator is able to induce the formation of hypodense eosinophils whose appearance may be involved in the pathogenesis of asthma. When mononuclear cells from umbilical cord blood were cultured for 3 weeks, low concentrations of IL-3 supported preferential growth of basophils, with eosinophils comprising a smaller proportion.[65] These basophils contained and released histamine by the IgE-dependent and independent stimuli. IL-5 increased the number and proportion of eosinophils in a dose-dependent manner without affecting the proliferation of other cell types in the IL-3-supplemented cultures. These cultured eosinophils could be activated by PAF.

Activation and release by different inflammatory stimuli, such as histamine, PAF, calcium ionophore, compound 48/80, LTB_4, PGs E_1 and E_2, heparin, and eosinophil-chemotactic factor, of enzymes, such as peroxidase, arylsulfatase B, β-glucuronidase, aminopeptidase, histaminase, cytochrome C oxidase, acid phosphatase, adenosine triphosphatase and glucose 6-phosphatase as well as that of the major basic protein from guinea pig peritoneal eosinophils obtained after repeated intraperitoneal injections of freeze-dried *Trichinella spiralis* was studied by Popper et al.[66] Eosinophils displayed a selective and stimulus-dependent enzyme and major basic protein reaction, providing evidence that these cells exhibit either inflammatory or cytotoxic, or even anti-inflammatory properties upon stimulation by various agents. In accord with this observation, eosinophils isolated from atopic individuals showed increased sensitivity to fMLP and PAF as assessed by chemoluminescence which is peroxidase dependent and of extracellular origin.[67] The response was inhibited by BN 52021 (**15**), and might reflect a "primed" state of eosinophils relevant for the pathogenesis of atopic disease.

In order to evaluate the role of calcium in the activation processes in eosinophils induced by PAF, the changes in cytosolic free calcium concentrations by using fura-2 assay were studied.[68] PAF caused a rapid and transitory rise in calcium levels which was specifically inhibited by WEB 2086 and EGTA, indicating the dependence of PAF response on external calcium. The dihydropyridine nimodipine had no effect. The PAF antagonist did not inhibit intracellular calcium rise induced by LTB_4 or fMLP. These findings suggest that calcium entry via receptor-operated calcium channels may be involved in PAF-induced degranulation of eosinophils.

The effect of nedocromil sodium on human eosinophil activation was studied by Moqbel et al.[69] Nedocromil sodium inhibited the increase of eosinophil activation induced by PAF. The effect was dose-dependent and paralleled that produced by BN 52021. In addition, the drug inhibited the increase in IgG-dependent release of LTC_4 from human eosinophils stimulated by fMLP. The same research group also found that BN was able to inhibit PAF-induced eosinophil chemotaxis assessed by a modified Boyden technique and cytotoxicity measured as percentage of schistosomula of *S. mansoni* coated with fresh untreated immune serum obtained from patients with *Schistosomiasis mansoni*.[70,71] The effect of BN 52021 was comparable to that of DSCG. The PAF antagonist was as effective against eosinophil chemotaxis as in reducing neutrophil chemotactic response. In addition, BN 52021 directly down-regulated PAF-induced enhancement of the ability of human eosinophils to adhere and kill opsonized schistosomula. More recently, BN 52021 was shown to prevent LTC_4 formation induced by A23187, opsonized zymosan, PAF, AA and PAF in combination with AA in purified human eosinophils.[72] This inhibition was however less expressed than that found on PAF-induced chemotactic response in eosinophils.

Factors responsible for *in vivo* eosinophil recruitment are poorly defined, although T-lymphocytes appear to be involved, since cyclosporin A (CsA) prevents eosinophilia induced by high dose cyclophosphamide prior to immunization.[73] In order to clarify this relationship Etienne et al.[74] studied the modulation of eosinophil mobilization in the rat induced by immune challenge after chronic treatment with BN 52021, BIM 23014, a somatostatin analog and CsA. CsA totally abolished both hypereosinophilia and peritoneal eosinophil infiltration. BIM 23014 significantly reduced the number of circulating eosinophils and cell infiltration. In contrast, BN 52021 decreased only peritoneal eosinophil recruitment but had relatively little effect on the number of circulating cells. It was concluded that PAF antagonists could decrease eosinophil infiltration in the peritoneum by inhibiting PAF-induced eosinophil chemotaxis. The chemotactic responsiveness of peripheral eosinophilic granulocytes isolated from patients with inflammatory dermatoses and healthy volunteers was determined.[75] Well characterized chemotaxins, the complement split product C5a, LTB_4, PAF and fMLP were used as chemoattractants. Eosinophils from healthy volunteers showed strong migratory responses towards C5a and PAF, but responded poorly to LTB_4 and fMLP. When patients were grouped by disease severity, eosinophil chemotactic responses to PAF were significantly enhanced in severely affected patients, but this was not true with C5a, LTB_4, or fMLP. The enhanced response to PAF was not related to a specific disease. No correlation between eosinophil chemotactic activity and peripheral eosinophil count was observed. The increased responsiveness of circulating eosinophils toward PAF may be related to altered receptor expression during cutaneous inflammation; this remains, however, to be determined by using specific PAF receptor antagonists.

PAF ANTAGONISTS AND ENDOTHELIAL CELLS

Endothelial cells exposed to various stimuli are very active in generating PAF.[77]

The role of calcium in the synthesis and accumulation of PAF in endothelial cells is well established. Alternatively, the lipid mediator has been shown to induce a transient increase of cytosolic free calcium in cultured human vascular endothelial cells as measured by the fura-2 loading assay.[78,79] The response appeared to be specific to PAF, since lyso-PAF was inactive and restimulation of the cells with PAF did not cause further increase in intracellular calcium, while the cells remained responsive to thrombin. These events could be produced in the absence of extracellular calcium. PAF-induced rise in intracellular calcium was completely blocked by BN 52021 **(15)**. These results suggest that receptor mediated increase in cytosolic calcium is an early event in PAF activation of human vascular endothelial cells.

PAF has been found to enhance or "prime" PMNL responses to subsequent stimulation with agonists, such as fMLP.[80,81] It was also tested whether thrombin-induced endothelial PAF production would prime responses of marginated PMNL. Endothelial monolayers of human umbilical vein were exposed to thrombin, then PMNL were layered on them. Later fMLP stimulation was applied and superoxide anion production, elastase release, adhesion to endothelium, capacity to cause endothelial cell lysis and detachment were assessed. Thrombin pretreatment significantly enhanced each of these responses through PAF release, since it enhanced incorporation of ^3H-acetate into endothelial PAF. BN 52021 blocked the enhanced neutrophil responses. This coagulation-fostered endothelial/PMNL interaction may underlie a paracrine response that may potentiate PMNL-mediated endothelial injury during sepsis and other thrombin-generating disorders. BN 52021 inhibited receptor-mediated activation of leukocytes to induce superoxide anion generation and eicosanoid release as well as bradykinin-, ATP- and A23187-induced PGI_2 generation of endothelial cells.[82]

Intact platelets and confluent human umbilical vein endothelial cells bound ^{3}H-PAF in the presence of bovine serum albumin.[83] WEB 2086 **(12)** inhibited this binding to a concentration-dependent manner. Various hetrazepines, such as WEB 2098, 2105, but not 2118 provided similar inhibition. According to these results the inhibition of PAF binding to these cellular elements by various hetrazepine derivatives occurs most probably at the PAF receptor level.

BN 52021, CV-3988 **(1)** and L-652,731 **(17)** were tested for their ability to prevent or reduce PAF-induced shape changes of large vein endothelial cells isolated from guinea pig's venae cavae.[84,85] BN 52021 produced a significant protective effect at small concentrations but had its own damaging effect at higher concentrations. CV-3988 and L-652,731 did not reduce PAF responses and at higher concentrations they induced shape change. Using electron spin resonance spectrometry the damaging effects of the latter two PAF antagonists were suggested to be due to their detergent properties. These results call attention to possible deleterious effects of some PAF antagonists to the vascular endothelium.

EFFECT OF PAF ANTAGONISTS ON CIRCULATION

Research devoted to the effect of PAF on circulation deserves high importance, since the phospholipid mediator induces drastic changes, especially as peripheral vasodilator. This effect had been discovered very early after characterization of PAF, and is still in the focus of interest. Apart from its characteristic effect on the vessels, PAF can influence the function of the heart, not only because the marked decrease in peripheral resistance could alter cardiac function, but also by a direct influence on coronary vessels, cardiac rhythm and myocardial contractility.

EFFECT OF PAF ANTAGONISTS ON THE HEART
Myocardial Function

In terms of myocardial function, the negative inotropic and coronary vasoconstrictor effects of PAF are well defined (see for review Reference 86). It was recently demonstrated that various alkyl chain homologs of PAF elicited a decrease in left ventricular contractile force with a rank order of potency that was similar, although not identical, to the order for their coronary constricting effects in isolated guinea pig hearts.[87] The relative potency in the heart did not correlate well with their relative potency in stimulating rabbit platelets and human PMNL. These data suggest that the occupation of PAF receptors by various alkyl chain homologs, initiating signal transduction and cell activation, could be governed by unique receptor specificities.

Experiments performed on isolated auricles of guinea pigs showed that PAF induced negative inotropic effect which reversed to positive inotropic action after washing.[88] Resting membrane potential was unaltered, while the amplitude and V_{max} of the upstroke of action potential were decreased and shortened, respectively. Calcium-induced action potential and contractions elicited in partially depolarized myocardium were depressed by PAF. Interestingly enough, these changes were inhibited by 4-aminopyridine, affecting "A" current in voltage dependent potassium channels. The results suggest that PAF effects on the membrane of cardiac cells could be related to a change in calcium and potassium conductance, and raise important consideration to further studies on PAF antagonists in the heart. Interaction of PAF with its antagonist, U-66985 was studied in isolated guinea pig atria.[89] PAF exhibited a marked cardiodepressive effect paralleling a lowering action potential duration. In depolarized preparations, PAF resulted in a decrease of the slow calcium potential amplitude. U-66985 led to the weakening of the PAF-induced depressing effects with a restoration of electrical and mechanical activities.

BN 52021 was shown to reduce myocardial depression induced by intravenous injection of bupivacaine, a local anesthetic agent, in various heart preparations of male Wistar rats.[90,91] BN 52021 (15) abolished PAF-induced cardiac rhythm disturbances in various experimental models.[92] Soloviev and Braquet[93] analyzed the response of isolated human and porcine coronary artery strips to hypoxia and found a biphasic contraction, i.e., an initial short fast phase followed by a long-lasting tonic shortening that seemed to be related to the release of intracellular calcium. Hypoxia-induced coronary constriction was increased by PAF and inhibited by BN 52021. Endothelium-deprived coronary strips responded with contraction when exposed to PAF. These studies indicate that hypoxia triggers PAF release from endothelial cells, activates PLC, facilitates IP_3 and diacylglycerol (DG) formation. In the presence of calcium and phospholipids, DG activates PKC which sensitizes the contractile proteins to calcium. PAF antagonists may inhibit this feedback mechanism, indicating an important locus for their mechanism of action.

The antianaphylactic effect of BN 52021 in the heart is well characterized. More recent studies confirmed the beneficial effect of ginkgolide B on passive cardiac anaphylaxis-induced functional disturbances of isolated working guinea pig hearts,[94] suggesting that PAF antagonists may have therapeutic value against cardiac symptoms during anaphylactic shock.

PAF Antagonists in Myocardial Infarction

Ischemic heart diseases are of interest as the major cause of sudden cardiac death and cardiac failure. Therapeutic interventions are basically focused on cardiac arrhythmias, coronary flow disturbances, and reduction of infarct size. Ventricular dysrhythmias are triggered by myocardial ischemia and reperfusion, coronary flow is regulated by the tone of vascular wall and blood homeostasis, while infarct size is related to cell injury and the capability of the cells for recovery.

PAF, synthesized rapidly especially by granulocytes upon hypoxic stimuli,[95] appears to be a particularly important mediator of myocardial ischemia.[96] Experiments conducted in anesthetized rabbits subjected to coronary artery occlusion and subsequent reperfusion provided evidence for the release of TXB_2 and LTs from infiltrating leukocytes interacted with PAF.[97]

Recent experimental data have indicated that PAF is generated during myocardial ischemia and reperfusion. Isolated rabbit hearts release PAF in a significant amount during the initial reperfusion after myocardial ischemia.[98] Lyso-PAF levels were found to be decreased in the plasma of patients with myocardial infarction and unstable angina, apparently because of the substrate depletion.[99-101] These findings suggest a new approach to the clinical management of ischemic heart diseases. Experimental evidence has accumulated that specific PAF antagonists provide prominent cardioprotective effect by preventing life-threatening arrhythmias during ischemia or reperfusion and by reducing infarct size.

Under *in vitro* conditions the isolated working heart preparation provides a possibility for studying regional ischemia- and reperfusion-induced arrhythmias. The antiarrhythmic effect of BN 52021 in comparison with metoprolol, a β adrenoceptor blocking agent, and diltiazem, a calcium channel blocker, on isolated rat hearts was studied.[102,103] The PAF antagonist produced a concentration-dependent antiarrhythmic effect during ischemia which was comparable to that of metoprolol and somewhat slighter than that produced by diltiazem. BN 52021 had no effect on heart rate, coronary flow, and myocardial function, while the β blocker induced slight bradycardia and the calcium channel blocker produced a negative inotropic effect. These observations are in favor of the concept that BN 52021 induces antiarrhythmic effect under ischemic conditions without influencing heart function. This effect seems to be valuable for the clinical management of cardiac arrhythmias during myocardial infarction. In accord, results obtained by Berti et al.[104] in isolated Langendorff rabbit hearts provided further evidence that BN 52021, and to a lesser extent BN 52063, a standardized mixture of BN 52020, BN 52021, and BN 52022 in a ratio of 2:2:1, displayed protective activity in acute myocardial ischemia by a mechanism different from that of calcium entry blockers, eventually involving an antagonism of cell membrane PAF receptors and release of PGI_2. In isolated guinea pig heart perfused with constant pressure, WEB 2086 (**12**) induced a dose-dependent inhibition of PAF-induced coronary vasoconstriction;[105] since BM 13505, a TXA_2 receptor antagonist induced the same protective effect, TXA_2 was thought to be responsible for this type of coronary constriction.

There is growing evidence that ginkgolide B and other PAF receptor antagonists may protect the heart against ischemia/reperfusion-induced tissue injury under *in vivo* conditions. Experiments performed in anesthetized open-chest rats by the occlusion and release of the main coronary artery showed that a solubilized, stabilized extract of *Ginkgo biloba* L. given intravenously as well as BN 52021 applied as a long-term oral pretreatment before coronary occlusion produce a significant antiarrhythmic effect in normal rats[106] and in obese Zucker rats,[107] respectively. Using the same method, Stahl et al.[108] demonstrated that the loss of amino-nitrogen and catepsin D as a consequence of myocardial tissue damage was significantly retarded by CV-6209 (**2**), a specific PAF antagonist injected after the occlusion of the main coronary artery. BN 52021 and CV-3988 (**1**) proved to be specific preventive agents against PAF-induced cardiac depression in isolated perfused rat hearts.[109]

It was recently demonstrated that BN 52021 and SRI 63-441 (**6a**) protected the heart of anesthetized greyhounds from ischemia- and reperfusion-induced arrhythmias.[110,111] PAF antagonists were capable of reducing ischemia-induced platelet count increase as well. In mongrel dogs, BN 52021 given in an intravenous bolus reduced ventricular arrhythmias in response to ischemia and reperfusion.[112,113] In anesthetized open-chest pigs subjected to a short occlusion of left anterior descending coronary artery then reperfusion, SRI 63-441 reduced myocardial dysfunction measured as depressed contractility during reperfusion.

The outcome of myocardial infarction is dependent on the duration of ischemia and the condition of tissue energy supply. These factors determine infarct size. Some of the antiarrhythmic drugs have no influence on infarct size; therefore, they are beneficial in saving the life of the patient only in the early phase, but do not protect the heart against the late consequences of myocardial infarction. This experience initiated studies with ginkgolide B on the extent of the infarcted area. Fontaliran et al.[114] described that in coronary artery ligated rats BN 52021 given before occlusion and two times daily during the observation period (1, 10, and 21 days) significantly reduced infarct size as measured after hemateine-phloxine-saffron dye by using a digitalization technique with Tandon computer image analysis (PCSOPE). In agreement with this finding, Gross et al.[115] and Maruyama et al.[116] reported that BN 52021 reduced infarct size in dogs subjected to 90 min coronary artery occlusion and 180 min reperfusion. In anesthetized rabbit, BN 52021 reduced the incidence of ventricular fibrillation and the extent of infarcted area, indicating a benefit of the PAF antagonist during acute coronary artery occlusion. These observations underline the potential offered by PAF antagonists in the prevention and treatment of myocardial infarction. It appears likely that their protective effect does not imply a simple delay of the ischemic insult but rather a salvage of the jeopardized myocardium via a cytoprotective effect. In conclusion, PAF antagonists may provide cardioprotective effect by preventing life-threatening arrhythmias or protecting myocardial tissue against ischemic cell damage. Ischemia/reperfusion-induced tissue injury is triggered by PAF as a consequence of a vicious circle among endothelial cells, circulating platelets, and leukocytes as well as cytokines released.[117] PAF antagonists are thought to cut off this vicious circle in a concentration which is highly specific, and do not cause any side effects; therefore these drugs may be used as safe intervention in clinical patients suffering from acute and chronic coronary heart diseases.

PAF ANTAGONISTS IN PERIPHERAL CIRCULATION
Shock Conditions

Three lines of evidence suggest the involvement of PAF in shock: (i) infusion of PAF in animals mimics shock state, (ii) increased levels of PAF are generated during shock, and (iii) specific antagonists of PAF inhibit or alleviate shock induced by various mechanisms. The potential role for PAF and its antagonists in peripheral collapse due to various shock conditions and trauma has been recently summarized.[118,119]

The hypotensive effect of PAF is well established and its mechanism has been analyzed. In open-chest pigs, PAF infusion induced increase in pulmonary resistance, with a concomitant right ventricular failure, fall in cardiac output and systemic blood pressure. U46619, a stable TXA_2 analog, and mechanical pulmonary constriction induced changes similar to PAF. Indomethacin and OKY-046, a specific TXA_2 synthetase inhibitor diminished all the hemodynamic effects of PAF; therefore it was suggested that TXA_2 release may contribute significantly to these events. Alternatively, acute right ventricular failure as a result of severe increase in pulmonary vascular resistance is the primary mechanism early in the course of PAF-induced shock in the pig.[120]

As determined by thin layer chromatography, high-pressure liquid chromatography, alkaline treatment, and bioassay on platelet aggregation, PAF release was detected in the blood of dogs who underwent mesenteric ischemia and reperfusion injury.[121]

The beneficial effects of BN 52021 and other PAF antagonists in shock states have also been well documented.[122-124] In conscious rats the effects of two PAF antagonists, BN 52021 and SDZ 63-441, on PAF-induced changes in blood pressure, heart rate, cardiac output, and hindquarters, renal and mesenteric blood flow were studied.[125] The hypotensive and cardiac effects of PAF were blocked, BN 52021 also attenuated the hindquarters and renal responses, but the mesenteric responses remained relatively unchanged. In the *in situ* mesentery of anesthetized rats, the effect of intraarterially injected PAF was shifted to the right by the concomitant infusion of SRI 63-441.[126] The effect of topically and systematically administered PAF on the arteriolar and venular diameter of rat mesenteric microvasculature was inhibited by BN 52021.[127] The ineffectiveness of lyso-PAF and fMLP as well as the lack of platelet and leukocyte accumulation suggest that PAF has a direct effect on microvessels. BN 52021 was efficient in blocking PAF-induced hypotension and biochemical parameters in rats.[128] In a recent study, PAF-induced hypotension in the rat was markedly inhibited by BN 50739 (**14**), a new potent PAF antagonist with a heptazepine framework.[16]

BN 52021 prevented the consequences of mesenteric artery occlusion/reperfusion induced shock in anesthetized dogs,[121-123] and attenuated serious hemodynamic alterations produced by tourniquet shock in dogs.[129] The protective effect of PAF antagonists against hypotension induced by intravenously injected PAF in the primate *Macaca fascicularis* was also demonstrated by prior administration of WEB 2086.[130]

In a recent study, the effect of endothelin-induced sudden death was investigated by using PAF antagonists, like WEB 2086 and CV-6209.[131] Both PAF antagonists protected the animals against sudden death, but CV-6209 did not prevent endothelin-induced blood pressure changes. This phenomenon was also observed in mice, and WEB 2086, diltiazem and dexamethasone increased survival rate, but aspirin was without effect. The conclusion may be drawn that PAF is involved in the sudden death caused by the toxic polypeptide endothelin.

Thermal injury releases inositolphosphates, DG, free AA, and lyso-PAF from eukaryotic cells.[132] PAF and eicosanoids are derived from lyso-PAF and AA, then induce formation of kinins. Activation of clotting and complement systems leading to clinical manifestation of edema, increased dermal temperature and pain. Using a well-established rabbit model of burn injury, known to induce shock conditions, the biochemical function of PMNL and especially their oxygen-derived species O_2-, together with PAF- and LTB_4-generating capacity were determined in groups treated with IPS 200, a non-toxic *Ginkgo biloba* extract.[133]

After burn injury, increase in hematocrit and red blood cell count reflected hemoconcentration with a short-lasting increase, then a rapid decrease in platelet count, while eicosanoid production and free radical generation increased. PAF and lyso-PAF production were also elevated. All these parameters were attenuated by the *Ginkgo biloba* extract, indicating a beneficial effect of this intervention on the vascular and biochemical consequences of burn injury. The effect of SRI 63-675 (**6b**) was also studied following thermal injury in rats.[134] Pretreated burned animals showed attenuated blood pressure fall, only a transitory hemoconcentration, a lower degree of hyperglycemia, hyperlactacidemia, glucagon and catecholamine concentrations in the blood as compared to untreated burned controls. Short-term survival was also markedly improved. These results suggest a mediator role for PAF and a benefit for PAF antagonists in burn injury.

Taken together, these observations are in favor of the suggestion that antagonists of PAF are of value in assessing the role of PAF in cardiovascular pathophysiological states and their clinical management in man.

PAF in Pulmonary Circulation

PAF is known to induce vasoconstriction in the pulmonary vessels. This effect has accounted for the right ventricular failure and venous congestion in the peripheral circulation,[120] and further studied in anesthetized, open-chest, newborn piglets.[135] Pulmonary pressure was increased by low doses of PAF, while cardiac function was ameliorated only after higher doses, indicating a primary effect of the lipid mediator on pulmonary vessels. Indomethacin and SQ 29458, a TXA_2 receptor blocker, prevented both effects of PAF. This finding suggests the role of TXA_2 as secondary mediator in the pulmonary vasoconstriction induced by PAF. These alterations were confirmed in large white pigs, and found to be uninfluenced by vagosympathectomy but blocked by prior intravenous administration of 5 mg/kg BN 52021,[137] suggesting that PAF receptor antagonists may have potential therapeutic value in severe pulmonary hypertension related to inflammation. Further studies in this field have indicated that PAF infused into the right pulmonary artery increased perfusion pressure and the ratio of wet-to-dry lung weight as an indicator of lung edema.[138] This method allowed an appropriate comparison by using the other lung infused with vehicle as an internal control. In addition, $PGF_{2\alpha}$ induced an equivalent increase in pulmonary pressure without causing similar increase in lung edema, thus suggesting that increased vascular permeability in the lung is mediated predominantly by specific PAF receptors. Two selective PAF receptor antagonists, BN 52021 and L-652,731 (**17**), inhibited these responses; therefore the experiments suggest that PAF antagonists can be implicated in the clinical management of lung edema.

Evidence for the possible role of PAF and TXA_2 in the genesis of group B Streptococcus-induced pulmonary hypertension was sought in anesthetized, ventilated piglets.[139] SQ 29548, a TXA_2 antagonist completely inhibited pulmonary hypertension, while SRI 63-072 (**5**) or SRI 63-441 (**6a**) had no effect. This finding indicates that Streptococcus-induced pulmonary hypertension involves TXA_2 rather than PAF in this species. McCormack et al.[140] have used WEB 2086 and BN 52021 to study the role of PAF in hypoxia-induced pulmonary vasoconstriction in isolated rat lung preparation perfused with blood. WEB 2086 produced a dose-dependent attenuation of pulmonary hypertension, but also decreased the effect of angiotensin II, while BN 52021 did not affect the response. These authors concluded that hypoxia-induced pulmonary hypertension is not mediated by PAF.

The definite role for PAF in pulmonary hypertension may be varied according to various tissue challenges. Therefore, further studies are needed for better understanding of the pathophysiological events in this pathology.

PAF Antagonists in Endotoxin-Induced Pathophysiological Changes

Endotoxin can induce pathophysiological changes in various cells and tissues. Its hypotensive effect and shock inducing capacity is summarized in the chapter dealing with peripheral circulation. The relationship of endotoxin to PAF is well documented.

The effect of endotoxic shock on the synthesis of PAF by the stomach, duodenum, and lung was examined in the rat.[141] Early after endotoxin treatment, all tissues synthesized PAF corresponding to the time when hypotension, hemoconcentration, and an increase in gastrointestinal vascular permeability were observed. It was also shown that administration of PGE_2 resulted in a significant reduction of endotoxin-induced cardiovascular complications, but did not affect PAF synthesis in the gastrointestinal tissues. It appears that PGE_2 exerts beneficial effect by affecting other pathways than PAF synthesis. In a study performed in conscious rats, the effect of BN 52021 was evaluated against PAF- and endotoxin-induced hypotension.[142] The results showed that conscious rats were extremely sensitive to PAF. BN 52021 significantly attenuated PAF-induced blood pressure drop, while it had no effect on the early hypotension induced by endotoxin. The late blood pressure lowering effect of endotoxin was however improved by the PAF receptor antagonist. These experiments emphasize the use of conscious animals for studying the effect of PAF antagonists. PAF applied topically and endotoxin given intravenously displayed similar effects on the diameter of rat mesenteric microvessels which could be inhibited by BN 52021 and WEB 2086;[143] thus PAF appears to be involved as mediator in endotoxin-induced microvessel changes. The effect of BN 52021 on survival in a resuscitated canine endotoxin model and the possible significance of PAF in endotoxemia-induced hemodynamic changes were examined.[144] BN 52021 improved survival rate and prolonged survival time, decreased hemodynamic changes in response to endotoxin, suggesting that endogenous PAF could have a central role in the pathophysiology of this entity. The significance of kinin system in endotoxin shock was studied in kininogen-deficient Brown Norway rats.[145] No difference was detected in the development of vascular collapse and plasma extravasation in the digestive tract characteristic to endotoxin shock when the responses of normal and kininogen-deficient rats were compared. The effects of endotoxin were blocked in both strains by BN 52021 and SDZ 63-675. There were some differences in endotoxin-induced changes in various tissues, indicating that the kinin system can be activated by endotoxin; this is however only secondary as a consequence of PAF release. No close relationship between PAF- and endotoxin-induced platelet aggregation *in vitro* could be obtained except when very small doses were compared which showed synergistic effects, presumably due to the involvement of AA metabolism.[146] The involvement of PAF in platelet pulmonary recruitment in response to aerosolized endotoxin in guinea pigs was suggested.[147,148] BN 52021, CV-3988 and brotizolam (**11**), but not indomethacin reduced endotoxin-induced platelet recruitment, suggesting the primary mediator role for PAF in the phenomenon. In conscious fasted rats chronically implanted with Nichrome electrodes in the duodenojejunum, intravenous endotoxin increased the interval between migrating myoelectric complex referring to motor disturbances in the intestine.[149] Intraperitoneal injection of PAF produced the same type of impairment of intestinal motility. BN 52021, indomethacin, and the PGE_2 antagonist SC 19220 reduced the effects of both endotoxin and PAF. The conclusion was drawn that both PAF and eicosanoids are involved in endotoxin-induced intestinal motor disturbances. The significance of TXA_2 biosynthesis in endotoxin-induced intestinal damage in the rat was studied by Boughton et al.[150] and a dose-related jejunal damage associated with PAF and TXB_2 release was found. Benzyl imidazole or OKY 1581, two TXA_2 synthetase inhibitors reduced tissue damage and TXB_2 release but not PAF formation. Administration of PAF in turn induced jejunal injury and TXB_2 release. These changes suggest the involvement of TXA_2 and the primary role of PAF in gastrointestinal damage.

It is known that PAF increases vascular permeability in the lung of awake sheep. The effect of BN 52021 in an ovine chronic lung preparation to determine its effectiveness in endotoxemia was recently studied.[151] BN 52021 prevented pulmonary hypertension and lung edema due to lymphatic flow disturbances induced by endotoxin. Interestingly enough, WEB

2086 did not block the early pulmonary hypertension produced by intravenous lipopolysaccharide bolus. This discrepancy calls attention to the diversity of PAF receptors in the lung and the selectivity of BN 52021 in the prevention of endotoxin-induced lung injury. The PAF antagonists inhibit endotoxin-induced hyperreactivity to histamine in guinea pig airways but not in coronary vessels,[152,153] pointing to the role for PAF in the endotoxin-induced hypersensitivity reaction of lung but not that of the coronary vessels in the heart. In female and postpartum rats, endotoxemic acute renal failures due to specific functional changes in glomerular hemodynamics were decreased by ginkgolide B,[154] indicating that, at least in part, PAF is a causal factor under these conditions.

RP 55778, a PAF receptor antagonist was shown to prevent endotoxin-induced hemo-concentration and TNF release in rats,[155] while dexamethasone proved to be ineffective. More recent studies indicated that BN 50739, a new heptazepine-type PAF antagonist was able to prevent endotoxin- and TNF-induced shock in rabbits[156] and conscious rats.[157]

Potential Role for PAF in Atherogenesis and Arterial Hypertension

More recently, PAF research has been extended to the field of degenerative, peripheral arterial diseases like atherogenesis and essential hypertension. Highly developed laboratory techniques have facilitated clinical studies. An increased activity of PAF acetylhydrolase, an enzyme that specifically inactivates PAF, in plasma low density lipoprotein from patients with essential hypertension was shown,[158] and the elevation seemed to be in correlation with the length of the history of hypertension. Patients suffering from obliterative arteriosclerosis of the lower limbs revealed hyperfunction of blood platelets expressed as increased sensitivity of platelets to ADP and PAF, increased levels of β-TG and TXB_2 as well as decreased levels of 6-keto-$PGF_{1\alpha}$ and cAMP.[159] Determination of the degradation of PAF to lyso-PAF indicated an increased PAF degrading capacity in the serum of patients having survived myocardial infarction as compared with that of healthy controls matched for age and body weight,[160] indicating an increased formation of the lipid mediator in this condition. The effects of dietary salt on circulating levels of C_{16}-PAF in patients with essential hypertension were also studied.[161] Basal levels of PAF were not different; however, net changes in circulating PAF levels significantly and positively correlated with changes in mean arterial blood pressure and creatinine clearance but not with plasma sodium and chloride concentrations or plasma volume in response to dietary salt restriction. These results suggest that C_{16}-PAF may play a compensatory antihypertensive role in essential hypertension.

Alternatively, Kawaguchi et al.[162] have demonstrated that exogenous PAF stimulated angiotensin converting enzyme activity in pulmonary artery endothelial cells. The stimulatory effect was suppressed by angiotensin converting enzyme inhibitors, such as enalapril and the PAF antagonists CV-3988. These results suggest that PAF may have an important role in regulating vascular tone by modulating angiotensin conversion. The significance of this finding in the genesis of chronic arterial hypertension remains however to be elucidated.

As mentioned in another chapter, PAF has been reported to induce endovascular surface lesions in animal experiments. Whole blood aggregation and TXB_2 production during aggregation were measured in cigarette smokers and non-smokers with or without major symptomatic peripheral vascular disease.[163] Plasma levels of lyso-PAF were measured using a bioassay with [^{14}C]-serotonin labeled rabbit platelets, after extraction and acetylation to active PAF. Aggregation induced by ADP and collagen was significantly less in non-smokers without vascular disease, but no difference in TXB_2 and lyso-PAF production was found between the groups studied. Thus PAF plasma levels do not seem to be consistently related to either smoking or vascular disease.

Recent studies in rabbits fed a normal or hypercholesterolic diet showed that one month-long peroral treatment with BN 52021 (20 mg/kg/day) significantly reduced accumulation of esterified cholesterol in the plasma and aorta of animals receiving atherogenic diet, while free cholesterol levels remained relatively unchanged,[164] since the PAF receptor antagonist showed no effect on cellular cholesterol esterification and liver acyl-CoA:cholesterol acyl-transferase activity. In normal and atherosclerotic cynomolgus monkeys, Lopez et al.[165] studied the possible role of leukocytes in the pathogenesis of vasospasm. Hind limbs were infused with fMLP, a peptide that activates leukocytes to release their vasoactive products. Infusion of fMLP did not alter resistance of large arteries in normal monkeys, but produced pronounced constriction in atherosclerotic animals. In parallel, LTs, PAF, and PGE_2 were also infused to determine their vasoconstrictor potencies in atherosclerotic arteries. LT_4 and PAF had minimal effects, while the constrictor effect induced by PGE_2 was greatly potentiated by atherosclerosis.

These results have put forward the hypothesis that PAF plays an important regulatory role in the maintenance of the integrity of arterial vessels wall. Further studies will clarify the exact mechanism of PAF action and the significance of PAF antagonists in hypertension and atherogenesis.

There is evidence that PAF can alter not only arterial tone but also induces contraction of the isolated rat portal vein.[166-168] BN 52021 and BN 52063 as well as salbutamol, forskolin, and theophylline inhibited PAF-induced contractile responses. These data suggest that rat portal veins possess specific PAF receptors through which the lipid mediator can modulate tissue cAMP levels.

It is known that endothelial cells can be damaged in the presence of activated poly-morphonuclear leukocytes. Since PAF activates neutrophils, its effect and that of PAF-activated leukocytes were studied in isolated rat aortic strips precontracted with $PGF_{2\alpha}$ to determine the alterations in acetylcholine-induced vasodilation.[28] PAF alone induced a small relaxation, while PAF-activated neutrophils elicited a marked vasodilation which was en-dothelium dependent and abolished by CV-3988 and catalase known to block the formation of certain oxygen-derived free radicals. This finding suggests that PAF and endothelial cell interaction plays a role in the regulation of vascular tone via neutrophil-induced formation of free radicals.

ROLE OF PAF IN THE CENTRAL NERVOUS SYSTEM

In ancient China, extracts from the leaves of *Ginkgo biloba* tree were used to increase cerebral circulation, thus inducing mental refreshment and delay in aging. This experience was adopted by modern medicine, and several natural extracts, e.g., the standardized prep-aration of Tanakan (IPSEN-Beaufour), are on the market in various countries. Recently, intensive research activity has been initiated to specify the pharmacological principal re-sponsible for the effect of these extracts on the central nervous system. As indicated in this chapter, it appears that ginkgolides, among others, may be responsible for the beneficial effect of the extracts on cerebral circulation. Paralleling this research, the effect of various synthetic PAF antagonists has also been investigated in cerebral ischemia and brain function. It has been revealed that both natural and synthetic compounds are able to influence important physiological regulatory processes in the brain.

PAF AND PAF RECEPTORS IN THE BRAIN

The presence of various homologs and analogs of PAF in a lipid extract of bovine brain was previously demonstrated. The synthesis of PAF in rat brain was evaluated using standard HPLC and TLC techniques and by correlation of the bioactivity with the acetylation state of the 2-position of the molecule.[169] PAF was quantified by bioassay and its ability to cause [^{3}H]serotonin release from washed platelets. The low basal level of PAF was greatly increased by intraperitoneal injection of chemoconvulsant drugs, picrotoxine and bicuculline as well as by electroconvulsion. When a [^{32}P]-labeled nerve ending (synaptosome) was challenged with synthetic PAF, accelerated turnover of polyphosphoinositides was observed, and an increased exchange in sodium/calcium was detected. PAF infused into the vasculature of isolated perfused rat brain caused changes consistent with an increase in blood-brain barrier permeability. These observations pointed to the multiple pathophysiological role of PAF in the brain. PAF production was measured by cultured rat cerebellar granule cells.[170] PAF was identified on the basis of its chemical and enzymatic characteristics, biological activities with washed platelets and behavior on thin layer chromatography and HPLC, and was detected both in the cells and incubation medium, indicating its release from cultured neurons. Since A23187 had only a mild stimulatory effect on PAF production, the conclusion was drawn that neuronal-generated PAF might be synthesized mainly by *de novo* pathway. Francescangeli and Goracci[171] observed that rat brain was able to synthetize PAF from 1-alkyl-2-acetyl-*sn*-glycerol and CDP-choline by a "DTT-insensitive" phosphocholine transferase, representing a *de novo* pathway for PAF biosynthesis. The microsomal enzyme is inhibited by calcium and requires magnesium.

PAF has been implicated as a critical mediator in neuronal cell damage, since it increased intracellular levels of free calcium in cells of the clones NG 108-15 and PC12.[172] The increase was dependent on extracellular calcium and inhibited by the antagonistic PAF analog CV-3988 (**1**) and calcium-influx blockers, such as prenylamine and diltiazem. These results suggest that PAF may play a physiological role in neuronal development and a pathophysiological role in the degeneration occurs when neurons are exposed to circulatory changes as a result of trauma, stroke or spinal cord injury.

PAF receptors are present in the brain together with PGE_2 and LTC_4 binding sites.[173] The presence of PAF receptor binding sites in gerbil brain and their occupancy with BN 52021 (**15**) have been described.[174] These receptors might be responsible for the anti-ischemic effect of this PAF antagonist. It was described that picomolar concentrations of PAF evoked the formation of inositol phosphates in primary astrocyte cultures. Lyso-PAF and down-regulation of PAF receptors with phorbol myristate acetate (PMA) abolished this accumulation.[175] The responsiveness of astrocytes to PAF was not additive with AA. These results provide further evidence for the activation of these cells in the central nervous system in response to trauma. PAF antagonists, BN 52021, BN 52111 (**7**) and BN 52115 (**8**) augmented benzodiazepine binding measured *in vivo* in hypothalamus, hippocampus, and possibly in cerebellum.[176] In cortical membrane preparations, there was no effect on benzodiazepine binding or chloride channel binding *in vitro*. These alterations suggest the hypothesis of a link between GABAergic system and PAF. The phospholipid mediator may serve as neuromodulator, enhancing the effects of neurotransmitters by altering receptor characteristics. PAF antagonists may increase neuronal inhibitory activity, with potential benefit in epilepsy, anxiety, and a number of other disease states.

PAF IN HYPOTHALAMIC HORMONE RELEASE

There are conflicting results with PAF and PAF antagonists on the hypothalamic neuropeptide release. Junier et al.[177] reported that PAF exerted an inhibitory effect on the secretion of luteinizing hormone-releasing hormone (LHRH) and somatostatin from rat median eminence *in vitro* and this phenomenon appeared to be well correlated with the presence of specific PAF receptor sites in the hypothalamus. These studies were extended to determine the mode of action of PAF on β-endorphin, corticotropin releasing factor (CRF), somatostatin, and LHRH release using specific PAF receptor antagonists, such as BN 52021 (**15**), L-652,731 (**17**) and kadsurenone (**16**).[178] In correlation with their specific binding to PAF receptor sites located on hypothalamic membranes, all the antagonists tested inhibited somatostatin and LHRH release and stimulated CRF and β-endorphin secretion. The authors put forward the hypothesis that there are two populations of PAF receptors in the rat hypothalamus in comparison with platelets that possess only one type of PAF receptor binding site.

The effects of PAF on the activity of hypothalamic-pituitary-adrenal axis *in vivo* and *in vitro* was studied by Bernardini et al.[179] PAF injected intravenously in rats caused a significant stimulation of pituitary corticotropin (ACTH) and adrenal corticosterone secretion. These changes were prevented by intraperitoneal administration of BN 52021. In explanted rat hypothalami maintained viable *in vitro,* PAF stimulated immunoreactive CRF secretion in a bell-shaped dose-response fashion. Alprazolam **(10a)** and BN 52021, two structurally different PAF receptor antagonists, inhibited this effect. Indomethacin, eicosatetraenoic acid and verapamil inhibited the PAF response, suggesting mediation by calcium influx and PLA_2 activation. These results are in favor of the concept that PAF is involved as activator of the hypothalamic-pituitary-adrenal axis and glucocorticoid secretion and can perhaps serve as a mediator in the interactions of the immune system with the central nervous system. This effect of PAF was further analyzed and assessed by prolactin formation in dispersed rat anterior pituitary cells *in vitro*.[180] PAF induced a dose-dependent rapid stimulation of prolactin release which was blocked by dopamine agonists and the PAF receptor antagonists L-652,731 and SRI 63-072 **(5)**. Inactive structural analogs of PAF, lyso-PAF and phosphatidylcholine were ineffective. α-Melanocyte-stimulating hormone (α-MSH) derives from a larger precursor molecule called proopiomelanocortin (POMC) which has the potential to generate ACTH and β-endorphin, from the anterior hypothalamus and septum, lipotropins (β- and γ-LPH), melanotropins (α-, β-, and γ-MSH) from the dorsolateral region of the hypothalamus in the rat. The levels of these PMOC-derived peptides and corticosterone were measured by radioimmunoassay in male Wistar rats after 5-day-long treatment with PAF using minipumps for intravenous infusion into the jugular vein and oral treatment with BN 52021 twice daily.[181] BN 52021 reversed the inhibitory effect of PAF, and, when it was simultaneously administered with PAF, a significant increase in ACTH concentration occurred. These data provided evidence that PAF and its antagonists could influence endocrine systems, and this influence might vary according to the application of PAF or its antagonists and the experimental conditions used. Therefore, further studies are needed for better understanding the role of the phospholipid mediator in hormone secretory function of the hypothalamo-hypophyseal axis.

The significance of PAF in the metabolism of astrocytes was recently studied[175] in cultures prelabeled with [³H]inositol. When the cells were exposed to AA, there was a dose-dependent accumulation of IP_3 which was abolished by EGTA. IP_3 formation evoked by carbachol or norepinephrine was additive with AA, whereas that produced by PAF or ATP was not additive with AA. These results suggest that AA released upon stimulation of astrocytes or other cells in the central nervous system could initiate and/or amplify intracellular signaling. The accumulation of IP_3 in NG108-15 neuroblastoma-glioma hybrid cells was stimulated by bradykinin, guanosine 5′-O-(3-thiotriphosphate) and the DG kinase inhibitor Ro 59022. Only the stimulation by bradykinin was inhibited by the bradykinin receptor antagonist (D-ArgO, Hyp3, Phe7, Thy5,8) bradykinin. Neither bradykinin nor Ro 59022 increased the labeling of the inositol phospholipids. The sulfhydryl-alkylating reagent *N*-ethylmaleimide abolished the stimulation caused by all three agents, possibly by preventing the binding of GTP to a guanine nucleotide-binding regulatory protein of as yet unknown size.

Recent results may further facilitate understanding the molecular mechanisms by which PAF contributes to long-term phenotypic changes in central nervous system.[182] PAF was shown to elicit a rapid and transient activation of the proto-oncogenes c-*fos* and c-*jun* in SH-SY5Y neuroblastoma cells, but only to a minor extent in Molt-4 T-lymphocytes. This effect was inhibited by the pretreatment of cells with BN 52021, suggesting the involvement of a specific PAF receptor. Moreover, PAF treatment was able to activate gene expression through an AP-1 element. It was proposed that genomic transactivation might occur in target genes containing a functional AP-1 transcription sequence.

EFFECT OF PAF AND ANTAGONISTS ON THE EAR AND EYE

The influence of minute doses of PAF on the inner ear potentials, especially on endolymphatic potential, showed a relationship of ion transport to the presence of specific PAF and TXA$_2$ receptors in this area, since the changes were affected by BN 52021 **(15)** and BM-13,177, a TXA$_2$ receptor antagonist.[183-186] Furosemide-induced changes of cochlear potential were also weakened by BN 52021 and TXA$_2$ synthetase inhibitors,[187] suggesting the involvement of PAF and TXA$_2$ receptors in the control of ion movements within the cochlea.

PAF produced dose-dependent depletion of the goblet cell population associated with the conjunctival epithelium.[188] This effect did not correspond to leukocyte infiltration and was consistent with a direct effect of PAF. In addition, PAF produced an increase in conjunctival microvascular permeability over an identical dose range. PAF-induced leukocyte emigration was small or absent and comprised a neutrophil infiltrate which exhibited no clear dose-dependent relationship. Lyso-PAF produced similar changes only at the highest concentration applied. PAF- and lyso-PAF-induced increases in conjunctival microvascular permeability were virtually abolished by CV-6209 **(2)**. The pronounced inhibitory activity of CV-6209 suggests that high doses of lyso-PAF may either weakly stimulate conjunctival PAF receptors or that there may be sufficient conversion of lyso-PAF to biologically active levels of PAF.

The involvement of PAF in the inflammatory response of the anterior segment of the rabbit eye after corneal injury by alkali burn was evaluated.[189] [^{14}C]AA was injected in the anterior chamber and the production of labeled PGs and hydroxytetraenoic acids (HETE) was monitored. Topically applied BN 52021 produced a delayed but specific inhibition of the formation of 5- and 12-HETE. The increased protein concentration in the aqueous humor after injury was not affected by the drug. BN 52021 exerted a protective effect in immune complex keratitis by inhibiting leukocyte infiltration and corneal edema.[190] Receptor binding studies conducted in the iris and ciliary body revealed the existence of high- and low-affinity binding sites of PAF. Local application of PAF on the rabbit eye caused a dose-dependent significant increase in intraocular pressure.[191,192] Prophylactic treatment with BN 52021 but not with indomethacin abolished the hypertensive phase. The PAF antagonists also decreased protein and PGE$_2$ contents in the aqueous humor elevated by laser irradiation of the iris. These results suggest a mediator role for PAF in the ocular inflammatory response.

Thierry et al.[193] have demonstrated saturable, specific, time-dependent, and reversible binding of [^{3}H]PAF in membrane preparations of the rat retina. Scatchard analysis revealed the existence of high affinity binding sites for the phospholipid mediator providing values comparable with membraneous PAF receptor sites in platelets, neutrophils, lung tissue, and brain. Therefore, PAF-induced disturbances in electroretinogram may be mediated via specific receptors located in the retina. In the chick retina acetylcholine and dopamine stimulated PAF production, while other neurotransmitters were ineffective.[194] Only muscarinic or D$_2$ receptors were involved in the response. Doly et al.[195] found that lithium used in concentrations corresponding to its therapeutically active doses significantly decreased electroretinogram amplitude which effect was abolished by cholera toxin and was partially inhibited by BN 52021. These results are in favor of the hypothesis that PAF may influence retinal function through the involvement of a G protein.

PAF ANTAGONISTS IN CEREBRAL ISCHEMIA
Effect of PAF on Cerebral Vessels

As a part of the vascular system, cerebral circulation is a particular area in vascular pathophysiology, since the response of cerebral resistant vessels, e.g., pial arterioles, has an important role in the regulation of blood flow in the brain. Pial arterioles were observed directly using a closed cranial window in chloralose-anesthetized piglets to determine the effect of the topical application of PAF.[196] The phospholipid mediator, norepinephrine, and U46619, a purported TXA$_2$ receptor agonist, produced a dose-dependent decrease in pial arteriolar diameter. After topical and intravenous administration of U-66985, a putative PAF antagonist, responses to PAF were attenuated significantly, but responses to norepinephrine and U46619 remained unchanged. Furthermore, PAF did not increase PG and LT levels in the cortical subarachnoideal fluid. These findings indicate that PAF is a potent constrictor of cerebral arterioles in newborn pigs and that its mechanism of action is independent of cyclooxygenase and lipoxygenase products of AA metabolism; furthermore, they suggest that U-66985 may be a selective PAF antagonist that crosses the blood-brain barrier. Using a closed cranial window, pial arterioles of newborn pigs were studied to test the hypothesis that prostanoids may play a permissive role in acetylcholine-induced constriction.[197] Acetylcholine-induced contraction was blocked by indomethacin but restored when it was coadministered with topical $PGF_{2\alpha}$, U46619 or PGH_2. The restored acetylcholine response was blocked by pirenzepine, a muscarinic-1 antagonist and the restoring ability of prostanoids was inhibited by SQ 29,548. PGE_2, PAF, and norepinephrine had no effect. Therefore, the activation of TXA_2/PGH_2 receptors appears to be necessary for acetylcholine-induced constriction, thus prostanoids play a permissive role in the contractile cholinergic response in pial vessels.

The effects of PAF on isolated feline basilar arteries and human pial arteries were also studied.[198] In high potassium medium PAF contracted both types of arteries, while in $PGF_{2\alpha}$ precontracted vessels it induced relaxation. These responses seemed to be independent of eicosanoid release. A decreased sensitivity of platelets to PAF in migraine patients during headache-free intervals was observed and briefly discussed.[199] It may be concluded that cerebral vessels respond to PAF in a particular manner; these phenomena, however, should be more intensively studied in forthcoming experiments.

Effect of BN 52021 and BN 50739 on Cerebral Ischemia

As mentioned above, PAF has been implicated as an important mediator of tissue injury in the brain. The basic observations that BN 52021 prevent ischemia/reperfusion-induced brain injury in gerbils[200,201] and PAF receptor blockade enhances early neuronal recovery after multifocal brain ischemia in dogs[202] have initiated further studies in this field. In comparison with WEB 2086 (**12**), the effect of BN 52021 on posttraumatic cerebral edema was investigated,[203] and found to have beneficial effects on edema formation and its time course. The role of PAF in cerebral ischemia and related disorders and the effect of BN 52021 have been recently reviewed.[204,205] The effect of BN 52021 on free fatty acid and DG accumulation and the loss of fatty acids from phosphatidylinositol-4,5-biphosphate (PIP_2) in mouse brain in response to electroconvulsive shock or decapitation ischemia was studied.[206] Electroconvulsive shock caused marked accumulation of free fatty acids and DG and loss of mainly stearic acid and AA from PIP_2 through activation. BN 52021 reduced injury-induced activation of PLA_2 and lysophospholipase, which mediate the accumulation of free fatty acids in the brain, while having negligible effect on PLC-mediated degradation of PIP_2. More recently, the effects of BN 52021 were studied in comparison with other chemically unrelated PAF antagonists, such as kadsurenone and brotizolam (**11**) applied either as pretreatment or posttreatment on cerebral metabolic and behavioral disturbances after bilateral carotid artery ligation and recirculation in Mongolian gerbils. It was found that PAF antagonists significantly improved behavioral disturbances characterized by stroke index, mitochondrial respiration, tissue water, and electrolyte contents in the post-ischemic phase, while the treatment did not modify the initial cerebral impairment. The results provide the first rationale for the use of PAF antagonists in the treatment of post-stroke syndrome. BN 52021 was recently found to reduce postischemic neuronal damage in the hippocampus of rat brain after forebrain ischemia. An isolated brain preparation of mongrel dogs was utilized to test the effect of BN 52021 on normoxic and post-ischemic complete brain ischemia, because it permitted delivery of a precise 14-min long complete ischemic insult and 60 min of reoxygenation in the virtual absence of PAF sources, such as platelets and leukocytes.[207] The PAF antagonist did not induce major changes in normoxic metabolic parameters, but significantly attenuated the ischemia-induced loss of ATP, ADP, phosphocreatine, and creatine from the brain tissue. Additional evidence in favor of the possible therapeutic potential of PAF antagonists in the management of cerebral ischemia has been provided by recent studies on the effect of BN 50739 **(14)** on brain edema, cortical microcirculation, blood-brain barrier disruption and neuronal death following focal brain injury.[208] A neodymium:yttrium-aluminum-garnet laser was used to induce highly reproducible focal cortical lesions in anesthetized rats. The severity of the lesion was assessed by progressive cortical hypoperfusion, edema and blood-brain barrier disruption in the vicinity of the hemispheroid lesion assessed acutely after injury. Histopathological evolution was followed up to 4 days, and secondary and progressive neuronal damage was revealed. BN 50739 ameliorated the severe hypoperfusion, reduced edema and progression of neuronal damage in the cortex and the CA-1 hippocampal neurons, thereby, indicating a marked beneficial effect of this new PAF antagonist in cerebral ischemia.

BN 52021 IN IMMUNE ENCEPHALOMYELITIS IN THE RAT

Intradermal injection of an encephalogenic adjuvant usually composed of spinal cord homogenate or myelin basic protein mixed to an emulsion with an equal volume of Freunds complete adjuvant induces experimental allergic encephalomyelitis in the rat which can be used as an animal model for multiple sclerosis. Rats developing encephalomyelitis were treated with intravenous PAF injection on day 5 and developed a more severe form of the disease at an earlier time point than did control animals.[209,210] Animals treated with BN 52021 did not develop the disease to any great extent. Treatment with vehicle had no effect compared to control. These results implicate PAF in the etiology of this model of multiple sclerosis and may suggest a role for PAF antagonists in the treatment of this disease.

PAF ANTAGONISTS IN AIRWAY HYPERSENSITIVITY

Heightened airway reactivity is a major characteristic of asthma. Inflammation developed as a consequence of immediate hypersensitivity reaction plays an important role in the characteristic bronchial hyperresponsiveness and symptoms of chronic asthma.[211] Several mediators have been implicated in the pathomechanism of airway hyperresponsiveness, but only PAF causes a prolonged increase in bronchial reactivity.[212] More recently, increasing attention has been paid to the late asthmatic response, because its treatment is still unsolved and only glucocorticoids offer alleviation. The acute and long-term pulmonary effects[213] as well as the role of PAF and PAF antagonists in the pathogenesis of asthma[214] have recently been reviewed. The significance of PAF, platelets, and eosinophils in bronchial hyperresponsiveness has been summarized by Page.[215]

AIRWAY HYPERREACTIVITY STUDIES *N VIVO*

A selective model for studying the IgE-mediated anaphylactic bronchoconstriction in the guinea pig was recently developed.[216] Guinea pigs were passively sensitized with mouse ascitic fluid containing dinitrophenol-specific IgE antibodies. Challenge of sensitized animals with dinitrophenol coupled to bovine serum albumin evoked a bronchoconstriction that was maximal 5 h after sensitization, and not blocked by mepyramine, FPL 55712, or BN 52021 **(15)** alone. However, when the sensitized animals were pretreated with the three drugs in combination, bronchoconstriction was specifically reduced. This model mimics human bronchial asthma in terms of the characteristic of bronchoconstriction and its pharmacological sensitivity. By using WEB 2170 **(13)**, a PAF antagonist of hetrazepine framework, the phospholipid mediator was found to be involved in active anaphylaxis in mice and guinea pigs.[217] The author has concluded that histamine release has to be minimized when the effect of PAF antagonists is studied in the guinea pig.

Bronchoconstrictor responses to PAF were analyzed in anesthetized guinea pigs[218] and cats.[219] Intravenous PAF injection caused dose-dependent increase in lung resistance and decrease in dynamic compliance and systemic arterial pressure. Sodium meclofenamate, a cyclooxygenase inhibitor, markedly reduced these parameters except the blood pressure response, so did SG 29,548, a TX receptor blocking agent. The responses were mimicked by a TX mimetic drug, U46619 or AA. CV-3988 (**1**) blocked all responses with the exception of that produced by U46619. These results show that, although airway and vasodepressor responses to PAF in the cat are mediated by different mechanisms, a similar PAF sensitive receptor is involved. A23187-induced airway constriction in the guinea pig was reversed by β_2 receptor antagonists, agents influencing arachidonate metabolism through lipoxygenase and cyclooxygenase pathways, but SRI 63-072 (**5**), a PAF receptor antagonist had only little effect, indicating that bronchoconstriction induced by calcium ionophore implies special characteristics.[220] The possible role of PAF in allergen-induced early airway responses in sheep was studied using WEB 2086 (**12**).[221] PAF responses contributed to antigen-induced bronchoconstriction. Inhaled PAF produced an increase in airway resistance which was inhibited by WEB 2086 and FPL 55712, but indomethacin and the H_1-antagonist chlorpheniramine were without effect, indicating that PAF acts indirectly through LT release. It was also found that PAF induced only incidental late airway response in the sheep, referring to important species differences.

PAF induces bronchoconstriction, leukopenia, and thrombocytopenia when injected intravenously in anesthetized guinea pigs. The effect of BN 52021 and BN 52111 (**7**) or BN 52115 (**8**), two dioxolan compounds with PAF antagonistic properties, were tested on these parameters.[222] All these compounds inhibited increased airway resistance and thrombocytopenia in a dose-related manner. BN 52111 applied in higher doses partially antagonized the decrease in the number of circulating leukocytes, but the other two compounds had no effect on leukopenia. The dioxolan derivatives proved to be more potent than BN 52021 in reducing PAF-induced bronchopulmonary alterations, while it induced a more expressed redution of TXB_2 generation, suggesting that the two phenomena are not directly related.

Airway hyperresponsiveness and inflammation assessed by bronchoalveolar lavage as well as neutrophilia in sheep challenged with carbachol and *Ascaris suum* antigen was blocked by WEB 2086.[223] This finding is in favor of the concept that PAF is involved in airway hyperreactivity and inflammation occuring after antigen challenge. Lung injury induced by intravenous infusion of purified human recombinant TNF in rats could not be reversed by two specific PAF receptor antagonists, WEB 2086 and SRI 63-441 (**6a**) suggesting that TNF-induced lung injury is mediated by eicosanoid rather than PAF.[224]

The effects of BN 52021 and CsA, either alone or in combination, on PAF- and antigen-induced bronchoconstriction were studied in passively sensitized guinea pigs.[225,226] Although a single administration of CsA alone had no effect on PAF-induced bronchoconstriction, a marked inhibition was found when CsA was combined with an inactive dose of BN 52021. This effect was in association with PAF-induced alterations in the number of leukocytes and platelets. The results strengthen the hypothesis that PAF and the immune system are involved in the regulation of bronchopulmonary reactions. In anesthetized guinea pigs PAF was shown to produce bronchial hyperresponsiveness to intravenous acetylcholine.[227] Pretreatment of guinea pigs with propranolol, a β-adrenoceptor antagonist, or indomethacin, a cyclooxygenase inhibitor, induced hyperreactivity to intravenous histamine. PAF-induced hyperresponsiveness was significantly attenuated by pretreatment with BN 52021, CV-3988, or WEB 2086, while these PAF receptor antagonists had no effect on propranolol- and indomethacin-induced bronchial hyperresponsiveness. Therefore, the latter response does not seem to involve PAF as mediator. The role of booster injection on capability of BN 52021 to block antigen-induced bronchoconstriction in ovalbumin-sensitized guinea pigs was recently investigated.[228,229] Irrespective of the titers of circulating immunoglobulins at various times after booster injection, BN 52021 was inactive against antigen-induced bronchoconstriction. However, when the PAF antagonist was tried in guinea pigs not subjected to booster injection, it inhibited bronchoconstriction induced by intratracheal installation of antigen or ovalbumin-induced contractions of lung strips. The booster injection may account for the loss of efficacy of BN 52021 as an inflammatory challenge, interfering with the pharmacologic modulation of the bronchopulmonary and secretory effect of PAF in the lungs.

IN VITRO STUDIES ON AIRWAY HYPERREACTIVITY

In isolated rat and guinea pig tracheal segments, PAF induced contraction and did not cause down-regulation of β-adrenoceptor.[230] In addition, PAF-contracted tracheal segments lost their ability to relax in response to isoprenaline. PAF increased the bronchoconstrictor response of mammalian airways to cholinergic agonists, and is thus implicated as a potential mediator of airway hyperreactivity. The phospholipid was employed in an *in situ* canine tracheal preparation which allowed differentiation of the effects on inducing airway edema and secretions.[231] PAF infused into the tracheal arteries induced a dose-dependent increase of the smooth muscle to parasympathetic stimuli. Regional stimulation by PAF did not render the lung more sensitive to vagus nerve stimulation, suggesting the role of locally released secondary mediators. Inoue and Kannan[232] showed that tracheal smooth muscle strips, excised from guinea pigs challenged *in vivo* with PAF for 7 days, 10 min/day, did not show increased sensitivity to acetylcholine and KCl but exhibited an increased sensitivity to histamine. Cimetidine, an H_2 receptor blocker, and indomethacin, a cyclooxygenase inhibitor, potentiated histamine-induced contractions both in control and PAF-treated animals to similar magnitudes. Under these conditions, an increased eosinophilic infiltration of the mucosa of the trachea was seen by histological examination. The results suggest a synergistic interaction between histamine and PAF in respect of smooth muscle reactivity and inflammatory response. Various LTD_4 antagonists exhibited a synergistic effect when applied together with L-652,731 (17), a PAF receptor antagonist in ovalbumin- and AA-challenged sensitized guinea pig tracheal strips,[233] indicating that PAF and LTD_4 may be considered as major mediators in this model of allergic bronchospasm. Pharmacological analysis of PAF-, LTB_4-, and LTD_4-induced contractions of tracheal, bronchial and lung parenchymal strips was carried out.[234] When the effluent of perfused lungs was superfused over the strips, the intraarterial injection of PAF caused a release of spasmogens which contracted all three tissues. Indomethacin inhibited these responses; however, treatment with indomethacin of the assay tissues did not block the contractile responses. Pretreatment of the lungs with indomethacin or aspirin did not block the release of spasmogens elicited by PAF but appeared to inhibit the release of cyclooxygenase products. Lipoxygenase inhibitors, NDGA or L-655,240, blocked the release of spasmogens from the perfused lungs. FPL 55712, an antagonist of slow reacting substance of anaphylaxis, did not block the PAF-response, while BN 52021 completely abolished spasmogen release by PAF from the lung. It appears likely that PAF induces LTB_4 release which then further generates cyclooxygenase products. The involvement of TXA_2 in the mechanism of action of PAF-induced contraction of guinea-pig parenchymal strips was analyzed by indomethacin, the TXA_2 synthase inhibitor OKY-046, the TXA_2 receptor antagonist L-655,240 or SKF-88046.[235] These compounds had no significant effects on PAF-induced bronchoconstriction, while NDGA and BW775c were inhibitory, indicating a major role for lipoxygenase products.

The interference of PAF with PAF antagonists, related structurally to the phospholipid, such as Ro 19-3704 (3c), Ro 19-1400 (4b) and CV 6209 (2) as well as agents structurally unrelated to PAF like BN 52021 and WEB 2086 were studied in isolated lungs from actively sensitized guinea pigs.[236] Both PAF antagonists inhibited PAF-induced bronchoconstriction in normal lung, but failed to influence that induced by PAF in actively sensitized animals. Ro 19-3704 and Ro 19-1400, at concentrations which abrogate the effects of PAF in the lungs of non-immunized animals, inhibited bronchoconstriction and release of histamine and LT-like material evoked by PAF injected intraarterially into lungs of sensitized animals. Interestingly enough, CV-6209 failed to block the responses induced by PAF in sensitized lungs. All antagonists suppressed edema formation induced either by ovalbumin or PAF. These results indicate the involvement of different mechanisms in allergic bronchoconstriction and inflammatory response; furthermore, sensitization provokes marked modification in PAF reactivity in the lung. In guinea pig parenchymal lung strips the effects of LTD_4, acetylcholine, histamine and KCl coadministered with PAF were studied.[237] There was no significant alteration in acetylcholine- and KCl-induced responses and in the PAF-induced inhibition of histamine response; however, PAF caused a marked, concentration-dependent decrease in LTD_4-induced contractions. BN 52021, cyclooxygenase and lipoxygenase inhibitors interfered with PAF-induced attenuation of LTD_4 contractions, suggesting a role of secondary TXA_2 generation. In histamine-contracted guinea pig tracheal preparations PAF induced relaxation and PGE_2 production.[238] WEB 2086 inhibited PAF-induced relaxation and PGE_2 release; BN 52021 markedly decreased the PAF response, but completely abolished PAF-induced PGE_2 release. These results are consistent with the presence of specific PAF receptors in the guinea pig trachea and the involvement of PGE_2 in PAF-induced relaxation.

More recently, human airways were used in culture to study the pathophysiology of pulmonary allergic reactions.[239] In this preparation PAF stimulated respiratory glucoconjugate release. The response was inhibited by Ro 19-3704, a PAF receptor antagonist, and LY 171,883, a specific LTD_4 receptor antagonist, while indomethacin had no effect, suggesting the involvement of lipoxygenase products. Interestingly enough, PAF response was augmented by atropine which finding makes unlikely that cholinergic receptors are involved in the effect of PAF. In guinea pig and human lung preparations, [^{3}H]WEB 2086 labeled specific PAF receptors, providing an excellent model for further studies on the involvement of PAF in airway hyperreactivity.[240]

It may be concluded that bronchial hyperresponsiveness due to immediate type hypersensitivity can be carefully divided into several subtypes whose pharmacologic sensitivity may be different, thus explaining the diversed clinical features and therapeutic interventions in bronchial asthma. Various PAF antagonists may be useful to select different types of hypersensitivity reactions in the lung.

PAF IN GRAFT REJECTION AND IMMUNE RESPONSES

GRAFT PROTECTION

The role of PAF in organ transplant rejection has been recently reviewed.[241,242] Eicosanoids and PAF can modulate the immune response *in vitro* and *in vivo*. PGs seem to attenuate, while TXA_2, LTs, and PAF potentiate the cell-mediated immune response. In addition, these compounds have non-immunological effects that may modify edema formation and decreased blood flow associated with the rejection process.

Studies on the rejection of murine tail skin allografts parallel with PAF-induced mortality in mice were conducted.[243] Daily peroral treatment with BN 52021 (**15**) significantly prolonged the survival time of the distal skin allografts. Dexamethasone prolonged the survival of either the proximal or the distal tail skin allografts. Intravenously administered PAF increased TXB_2 concentration in the intact skin, while in the transplantation group BN 52021 lowered TXB_2 content both in intact and regenerated skin. However there was no correlation between skin TXB_2 content and allograft survival, showing that this eicosanoid may not be involved as mediator of the PAF effect during transplantation. In parallel experiments, the PAF antagonist significantly reduced mortality rate induced by the same dose of PAF injected intravenously that increased TXB_2 content in the skin. The conclusion may be drawn that PAF-induced shock is an inappropriate model as a screening test to select specifically effective PAF receptor antagonists against graft rejection. In a further study, starting from the observation of Kagawa et al.[244] that rat cardiac allograft survival could be prolonged by inhibitors of AA metabolism, Becker et al.[245] made an attempt to specify the role of eicosanoids, using PG analogs, the specific TXA_2 receptor antagonist, BM-13177 and the specific

TXA_2 synthase inhibitor Hoe-944 as well as aspirin in combination with BN 52021 with respect of the allograft survival of mouse tail skin. Besides determining local prostanoid concentrations in the regenerated skin, *in vitro* experiments with human granulocytes were carried out to reveal correlation between eicosanoid changes in skin and in circulating granulocytes after treatment with the drugs used. They concluded that, in contrast to other immunological processes, like anaphylactic bronchoconstriction, TXA_2 may not account for graft rejection. This is reflected by the lack of relationship of graft survival to skin and granulocyte eicosanoid contents under the influence of drugs studied. Heterotopic heart xenografting or orthotopic liver xenografting from guinea pig to rat confirmed that BN 52021 could prolong graft survival time.[246]

An attempt has been recently made to prolong organ preservation by using BN 52021.[247] It was shown that the application of the PAF antagonist in traditionally used perfusion solutions significantly improved preserved pulmonary function as compared to that of control animals. Thus, BN 52021 may be applied to lung transplant donors and recipients in order to make lung transplantation possible even with long physical distances between donor and recipient.

IMMUNE AND CYTOTOXIC PROCESSES

The role of PAF in immune and cytotoxic processes has been briefly summarized.[248]

The significance of PAF in the mediation of pathophysiological responses to aggregated immunoglobulins using BN 52021 was studied in Sprague-Dawley rats.[249] Infusion of soluble aggregates of IgG significantly and rapidly reduced the time of lysis of diluted blood clot which paralleled the appearance in plasma of tissue-type plasminogen activator and serum levels of N-acetylglucosaminidase as well as blood neutrophil count. In trials with rats previously depleted of circulating PMNL by treatment with vinblastine, no change in N-acetylglucosaminidase was detected. When the animals were given BN 52021, alterations induced by challenge with immune complexes were suppressed, suggesting a role for PAF in immune complex diseases. By contrast, BN 52021 did not interfere with the clearance of the aggregates from the circulation. The involvement of eicosanoids and PAF in immune-complex alveolitis was demonstrated in the rat lung.[250] An increase in the release of PGE_2, TXA_2, and LTB_4 into the bronchoalveolar space and a decrease in the number of circulating platelets were observed. Thrombopenia was inhibited by indomethacin, BN 52021 and econazole, a TXA_2 blocker, but remained unaffected by NDGA. These results may be explained by an interaction between PAF and TXA_2 in this immune complex hypersensitivity reaction.

The influence of BN 52021 and BN 52063 on the immunosuppressive effect of CsA was studied on lymphocyte proliferation and IL-1 and IL-2 production.[251] CsA inhibited in a dose-dependent manner the proliferation of rat spleen cells. Submaximal doses of CsA in association with BN 52021 showed potentiating effect. This synergistic effect was also seen when *in vitro* cytokine generation was determined. These alterations could be reproduced *ex vivo* after 4-day-long treatment of rats with BN 52063. This finding is promising for using PAF antagonists in association with CsA to prevent graft rejection. Studies are in progress to determine whether PAF antagonists could decrease CsA-induced nephrotoxicity without altering its immunosuppressive effect. BN 52021 was studied on human natural killer activity against K 562 target cells by using ^{51}Cr-release as a measure of cytotoxicity.[252] The PAF antagonist significantly reduced natural killer activity which was not due to the impairment of binding of effector cells to target cells. Preincubation of target cells with BN 52021 induced a higher reduction in cytotoxicity than that of effector cells. Moreover, the increase in cytotoxicity induced by interferon was less pronounced when BN 52021 was added in the incubation medium. The natural killer activity of platelet-depleted large granular lymphocyte-enriched effector cell population was inhibited in a similar manner. Two other structurally unrelated PAF antagonists, BN 52111 (**7**) and WEB 2086 (**12**), showed similar action on natural killer cells as did BN 52021, indicating the presence of specific PAF binding sites responsible for the phenomenon. Finally, it was also demonstrated that synthetic PAF induced a dose-dependent cytotoxic action on K 562 cells which was effectively suppressed by BN 52021; thus these results provide indirect evidence for the involvement of the lipid mediator in natural killer activity.

PAF AND ITS ANTAGONISTS IN INFLAMMATION AND ARTHRITIS

The search for the possible significance of PAF as mediator of the acute and chronic inflammatory reactions has become of great interest. Silva and colleagues[253] described how subcutaneous injection of PAF into the footpad of rats led to a local inflammatory response followed by desensitization after repeated injections. Desensitization was not affected by previous adrenalectomy but the acute response was exacerbated. LY 171883, an LTD_4 inhibitor, suppressed PAF-induced edema formation, suggesting a role for this eicosanoid in the pro-inflammatory mechanism. PAF does not appear to be involved as mediator in the inflammatory process induced by *Bothrops jararaca* venom,[254] while it has a minor role in the mouse paw edema induced by PLA_2 derived from the snake venom *(A. piscivorus piscivorus)* since this reaction was only partially reduced by kadsurenone **(16)**, a PAF receptor antagonist.[255]

Changes in vascular permeability to FITS-dextran 150 associated with topical application of PAF in the hamster cheek pouch preparation were calculated using a mathematical model.[256] The best-fit estimate of apparent interstitial diffusion coefficient remained constant at various PAF concentrations, implying PAF as a potential modulator of macromolecular permeability in the microcirculation. This was the first study which quantified the changes in permeability-surface area product of FITC-dextran 150 as a function of PAF concentration. The role of PAF in systemic vascular permeability in selected tissues was studied by using Evans blue dye as a marker.[257,258] Increasing doses of the phospholipid were injected into the caudal vein and the dye was extracted by formamide and measured photometrically. Extravasation of the dye varied markedly from one tissue to another (peak extravasation was seen in the pancreas and duodenum) and increased as a function of time (from 0 to 60 min). BN 52021 **(15)** and L-655,240, a TXA_2 antagonist, inhibited PAF response.

Experiments were performed to study the role of PAF in zymosan-induced pleurisy in the rat.[259] BN 52021 injected intraperitoneally significantly inhibited pleural exudation and cell migration induced by zymosan. When PAF was injected intrapleurally twice a day, a selective and progressive desensitization developed.[260] It was noted that, in PAF desensitized animals, both exudation and cell infiltration induced by zymosan were blocked, whereas the responsiveness to serotonin remained unchanged. This study suggests that zymosan-induced pleurisy may be largely dependent on PAF release. PAF could be involved as mediator in PMA-induced rat pleurisy[261] as well. Inflammatory exudate induced by Arthus reaction in the rat peritoneal cavity was analyzed for PGE_2, and TXA_2 by enzyme immuno-assays and LTB_4 by radioimmunoassay.[262,263] All the eicosanoid levels were increased by antigen challenge. Indomethacin inhibited PGE_2 and TXA_2 release and increased LTB_4 formation, BN 52021 suppressed LTB_4 production and increased PGE_2 release, whereas TXB_2 production was not affected. This finding is in favor of the concept that PAF-eicosanoid interaction is involved in Arthus reaction.

Aggregation of washed rabbit platelets was used as a measure of the biological activity of a lipid prepared from inflamed gingiva.[264] The mobility of active lipid was coincident with that of authentic PAF on thin layer chromatography. Aggregation was dose-dependent and inhibited by pretreatment with ONO 6240 **(3b)**, a specific PAF antagonist, but not by indomethacin or creatine phosphate/creatine phosphokinase which inhibit platelet aggregation induced by AA or ADP, respectively. Normal gingival tissue contained less active lipid than the inflamed tissue, suggesting that PAF may be involved in the occurrence and maintenance of periodontal disease.

BB rats spontaneously develop insulin-dependent diabetes mellitus in association with a marked inflammatory reaction in the Langerhans islets as indicated by light microscopical observation. BN 52021 was used for daily treatment of these rats for a longer time period.[265] The PAF receptor antagonist dramatically diminished the degree of insulitis exemplified by an increased ratio of insulin/glucagon cells and a dose dependent reduction of eosinophil infiltration in the tissue. These changes were not accompanied by alleviation of diabetic symptoms. PAF inhibitors may prove to be a useful immunomodulator therapy for insulin-dependent diabetes since β cells are preserved.

Antigen-induced arthritis in the rabbit was used to analyze the possible role of PAF in the acute inflammatory response.[266] Antigen-induced arthritis was reduced by BN 52021. For suppressing exudation the PAF antagonist overcame the activity of non-steroidal anti-inflammatory agents, while the blocking effect was reversed when synovial fluid was assessed for PGE_2 content. BN 52021 suppressed cellular infiltration as well. A PAF-like lipid extracted from the synovial fluid of patients with arthritis was also detected. It was identified as PAF by thin-layer chromatography and bioassay on rabbit platelet serotonin secretion assay. The effect of lipid mediator was inhibited by BN 52021 and WEB 2086 (12). These results are in agreement with the concept that PAF may have a mediator role in arthritis and its antagonists can be applied as therapeutic intervention in human rheumatoid arthritis. Femoral head cartilage was removed from male Wistar rats and implanted into the subcutaneous tissue of female Wistar rats.[267] PAF was constantly infused in minute doses by a minipump, and BN 52021 was administered orally twice a day as a long-term treatment. Glycosaminoglycan loss from the implanted cartilage was assayed and the data obtained were compared to age-matched nonimplanted cartilage. Glycosaminoglycan was lost from the implanted cartilage and this was unaffected by PAF or BN 52021 treatment. There were no differences in body weight and serum haptoglobin levels in response to treatments. However, when cartilage was cultured in a medium that contained PAF and IL-1, there was a greater loss of glycosaminoglycan than in a medium which contained the mediators separately. This synergism between PAF and IL-1 in arthropathies refers to a possible interaction of these mediators in human pathology.

More recently, Montrucchio et al.[268] provided evidence for the role of PAF in the inflammatory process, showing that it could be isolated and identified from the peritoneal fluid of patients who develop peritonitis after serial peritoneal dialysis. This suggests that the phospholipid mediator may contribute to increased permeability of the peritoneal vascular bed in response to inflammatory stimuli.

INFLAMMATORY SKIN DISORDERS

Intensive research has been continued on the possible role of PAF in various inflammatory skin disorders. Release of the phospholipid mediator and its precursors was demonstrated during allergic cutaneous reactions. In pollen sensitive patients, sterile skin chambers over-lying blister blase sites were filled with pollen diluted Hanks solution, then samples withdrawn were processed and assessed for PAF by platelet aggregation bioassay.[269] After incubation with PLA_2 the responses obtained were inhibited by specific PAF receptor antagonists, BN 52021 and L-652,731 (17). Cultured human skin keratinocytes, but not fibroblasts activated by PAF, accumulated inositol phosphates while precursor and lyso-PAF had no such effect.[270] Stimulation by PAF also resulted in accumulation of DG and PGE_2 release. For differentiating the sensitivity of rabbit skin to PAF-induced edema formation, the effects of several PAF antagonists were studied.[271] SRI 63-675 (6b) and CV-3988 (1), two structurally related antagonists, produced partial inhibition of the PAF response but the effect of other agonists was also reduced. 48740 RP (9a) induced a partial but selective inhibition. BN 52021 markedly inhibited PAF response in a selective manner, especially when administered intravenously. Kadsurenone and its synthetic derivatives blocked the responses selectively. The order of magnitude in efficacy was L-659,989 (**18**) > L-652,731 > kadsurenone. WEB 2086 given either intradermally or intravenously showed a selective activity similar to that of L-659,989. These results suggest that the model of skin lesion for studying PAF antagonists should be rigorously selected. Dithranol-induced dermatitis in mice was found to involve PAF as mediator, since BN 52021 was inhibitory, the coinvolvement of other mediators like PGs, histamine, and reactive oxygen free radicals was also demonstrated.[272,273] The effect of BN 52063, a mixture of ginkgolides, was studied on contact dermatitis in the mouse.[274] The response was inhibited in a dose-dependent fashion and was found to be additive when the PAF antagonist was given together with betamethasone, suggesting a new therapeutic approach for the clinical treatment of allergic skin reactions. IL-1 was released from guinea pig keratinocytes incubated in the presence or absence of endotoxin.[275] The lipopolysaccharide induced a dose-related increase in IL-1, while PAF alone was without effect. However, PAF potentiated endotoxin-induced cytokine generation. This finding suggests that under various stimuli PAF may possibly modulate local immune reactions in the skin. IL-1 release from human epidermis cells was stimulated when the cells were exposed to UV irradiation.[276] Since this augmented response was inhibited by BN 52021, indirect evidence for the involvement of PAF in cutaneous reaction was provided.

PAF AND PAF ANTAGONISTS IN THE GASTROINTESTINAL TRACT

The role of PAF in various kinds of tissue injury in the gastrointestinal tract has been extensively studied. It is now well established that the phospholipid mediator is involved in gastrointestinal ulceration, necrotic, and ischemic processes. Intensive research is still in progress in this important field.

GASTROINTESTINAL ULCERATION

Microcirculation plays an important role in the maintenance of functional integrity of the stomach and in the provision of its defense mechanisms against damage.[277,278] Changes in blood flow in the gastroduodenal mucosa, brought about by the local release of vasoactive or cytotoxic mediators, including oxygen-derived free radicals, eicosanoids, and PAF have been implicated in the pathogenesis of various forms of peptic ulceration and erosive gastritis. Damage to microvessels and vascular endothelium, leading to disruption of microcirculation is considered to be an initial event in the development of such lesions.

Using continuous monitoring by laser-Doppler flometry and reflectance spectrometry of gastric mucosal hemodynamics, the effect of intravenous PAF infusion was studied.[279] Gastric mucosal damage was assessed by microscopical scoring and measurement of thiobarbituric acid reactants as an index of lipid peroxidation. PAF induced hypotension and gastric mucosal injury which was related to congestion, elevation of thiobarbituric acid reactants and oxygen-derived free radicals. This effect of intravenous PAF was confirmed by using superoxide dismutase plus catalase.[280] The reduction in the number of circulating PMNL paralleled the gastric mucosal damage and thiobarbituric acid reactants, indicating the important role for oxygen free radicals in PAF-induced gastric ulceration. The significance of PAF in inducing gastric damage was underlined by the observation that the activity of acetylhydrolase, which converts PAF into inactive lyso-PAF, was increased in rats with gastric ulcers induced by water-immersion stress.[281] Alternatively, the PAF antagonist CV-3988 (**1**) and hydrocortisone acetate inhibited distinct bleeding and a remarkable increase in mucosal vascular permeability observed by dye leakage assessment induced by acid perfused stomach in anesthetized rats.[282]

In isolated normal rat jejunum, PAF induced immediate and late dose-dependent increases in short-circuit current when the experiments were conducted at or before approximately 9 A.M.[283] These responses were reduced in chloride-free buffer and inhibited by the chloride channel blocker, diphenylamine-2-carboxylate. Early phase responses were blocked by BN 52021 (**15**) and WEB 2086 (**12**) as well as by the neurotoxin, tetrodotoxin. The conclusion was drawn that PAF receptors are involved in a chloride secretion process which follows a circadian rhythm.

The role of PAF in endotoxin-, restraint-stress-, and ethanol-induced gastrointestinal ulceration was studied in rats.[284] BN 52021 and BN 52063 markedly reduced the deleterious effects of PAF and endotoxin. BN 52021 and triazolam (**10b**), a structurally unrelated antagonist for PAF, partially reduced restraint-stress-induced gastric damage in young female but not male rats. Similar partial protection was obtained in rats with ethanol-induced gastric damage. In contrast to atropine and ranitidine, BN 52021 did not affect the gastric hypersecretion in pylorus-ligated rats nor aspirin-induced gastric ulcerations. In a further study,[285] BN 52021 was more effective against PAF-induced gastric lesions than in reducing endotoxin-induced gastrointestinal damage. In the cold restraint stress model, BN 52021 decreased both gastrointestinal lesions and plasma transaminase activity. These results indicate that PAF plays a major role in the gastric damage induced by endotoxin and may partially contribute to the gastric lesions induced by ethanol and stress, providing evidence for a potential therapeutic use for PAF antagonists in certain types of gastrointestinal lesions in man.

Tetrodotoxin did not affect the rise in intragastric pressure induced by the TXA_2 mimetic U46619. Endotoxin-induced increase in intragastric pressure was inhibited by L-652,731 (**17**), indicating an important role for PAF in this response.[286,287] LTC_4 and PAF, affecting gastric microcirculation, caused mild gastric mucosal injury and greatly augmented mucosal lesions produced by other irritants such as absolute ethanol, taurocholate, aspirin, or stress.[288] These lesions were accompanied by mucosal LTC_4 generation which was further increased by PAF.[289,290] BN 52021 abolished PAF-induced gastric lesions and reduced LTC_4 generation when PAF and ethanol were given together.

The amplificative role of PAF in the oxidative stress following reperfusion of ischemic stomach was also detected.[291] As assayed by extraction, purification, and platelet aggregation, PAF production was increased in the gastric mucosa after dexamethasone treatment,[292] and this increased PAF generation appeared to have a mediator role in dexamethasone-induced gastric ulceration, since BN 52021 showed a gastroprotective effect under these conditions. These results are in accordance with those published by Eliakim et al.[293] who studied the involvement of PAF in ulcerative colitis, and demonstrated that sulfasalazine and prednisolone produced enhanced production of the phospholipid mediator.

In contrast to these findings, pretreatment with dexamethasone resulted in a significant attenuation of endotoxin-induced hemoconcentration, hypotension, and damage in the duodenum and stomach.[294] It also significantly reduced PAF synthesis by the lung but had no effect on endotoxin-induced increase in PAF release and vascular permeability in the gastrointestinal tissues. These authors suggest that dexamethasone-induced protection may be related to inhibition of PAF release from the lung; moreover, PAF release from gastrointestinal tissue likely contributes little to the systemic disturbances in endotoxic shock. The conclusion may be drawn that PAF release from different tissues varies with the types of challenge used, and this point should be taken into account when the therapeutic efficacy of PAF antagonists is under investigation.

As indicated before, when given peripherally, PAF induces severe gastric mucosal damage. Since PAF and PAF metabolizing enzymes are present in the brain, Cucala et al.[295,296] studied rat gastric acid secretion and gross mucosal integrity in response to intracerebroventricular PAF and compared it with that to thyrotropin releasing hormone (TRH), a known central gastric secretagogue. Centrally applied TRH and intravenous pentagastrin increased gastric acid output. In contrast, acid output decreased after intracerebroventricular PAF and the lipid mediator reduced pentagastrin-stimulated gastric acid secretion. Morphological changes were found to be opposite when TRH and PAF were compared. Thus, it appears likely that a gastric secretion modulatory system exists at the central level in which PAF initiates gastroprotective mechanisms.

INTESTINAL ISCHEMIA-INDUCED MUCOSAL DAMAGE

PAF release, assessed by extraction of plasma samples obtained after mesenterial artery occlusion and reperfusion, then extracted and separated first by thin layer chromatography followed by high pressure liquid chromatography and alkaline treatment, bioassayed by platelet aggregation, was demonstrated in an anesthetized dog model.[297]

Otamiri et al.[298] observed that intestinal permeability, lysosomal enzyme release, as well as malondialdehyde content in the rat ileum after ischemic insult, were inhibited by quinacrine and NDGA, while BW755C had no effect and indomethacin potentiated the response. BN 52021 did not influence the myeloperoxidase activity but decreased the formation of malondialdehyde and the increase in mucosal permeability and N-acetyl-β-glucosaminidase release, indicating a role for activation of specific PAF receptors in ischemia-induced intestinal mucosal damage. Ischemia-reperfusion induced extensive gastric mucosal injury and an increase in chemoluminescence activity of neutrophils obtained from the portal vein in hemorrhagic shock rats.[299] CV-3988 significantly reduced the gross and histologic gastric damage, and the increase in chemoluminescence activity of PMNL, suggesting that PAF-generated hypoxia might stimulate oxygen free radical production, resulting in gastric injury.

Bowel Disease and Necrosis

Several candidate mediators of acute inflammation, such as E-type PGs, histamine, and bradykinin are potent pro-diarrheal colonic secretagogues. They act to increase serosal to mucosal transport of chloride and passive water efflux. The effect of PAF was studied on transepithelial potential difference and, under voltage clamp conditions, short circuit current in muscle-stripped rat colon.[300] PAF induced dose-dependent increases in transepithelial potential difference and short circuit current. Lyso-PAF had a much smaller but discernible effect. PAF displayed 'sidedness' with serosal application effective and mucosal application ineffective. Inhibitor studies suggested that chloride was the principal ion carrier but PAF antagonists such as kadsurenone, CV-3988 and WEB 2086 did not block the response. Unlike bradykinin, PAF did not cause the release of PGE$_2$ into the serosal bathing fluid, and its action was not attenuated by cyclooxygenase inhibitors, like piroxicam, mefenamic acid, or flurbiprofen. This suggests that PAF has a powerful pro-diarrheal secretory action on colonic epithelium which is not mediated by previously defined PAF receptors and seems independent of prostanoid generation.

Sun and Hsueh[301] have demonstrated that rats treated with PAF or endotoxin develop ischemic bowel necrosis associated with shock. In this model, the morphological changes of TNF-induced bowel lesions were indistinguishable from those caused by PAF. TNF could induce PAF production in bowel tissue, and the effects of TNF and endotoxin on PAF production in the intestine were additive. Furthermore, TNF and endotoxin are synergistic in inducing bowel necrosis, and TNF-induced bowel necrosis was due to PAF release, since SRI 63-119 (**3a**), a PAF receptor antagonist offered protective effect.[302] Rats pretreated with allopurinol or superoxide dismutase together with catalase markedly improved the lesions induced by administration of PAF into the mesenteric vasculature, indicating that most of the intestinal damage was due to the release of oxygen free radicals.[303] The major source of oxygen free radicals is xanthine oxidase, as allopurinol ameliorated small bowel lesions. Allopurinol reduced PAF-induced hypotension as well. Superoxide dismutase/catalase did not alter hypotension induced by PAF but improved hemoconcentration and leukopenia induced by the phospholipid mediator. The direct effect of PAF on enterocytes was determined in a human rectal adenocarcinoma cell-line HRT-18 by studying the production of cAMP and stimulation of electrogenic chloride secretion as its functional counterpart.[304] In this model, PAF applied at very low concentration increased cellular cAMP level, while at high concentration it did not. This effect and the absence of an apparent specific inhibition by BN 52021 and forskolin may indicate that PAF may not affect adenylate cyclase. Low doses of PAF did not influence short-circuit current either, while forskolin induced a substantial rise in its activity. These results suggest that at low concentrations PAF may act at different functional sites on chloride secretion in HRT-18 cells.

The mediator role of PAF in intestinal inflammation and ulceration was further investigated.[305] Using the rat colitis model, the effects of treatment with BN 52021 in comparison with WEB 2086 and WEB 2170 (13), two structurally dissimilar PAF antagonists, were studied in endotoxin-induced ulceration by measuring PAF biosynthesis and changes in vascular permeability. In agreement with previous findings,[306,307] PAF antagonists and inhibition of LT synthesis[308] were found to accelerate healing of chronic colitis, thereby suggesting a role for PAF in the mechanism of intestinal ulceration induced by endotoxin shock. Long-term treatment with BN 52021 or 5-aminosalicylic acid given intracolonically to rats after induction of chronic colitis did not affect colonic damage; however, after intraperitoneal administration BN 52021 reduced the incidence of adhesions and diarrhea, while 5-aminosalicylic acid did not.[308] Using an *in vitro* superfusion system, the effects of PAF on contractility segments of ascending colon were assessed. Tissue segments from normal rats contracted to PAF; however, non-inflamed segments derived from rats subjected to colitis 2 weeks before were relatively insensitive to the lipid mediator. These results are in opposition to the concept that PAF plays an important role in the acute inflammatory response in this model, but may be important in the prolongation of inflammation and ulceration. The contractility changes in the ascending colon may occur as a consequence of inflammation.

EXPERIMENTAL PANCREATITIS

A recent study indicated that a single injection of PAF into the superior pancreatico-duodenal artery of rabbits induced dose-dependent morphological alterations in the pancreatic tissue and increased serum amylase activity, both characteristic of an acute pancreatitis.[309] Two or 3 days after injection, tissue edema and infiltration with PMNL, cell vacuolization and acinar cell necrosis developed. By electron microscopy an increase in the number of zymogen granules in the apical region of acinar cells was observed as an early sign of PAF-induced tissue damage. CV-3988 antagonized the effect of PAF; in addition, the significant protection provided by atropine suggests a potential role for cholinergic mechanisms in PAF-induced pancreatic alteration. The preventive effect of BN 52021 on the formation of oxygen free radicals in cerulein-induced acute pancreatitis in rats also suggests a therapeutic value of PAF antagonists in acute pancreatitis.[310]

EFFECT OF PAF AND ITS ANTAGONISTS ON LIVER CELLS

Parenchymal cells (hepatocytes) are the sites at which the principal metabolic functions of the liver are located. In the perfused liver, responses, e.g., vasoconstriction and glycogenolysis, to stimulating agents such as zymosan, PAF and AA, are inhibited by indomethacin and bromophenacyl bromide, inhibitors of cyclooxygenase and PLA_2, respectively.[311] Since cultured Kupffer and endothelial cells, but not hepatocytes, produce eicosanoids, and eicosanoids, especially PGs, induce a similar pattern of responses when added directly to the perfused liver, an involvement of these non-parenchymal cells in mediating the above responses is considered likely.

Ligand binding studies indicate that PAF down-regulates its own receptors on the plasma membrane of isolated rat Kupffer cells but has no significant effect on the binding affinity of the receptors for PAF. Exposure of isolated rat Kupffer cells to PAF resulted in a rapid, time-dependent reduction in the number of cell surface receptors to a new steady state concentration.[312] With receptor synthesis inhibited by cycloheximide in the absence of PAF, the half-time of the surface PAF receptor was about 4 h, suggesting that PAF receptors are not recycled and that the loss of PAF receptors from the plasma membrane is accelerated by PAF binding. Under the same conditions, BN 52021 or U66985 alone had no effect on the number of surface PAF receptors; however, the PAF antagonists inhibited PAF-induced down-regulation of PAF receptors in a concentration-dependent manner, suggesting that PAF-induced down-regulation is a receptor-mediated process. This process is reversible, and prevented by cycloheximide. These observations suggest that the restored PAF receptor is newly synthesized rather than recycled.

Cultured rat Kupffer cells synthesized and released PAF when stimulated with calcium ionophore A23187 in a concentration- and time-dependent manner as measured by the [^{3}H]serotonin release assay.[313] It is suggested that Kupffer cells are important cellular components which produce and release PAF in order to facilitate communication between hepatic sinusoidal and parenchymal cells. Further, it was also suggested that PAF production in response to reticuloendothelial cell stimulation was responsible for hepatic glycogenolysis in the isolated rat liver. PAF stimulated production of PGI_2, PGE_2, and $PGF_{2\alpha}$ by rat liver cells.[314] The stimulation was inhibited by L-659,989 **(18)**, kadsurenone **(16)**, L-652,731 and BN 52021.

PAF is known to stimulate hepatic glycogenolysis, causes hepatic vasoconstriction and stimulates the production of cyclooxygenase-derived metabolites of AA, primarily PGD_2. Ibuprofen abolished PG release but did not affect hepatic glygogenolysis.[315] Thus, in contrast to previous observations, the two responses are not causally related. There was an inhibition of PAF response by prior exposure of the cells to PAF or TPA-type tumor promoter TPA, teleocidin and aplysiatoxin, as well as with the second stage tumor promoter mezerein, all of which activate the calcium/phospholipid-dependent PKC, indicating a homologous and heterologous desensitization. Application of PAF to [^{3}H]-inositol-labeled Kupffer cells produced dose-dependent increases in labeled inositol phosphate levels, demonstrating a response which was inhibited by SRI 63-675 **(6b)**, stimulation of PKC and PMA.[316] Concomitantly, PAF induced an increase of cytosolic free calcium concentrations in single Kupffer cell loaded with fura-2, thus interactions of PAF with Kupffer cells may result in hemodynamic and metabolic responses to the phospholipid mediator in the liver. PAF but not lyso-PAF stimulated PGI_2 production in isolated rat liver cells (the C-9 cell line) which could be blocked specifically with several PAF antagonists, such as L-659,989, SDZ 63-675, kadsurenone, L-652,731, WEB 2170, WEB 2086, and BN 52021.[317] The latter drug specifically inhibited PGI_2 release induced by PAF in a study applying several stimulators; therefore the stimulus appears to be mediated by occupancy of a PAF receptor. Using microsphere method with reference sample in conscious rats with cirrhosis due to bile duct ligation, the effects of BN 52021 on systemic and splanchnic hemodynamics were examined.[318] BN 52021 significantly reduced portal pressure when given intravenously as compared to placebo controls. Cirrhotic rats given BN 52021 exhibited significantly lower cardiac index, higher systemic vascular resistance and lower portal tributary blood flow than controls. These results are in favor of the concept that PAF might be one of the mediators responsible for the hyperdynamic circulation observed during cirrhosis. Systemic endotoxemia was observed in patients with acute and chronic liver failure, and bacterial endotoxin is known to increase vascular permeability. Intraportal endotoxin administration was applied in normal rats to study the rapid ascites formation, systemic hypotension, hemoconcentration, and the formation of acute erosions of the gastrointestinal mucosa as well as an increased generation of PAF.[319] Two PAF antagonists, L-652,731 and CV-3988, reduced these symptoms, supporting the view for the involvement of PAF as mediator in these responses.

PAF AND PAF ANTAGONISTS IN KIDNEY PATHOLOGY

In the last years, increasing attention has been paid to the role of PAF in kidney function and pathology. Systemic and renal hemodynamic responses to PAF[320] as well as the role of the lipid mediator in nephrology[321] have been briefly overviewed.

CELLULAR AND HEMODYNAMIC CHANGES

Results obtained in isolated glomeruli of normal rats incubated with PAF and the PAF antagonist BN 52021 (**15**) suggested that PAF could modulate glomerular filtration rate not only by inducing changes in systemic or intrarenal hemodynamics, but also by modifying the filtration surface, thus reducing ultrafiltration coefficient.[322] In cultured mesangial cells, angiotensin II stimulated PAF production, indicating a possible involvement of the lipid mediator in the angiotensin II-induced progression of renal glomerular disease.[323] Continuous infusion or bolus injection of PAF induced marked reduction of renal plasma flow, glomerular filtration, and urinary sodium excretion parallel with systemic hypotension.[324] When given alone, L-655,240, a TXA_2-PG endoperoxide antagonist, had no influence on blood pressure, renal blood flow, and filtration rate, but slightly elevated diuresis. On the other hand, the effect of PAF on hypotension was blocked. In small doses these drugs failed to prevent PAF-induced renal plasma flow and filtration rate, but attenuated PAF-induced effect on urinary sodium excretion in a dose-dependent manner, suggesting a role for eicosanoid release in the renal effect of PAF. It is known that renal vascular escape is induced by norepinephrine, a phenomenon in which PGs have been implicated. In a recent study, Fontales and Ferreira[325] demonstrated that BN 52021 could block norepinephrine-induced escape and reversed entirely tachyphylaxis promoted by repeated administration of the sympathomimetic amine.

PAF AND PAF ANTAGONISTS IN KIDNEY INJURY

PAF produced by various cells and organs may be involved in the mechanism of proteinuria and many other nephropathies. The beneficial effect of specific PAF antagonists in the treatment of such disorders was recently reviewed.[326]

A single injection of BN 52021 offered marked protection against the sharp decrease in glomerular filtration rate and renal blood flow induced by intramuscular injection of glycerol in rats.[327] Under these conditions, an increased release of PAF was also demonstrated. These findings indicate a role for PAF in the pathomechanism of glycerol-induced acute renal failure. Evaluation of the eventual role of PAF in post-ischemic recovery of renal function by using BN 52021 was recently published.[328] In anesthetized rats with 30 min occlusion of their left renal artery, the PAF antagonist given after the release of occlusion, induced an immediate increase in urine flow, glomerular filtration and sodium excretion. In the anesthetized male rat, acute endotoxin infusion induced renal vasoconstriction and decreased glomerular filtration rate in the absence of systemic hypotension.[329] Renal blood flow, glomerular filtration rate and urine flow rate were significantly improved by BN 52021 and SRI 63-675 (**6b**). In the rat kidney inner medulla, renal necrosis induced by 2-bromoethyl-amine hydrobromide increased PAF production due to a triggered *de novo* synthesis by activation of cholinephosphotransferase was observed.[330]

INVOLVEMENT OF PAF IN RENAL IMMUNE INJURY

In an anaphylaxis model of perfused guinea pig kidney, ovalbumin challenge induced release of histamine and eicosanoids, such as TXA_2 and LTD_4. BN 52021 produced a dose-related reduction in release of anaphylactic mediators, suggesting a regulatory role for PAF in kidney anaphylaxis.[331,332] Alternatively, it was also demonstrated that PAF induced release of IL-1 and TNF with a coincidence of maximal proteinuria.[333] BN 52021 produced a marked diminution of cytokine production and proteinuria.

CsA represents the most important therapeutic tool which has taken place in recent years in the field of kidney transplantation; however, its nephrotoxicity remains a relevant clinical problem. Therefore, a considerable effort has been made to reduce CsA-induced nephrotoxicity. In cultured rat mesangial cells and glomerular cross-sectional area of isolated rat glomeruli, the effect of BN 52021 was studied.[334] CsA produced amelioration of both parameters measured, while some of its toxic effects were prevented by the PAF antagonist, indicating a role for PAF in CsA-related nephrotoxicity. Using this model, not only BN 52021 but also verapamil was found to be effective.[335] In order to evaluate the effect of BN 52021 on CsA-induced nephrotoxicity, euvolumic Munich-Wistar rats were subjected to micropuncture studies.[336,337] BN 52021 alone did not change the total or single nephrone and glomerular filtration rate; however, CsA caused a decline in these parameters. Previous administration of BN 52021 in CsA-treated rats blunted the effects of the nephrotoxic agent on superficial nephrons, while the total renal function was not prevented. This study calls attention to the role of PAF and the clinical applicability of BN 52021 in CsA-induced nephrotoxicity. Egido et al.[338] studied the effect of BN 52063 on a rodent model with several features of chronic CsA nephrotoxicity and its relation to the involvement of eicosanoids and PAF in this process. Four-week-long administration of CsA produced a significant amelioration of kidney function and patchy interstitial fibrosis. Treatment with BN 52063 resulted in a marked improvement of these parameters. A combined effect of BN 52021 and WEB 2086 (**12**) was found to be effective. Recent observations have indicated that BN 52021 and BN 52063 could prevent not only CsA- but also cis-diammine-dichloroplatinum-induced glomerular hemodynamic alterations[339] and nephrotoxicity in the rat.[340] These results are in accordance with the findings obtained by CsA, i.e., PAF might be involved in tissue injury caused by various agents, and PAF antagonists may be candidates as therapeutic intervention in reducing nephrotoxicity.

PAF AND PAF ANTAGONISTS IN THE REPRODUCTIVE SYSTEM

More recently increasing attention has been paid to the role of PAF in the biology of reproduction. The results were briefly reviewed by Page and Abbott.[341]

OVULATION AND PREIMPLANTATION

Follicle rupture during ovulation is associated with inflammation-like changes; therefore the effect of BN 52021 (**15**) was tested in rats whose ovulation was stimulated with administration of human chorionic gonadotropin.[342,343] The PAF antagonist given locally inhibited follicle rupture and the hormone stimulated increase in ovarian collagenolysis and vascular permeability; furthermore, its effect could be reversed by simultaneous administration of PAF. At 2-h intervals during the ovulatory process in gonadotropin-primed 25-day-old Wistar rats the ovaries were extirpated, homogenized and extracted for lipids.[344] The extract was then separated by thin layer chromatography, and the portion of the silica gel that comigrated with authentic PAF was measured by a rabbit platelet [³H]serotonin assay. The ovarian level of PAF decreased by 2 h after treatment with human chorionic gonadotropin. Preliminary tests showed that the lipid extracts from the ovaries also contained PAF inhibitor(s) that comigrated with PAF. Their levels were also decreased in response to gonadotropin treatment. These results emphasize the involvement of PAF in ovulation. In this context, Harper[345] published that PAF levels in the uterus were hormonally controlled, being elevated by progesterone and PGE_2. Antagonists of PAF therefore can interfere with sperm function, ovulation, and implantation, resulting in a physiological regulation of reproduction. PAF together with early pregnancy factor, a glycoprotein are early signals of pregnancy. In rabbits PAF could induce the production of ovary and oviduct early pregnancy factor.[346]

The *in vitro* inhibition by CV-3988 (**1**) of the stimulatory effect of PAF in mouse oocytes indicates the involvement of specific PAF receptors in the fertilization process.[347]

PAF IN PREGNANCY AND EMBRYONIC TISSUE

The soluble PAF produced by mouse embryos was shown to possess properties similar to authentic PAF.[348-351] The embryo-derived lipid was extracted and assayed by monitoring the decrease in the porportion of single platelets in rabbit whole blood due to aggregation. SRI 63-441 (**6a**), SRI 63-412 (**6b**), WEB 2086 (**12**) and BN 52021 inactivated the release of PAF produced by embryos in response to PLA$_2$. Kodama et al.[352] reported successful isolation of PAF in mouse embryos, while Ryan et al.[353] found that *in vitro* production of PAF could influence embryonic metabolism as indicated by an increased production of CO$_2$ from carbon-1 position of lactate. In an *in vitro* study, PAF induced fertilization assessed by a positive β-human chorionic gonadotropin per oocyte retrieval. The increase in number of positive pregnancy tests referred to a PAF-mediated support of pre-embryo development. In rat embryos the rank order of cyclooxygenase arachidonate products was 6-keto-PGF$_{1\alpha}$ much greater than congruent to PGF$_{2\alpha}$ congruent to TXB$_2$, while no lipoxygenase products were detected.[354] PAF production was also detectable in early post-implantation rat embryos. A luteotrophic, small molecular weight, heat labile, dextran-coated charcoal-absorbable, lipid soluble factor derived from platelets that did not appear to be PAF, was isolated from bovine conceptuses.[355] These results demonstrate an increased extent of lipid metabolism and a role for various lipid mediators, including PAF, during initiation and maintenance of pregnancy. These early pregnancy signals were demonstrated in all domestic animals.[356] Injection of PAF but not lyso-PAF into the left uterine horn induced a dose-dependent decidua-like reaction in the pseudopregnant rat.[356,357] BN 52021 inhibited the effect of PAF on decidua-like reaction indicating the involvement of specific PAF receptor sites in the phenomenon. These specific PAF receptor sites were than characterized in purified uterine membranes from pregnant rabbits, and relative potencies of PAF and its antagonists in displacing ^{3}H-PAF were determined and found to be lyso-PAF > CV-3988 > PAF > U 66985 > A 02405 > BN 52021 > U 66982.[358] Kudolo and Harper[359] described the presence of unique PAF receptor subtypes in the uterus of pregnant rabbits using specific antagonists and PAF analogs, and emphasized the importance of species specificity in receptor binding.

ANTIFERTILITY EFFECT OF PAF ANTAGONISTS

CV-3988, U 66985 and SRI 63-441, all structural analogs of PAF inhibited fertilization *in vitro* and *in vivo* in rabbits when added to the ejaculate before insemination. Antagonists that were not structural analogs were ineffective. When SRI 63-441 was given intravenously prior to ovulation, no effect on fertilization was seen. On the other hand, when the PAF antagonist was instilled into the vagina immediately before insemination, a highly significant reduction in the fertilization rate was achieved. It is concluded that PAF antagonists can influence directly the sperm membrane rather than antagonize the effect of PAF. To verify these results, other PAF antagonists should also be tried. The effects of synthetic PAF on the motility of human spermatozoa were recently investigated using videomicroscopy.[360-362] PAF resulted in a statistically significant increase in motility, while lyso-PAF had no such effect. The results suggest that treatment of spermatozoa with PAF in severely astheno-zoospermic males may be of therapeutic value.

CLINICAL STUDIES ON THE EFFECT OF PAF ANTAGONISTS IN VARIOUS DISEASES

Apart from the abundance of experimental studies, relatively few papers have been published on the clinical pharmacology of PAF receptor antagonists.

Platelet aggregation induced *ex vivo* by adrenalin, ADP, collagen, or PAF may be useful as a model describing effects in humans.[363] In intravenous and inhalative single rising dose tolerance trials this method proved to be useful for monitoring the pharmacological effect of WEB 2086 (**12**) whose oral administration resulted in a clear, dose-related inhibition of PAF-induced platelet aggregation. The safety, tolerability, and pharmacological activity of WEB 2086 were examined in two double-bind, placebo-controlled, within subject crossover studies.[364] Pharmacological activity of the compound was monitored with *ex vivo* PAF-induced platelet aggregation which showed a continuous, almost complete inhibition in response to multiple administration of the compound. No clinically significant drug-related effects on vital and laboratory parameters or obvious drug-dependent adverse reactions were observed. These results indicated that WEB 2086 is an effective PAF antagonist in human beings and showed no side effects that would raise objections against further clinical trials with this substance in patients.

Ginkgolides, especially BN 52063, a standardized mixture of various ginkgolides and BN 52021 (15) also underwent clinical trials. Bonvoisin and Guinot[365] performed multicenter, short-term clinical trials with a strategy to demonstrate safety, confirmation of PAF antagonistic property, pharmacokinetic and pharmacodynamic profile, possible bronchodilator activity, single and multiple-dose investigation on the effect on nonspecific bronchial provocation tests in asthmatic patients and atopic patients during specific allergic challenge. The results obtained seem encouraging and are the first clinical demonstration of the possible usefulness of a PAF antagonist in asthma. As expected, similar to glucocorticoid treatment, changes need some time, about 2 weeks, to occur. Longer-term studies, particularly on more severely affected asthmatic patients, may provide further evidence for the benefit of BN 52063 in the clinical management of asthmatic patients.[366] It is suggested that the use of PAF antagonists in combination with other mediator antagonists would be useful, since not only a single mediator is involved in the pathophysiology of asthma. BN 52063 was also evaluated in clinical studies by Robert and Barnes[367] using a protocol for prevention of allergic bronchoconstriction and allergic dermal responses modelized with dose-related increases in wheal and flare reactions induced by intradermal injections of allergen. Randomized, coded BN 52021 and identical placebo capsules were given to subjects in a double-blind fashion. Airway challenge was made by inhalation of metacholine and PAF. The data obtained indicate that BN 52063 is an active and relatively selective PAF antagonist in man; however, in contrast to the skin where it produced an inhibition by approximately 50% of the PAF-induced wheal and flare response in both normal and atopic subjects, the bronchoconstriction induced by PAF in normal volunteers was only partially affected. In a further paper, Charpentier et al.[368] described the results of randomized double-blind clinical studies on the tolerance and immunological effects of BN 52063 in healthy volunteers using various immune functions, including changes in lymphocyte subsets, mitogen-induced lymphokine production, natural killer cell activity and neutrophil bactericidal responses. These results demonstrated that PAF modulated T-cell activity and membrane antigen expression. Studies on the cardiovascular and neurological tolerance, and effects of BN 52021 on *ex vivo* PAF-induced platelet aggregation and skin reactivity, notably the wheal and flare reaction evoked by PAF as well as its effects on bleeding time in healthy volunteers after intravenously administered drug were also performed[369] and proved that BN 52021 was well tolerated and resulted in a sustained antagonism on PAF-induced platelet aggregation, while that induced by ADP remained unchanged. The efficacy of BN 52021 on the biological tests studied was higher than that of BN 52063.

The effect of aerosolized BN 52021 on immediate bronchoconstriction and change in total white blood cells and eosinophils in peripheral blood following exposure to inhaled PAF in normal and asthmatic children was examined.[370] Airways of asthmatic children were more sensitive to PAF than those of normals. Previous inhalation of BN 52021 could block both the bronchoconstriction and decrease in white and eosinophil blood cells induced by PAF aerosol. Therefore, PAF appears to be involved as mediator in the pathogenesis of asthma in man, and BN 52021 may have a potential effect in the prevention and treatment of bronchial hyperreactivity. In a recent report by Hopp et al.,[371] an attempt was made to further elucidate the role of PAF on nonspecific bronchial reactivity in non-asthmatic human volunteers. PAF did not increase significantly metacholine-induced airway responsiveness, thus the authors called attention to the necessity to further elucidate the potential role of PAF in airway reactivity.

BN 52063 was effective in reducing clinical and histological effects of PAF when compared to intradermal injection of human serum albumin in atopic skin of clinical patients.[372] The time course of action of BN 52063 was determined on PAF-induced platelet aggregation in whole blood over 10 h in a randomized, double blind, placebo-controlled crossover study in male healthy subjects.[373] After placebo, platelets showed a marked and previously unreported diurnal rhythm in their sensitivity to PAF, being most sensitive in the first blood sample withdrawn at 8:30 A.M. and least sensitive at 4:30 P.M. with a threefold difference between these times. The diurnal change in platelet responsiveness to PAF needs to be taken into account when designing studies which include measurement of platelet aggregation. BN 52063 inhibited platelet aggregation throughout the 10 h; its effect was maximal 4 hours after oral administration, when the concentration of PAF required to induce aggregation was increased threefold.[374] Tanakan, a natural extract of *Ginkgo biloba* leaves, possessing PAF antagonist activity, was investigated in an open study on healthy male volunteers.[375] *Ex vivo* platelet aggregation induced by adrenalin, ADP, collagen, and PAF in platelet-rich plasma samples from blood taken before and after a single oral dose of Tanakan was reduced. No concomitant changes in coagulation, skin bleeding time, hematological and biochemical laboratory tests, blood pressure or pulse were observed. The results provide a possible explanation for the clinical efficacy of Tanakan in the treatment of peripheral vascular disease, and confirm previous findings that the extract is well tolerated.

Finally, an interaction of BN 52063 and flunitrazepam, a benzodiazepine derivative, by the technique of quantified electroencephalography was demonstrated in young healthy volunteers.[376] BN 52063 alone did not result in any statistically significant change in the α and β waves. Flunitrazepam induced an increase in β 2 rhythm and a decrease in α rhythm. These changes were less pronounced when the benzodiazepine was co-administered with BN 52063. This finding suggests a possible implication of PAF in memory processes in man.

PAF/CYTOKINE INTERACTION AS A BASIC CONCEPT FOR THE ROLE OF PAF IN VARIOUS PATHOLOGICAL CONDITIONS

Recent progress in PAF research at the cellular level has explored a unique role for the phospholipid mediator in a great variety of pathophysiological conditions. It has become apparent that endotoxin, in addition to PAF, induces the release of other mediators, particularly cytokines such as TNF.[377] Indeed, the injection of endotoxin is associated with extensive production of TNF, while TNF administration induces a shock-like condition often resulting in death by multiorgan failure. These effects can be prevented if the animals are pretreated with a neutralizing monoclonal antibody against TNF,[378] indicating an important role for TNF in endotoxemia and other shock states. We have recently proposed that a complex interaction between PAF, proteases, TNF and other cytokines is of fundamental importance in initiating the pathological changes not only in shock and sepsis, but also in trauma and diverse ischemic disorders.[117,379,380]

Ischemia, shock, atherosclerosis, and related disturbances are characterized by endothelial injury, bleb formation, plasma leakage, hemodynamic alterations and eventually vascular collapse and end-organ failure. The primary event in this train of events is cellular activation leading to the adherence of blood cells, such as platelets, PMNL, eosinophils and monocytes to the endothelial surface followed by their aggregation, infiltration, and degranulation. Such phenomena, which are also observed in pathologies, such as asthma and graft rejection,[1-4] can be directly induced by administration of PAF itself. Infusion of PAF in the mesenteric bed of anesthetized guinea pigs causes severe microvascular damage, which can be inhibited by various structurally unrelated PAF antagonists. Interestingly, concomitant administration of TNF or lipopolysaccharide with a nonthrombogenic dose of PAF also causes enhanced thrombosis, this again being inhibited by PAF antagonists.[379]

As we have seen, tissue damage mediated by oxygen free radical production is also a major component of ischemia/reperfusion injury and is undoubtedly of considerable importance.[117] Neutrophils appear to be a crucial cell type with regard to free oxygen radical generation. In the inflammatory microenvironment these cells become activated by various agonists, adhere to the endothelial surface and release lysosomal proteases. Activated neutrophils also undergo a "respiratory burst", which results in the reduction of molecular oxygen to superoxide anion.[381] This latter product is rapidly converted to hydrogen peroxide and toxic free radicals which damage the endothelium. PAF is known to be a potent chemotactic agent for neutrophils, inducing superoxide release, aggregation and degranulation in this cell type.[1-4,117,379,380] PAF is also one of the most active chemotactic factors for eosinophils,[382] cells from which it elicits the release of major basic protein, free radicals and LTC_4, products extremely damaging to microvascular integrity.[379,380] Eosinophil infiltration is another prominent feature of certain inflammatory lesions and may play a particularly important role in asthma and graft rejection.

In addition to directly eliciting cell chemotaxis and oxygen free radical production, PAF can also induce the release of various inflammatory cytokines, such as TNF. We have shown that PAF stimulates TNF production from peripheral blood derived monocytes and at picomolar concentrations amplifies lipopolysaccharide-induced TNF production, and all these effects can be inhibited by various PAF antagonists.[50-52,383,384] PAF also acts synergistically with γ-interferon to increase the monocyte cytotoxicity. PAF can modulate the production of both IL-1[162-168] and IL-2[385-393] from rat monocytes and lymphocytes, respectively, cytokines which in turn elicit the release of other mediators and growth factors.

Similar to PAF, TNF also enhances neutrophil superoxide anion production and adherence.[394] TNF may also indirectly regulate eosinophil cytotoxicity via its effect on the release of other cytokines and growth factors. In addition to directly modulating neutrophil activity, at very low concentrations both PAF and TNF can "prime" neutrophils to respond in an enhanced manner to subsequent agonistic stimuli that would otherwise be ineffectual. Amplified responses including aggregation, adhesiveness, superoxide anion production and elastase release have been reported using fMLP as the inducing agonist following priming with PAF.[30,394] Furthermore, we have recently shown that TNF can prime the PAF-induced superoxide anion generation by human neutrophils, the enhancing effect of the mediator being completely abolished by ginkgolides and various PAF antagonists. These compounds also decreased by 50% the superoxide production elicited solely by TNF, indicating that this effect of TNF is partially mediated by a mechanism involving endogenous PAF.[380]

Apart from inducing vascular damage via infiltration and degranulation of various blood cells, PAF,[380] IL-1, and TNF[395,396] also exert direct effects on the vascular system, causing hypotension when administered *in vivo*. Furthermore, while it has been known for some time that endothelial cells produce PAF when stimulated with various agonists such as thrombin,[397] it has recently been established that TNF, IL-1, and lymphotoxin, but not IL-2, IL-3, IL-6, γ-interferon, and colony stimulating factors, induce cultured endothelial cells to synthesize PAF, the majority of which remains associated with the cells.[398] GM-CSF, another cytokine produced by activated T cells, endothelial cells and fibroblasts stimulated by TNF, is also able to prime the PAF-induced production of both superoxide and LTs[399-401] from human PMNL. This suggests that GM-CSF may also be involved in the PAF/cytokine interactions during various pathological states such as shock and ischemia.

Thus it seems that in these conditions complex interactions may arise between mediators and cells which eventually give rise to microvascular damage. The fact that PAF and various cytokines can not only induce the release of each other, but also their own generation *in vivo* indicates that self-generating positive feedback cycles may become established. We propose that PAF and TNF play pivotal roles in the formation of initial loops, which subsequently recruit other cytokines and growth factors into the feedback network.[117,379,380] For example, a situation can be envisaged where in the inflammatory microenvironment PAF primes the release of IL-1 and TNF from activated monocytes and LT and oxygen free radical production from stimulated PMNL. PAF also activates platelets to form thrombin and ATP which in turn, as IL-1 and TNF, act on the endothelium to produce more PAF resulting in increased neutrophil chemotaxis. These cells may then be primed by TNF for PAF-induced superoxide anion generation. In addition, PAF generated by the endothelium may amplify the TNF- and IL-1-activated production of IL-6 and GM-CSF from endothelial cells. This latter growth factor which is also produced by stimulated monocytes, potently enhances release of superoxide anion and LTC_4 by eosinophils.[402] Furthermore, in combination with IL-3, it elicits monocyte cytotoxicity by inducing TNF secretion from this cell type.[403]

The priming ability of these mediators indicates the extreme sensitivity of the inflammatory process and the rigid controls which must usually operate to stop excessive inflammatory responses. It may be that an equilibrium exists between the mediators involved in the priming and feedback processes and internal mechanisms which down-regulate these loops and confine cytotoxic reactions to a specific site. Indeed, several endogenous inhibitors of PAF, TNF, IL-1, and IL-2 have been reported.[380] Under normal physiological conditions a balance may be maintained between cytotoxic and inhibitory mechanisms, which would strictly control the inflammatory process and prevent endothelial injury. In contrast, in pathologies such as ischemia and shock where there may be an overloading of the system by excessive mediator production or a critical reduction in inhibitory factors, the feedback cycles may become unregulated and the toxicity converted into a systemic process, resulting in oxygen free radical production, endothelial damage, cell infiltration, vascular leakage and microcirculatory collapse. This fine balance between the protection and destruction of the processes maintaining life is reminiscent of the catastrophe theory proposed by Thom[404] and Zeeman[405] in the early 1970s. In several recent publications we have developed the application of this theory to the control of PAF/cytokine interactions and the regulation of microvascular integrity.[117,379,380]

Support for the potential importance of the PAF/cytokine feedback system in various pathophysiological conditions is not only provided by our *in vitro* data demonstrating that PAF antagonists drastically reduce TNF-stimulated neutrophil superoxide anion generation,[380] but also by the *in vivo* observations of Sun and Hsueh[301] who found that the PAF antagonist SRI 63-119 prevents TNF-induced bowel necrosis in the rat. In addition, Heuer and Letts[406] showed that pretreatment of mice with either *S. typhosa* endotoxin or TNF significantly enhanced the mortality induced by PAF. This effect occurred at dose levels where PAF, endotoxin, or TNF given alone did not significantly affect these parameters. Similar to the situation observed *in vitro* with PMNL responses,[30] the enhancing effect was not recorded when PAF was given prior to TNF. Furthermore, in studies where rats received an injection of TNF prior to the injection of a low and inactive dose of PAF, a marked amplification of the vascular escape was recorded, mainly in the trachea, bronchi, lung parenchyma, pancreas, kidneys, and duodenum.[407] A similar potentiation of cytokine/PAF effects has also been observed in models of cartilage breakdown where the combination of inactive individual doses of TNF and PAF caused a significant loss of glycosaminoglycans.[408]

In conclusion, it appears that there are complex interactions between PAF, proteases and cytokines in the evolution of shock and ischemic states. The fact that PAF is part of a multicomponent system may explain why PAF antagonists, which inhibit both the direct and amplification as well as priming effects of the mediator, are effective in diverse pathological models of these conditions. Indeed, PAF antagonists are currently being evaluated clinically and may constitute valuable drugs in diseases, where control of the inflammatory response has to be reinstated therapeutically. In common with the numerous other drugs already employed for the treatment of inflammation, the end result of PAF antagonist action is protection of vascular integrity. While PAF inhibitors probably achieve this result by inhibiting the priming, amplification and feedback processes described above, other agents effective in shock and ischemia may produce a similar vascular protection via their own individual mechanisms of action.

However, with regard to the development of potential therapeutic regimes for shock and ischemia, it should be emphasized that PAF antagonists alone are only capable of blocking the pathological processes directly or indirectly dependent on PAF, no matter how diverse these may be. The vast majority of other anti-inflammatory drugs also only act through inhibition of a single mediator, synthetic pathway or process. As proposed in this article, the complex multi-component nature of the deleterious processes operating in shock and ischemia suggests that more successful therapeutic regimes may consist of a combination of drugs possibly including protease inhibitors, calcium antagonists, PGI_2 analogs, inhibitors of ILs and growth factors, anti-TNF anti-bodies, and PAF antagonists.

It is also extremely important to note that any drug therapy should endeavor to offer vascular protection as rapidly as possible. This is not only of critical importance for the immediate outcome of the condition but also for the future prognosis. Indeed, endothelium that has sustained previous damage may be particularly prone to future injury. Recently, it has been shown that the recovery of balloon denuded pig endothelium is not complete as the cells lose the ability to produce EDRF and possibly other relaxant agents.[409] EDRF also reduces platelet aggregation and the inability of previously damaged endothelial cells to produce such factors suppressive to the activity of the feedback mediators, makes regenerated endothelium markedly more susceptible to further inflammatory damage.

In addition to combinations of drugs, another possible pharmacological approach to the treatment of various pathological states such as shock and ischemia is the design of compounds which possess a dual or multi-inhibitory activity. Our laboratory is currently developing such drugs and studies on animal models with compounds acting as PAF antagonists/anti-proteases or PAF antagonists/5-lipoxygenase inhibitors have produced very encouraging results. Despite the technical difficulties of combining drugs with various inhibitory properties, application of compound having multi-inhibitory effect in one molecule may offer a great potential for the therapy of shock, ischemia and other inflammatory diseases.

ANTIPROTEASE ACTIVITY OF BN 52021

Apart from its specific PAF antagonistic property, BN 52021 (**15**) has been described as a nonspecific inhibitor of proteases. Indeed, several investigations have demonstrated that BN 52021 displays some inhibitory effect on both seryl and aspartyl proteases. Using bovine and human trypsin, Deby-Dupont et al.[410] found that low concentrations of BN 52021 inhibited enzyme activity even when trypsin was bound to α_2 macroglobulin.

In addition, Montagné et al. (unpublished observations) demonstrated that treatment with BN 52021 of HIV-1 infected lymphocytes, dramatically increases the survival rate of the cells (3000% increase in survival against 2000% for azathioprim). This effect is independent of both (i) PAF antagonist properties, since other potent PAF antagonists like BN 50730 or BN 50739 (**14**) do not increase survival, and (ii) reverse transcriptase inhibitory effect, since this enzyme is not affected by the treatment. In contrast, BN 52021 and some more simple lactonic structures, like BN 50548 or BN 50743 inhibit syncytium formation and expression of HIV core proteins P 17 and P 24.

The effect of BN 52021 and BN 52063 given orally on plasma protease activity was studied in rats parallel with the assessment of endotoxin-induced lethality.[411] Endotoxin induced a long-lasting increase in plasma trypsin-like activity which overcame that of PAF. Both ginkgolide preparations and dexamethasone inhibited plasma trypsin-like activity, while aprotinin was ineffective. Since the ginkgolides also reduced the endotoxin-induced lethality, their antiprotease activity appeared to be as a consequence of their PAF antagonistic effect. However, the existence of such an effect calls attention to the pathophysiological significance of the antiprotease property of ginkgolides in various pathophysiological processes in which they exhibit a protective effect.

The antiprotease property of BN 52021 may be explained by the presence of the lactone ring in the molecule which may covalently bind to the serine hydroxyl group of the enzyme, and through a formation of a tetrahydral intermediate, such interaction may lead to an inactivated acyl enzyme. A similar mechanism may be involved between the carbonyl group of the enzyme and the lactone in the aspartyl protease system.

The antiprotease activity of the molecule may contribute to its beneficial effect demonstrated in a series of pathophysiological conditions, and even in the effect of PAF as a signal molecule in some physiological feedback mechanisms.

CONCLUDING REMARKS

In the last 2 years considerable progress has been achieved in the research of ginkgolides. A rather bulky mass of information has become available concerning the effect of these specific PAF receptor antagonists in a great variety of tissues, indicating that, similarly to eicosanoids, PAF plays an important mediator and modulator role in various pathophysiological events.

In contrast to previous research activities devoted predominantly to inflammation, allergic states, such as immediate and delayed hypersensitivity reaction, immune complex diseases and hemostasis, increasing attention has been paid to the involvement of PAF in circulatory disorders, such as ischemic states in the brain, heart and gastrointestinal tract which are due to acute and chronic failure of peripheral circulation. A great deal of evidence has been provided to the role of PAF in various shock conditions. As a result of a considerable effort, it is obvious now that natural and synthetic PAF antagonists are candidates for the clinical management of stroke, myocardial infarction, gastrointestinal ulceration, and different pathological conditions related to peripheral circulation. The indication that PAF might be involved even in atherogenesis is remarkable. Recognition of the role of PAF in reproductive physiology might be an initial step in developing new contraceptives.

Studies on the physiological feedback mechanisms involved in the regulation of hormone release in the brain are of great interest. These results emphasize the significance of cell membrane processes, particularly the release of PAF, as an important signal for triggering troph hormone secretion. These mechanisms may be active also at the peripheral level triggering opposite effects in hormone secretion thus suggesting highly sensitive control mechanisms through which PAF can modulate feedback control of hormonal homeostasis. These results call attention to the complexity of an eventual therapeutic effect of PAF antagonists. This awaits however better elucidation by forthcoming research activity.

Intensive research has been conducted in allergic states as well. This has led to a better understanding of the role for PAF in the complex pathology of asthma and other allergic conditions. Basic knowledge on the graft protecting effect of PAF antagonists was extended to the possible usefulness of ginkgolides in organ preservation.

Studies on the relationship between the basic molecular structural framework and the PAF receptor antagonistic properties have led to several definitive conclusions which might be useful for future studies to develop more and more effective compounds with PAF antagonistic properties. In this respect, particular attention should be paid to the diversity of PAF receptors in various organs. The specification of these binding sites by the aid of more and more specific antagonists may result in better understanding of diverse pathophysiological events and more specific therapeutic approach to various diseases. This process may lead to the solution of the greatest problem in PAF antagonist research, notably the correct specification of the indication for a particular drug to a well determined pathological condition or disease. Such theoretical and practical research activity may accelerate the development of PAF antagonists for the treatment of clinical patients. At the moment, PAF antagonists appear to be appropriate for the treatment of various ischemic disorders, especially cerebral ischemia.

As usual, the intensive research on PAF and PAF antagonists has led to contradictory results, as well. These are however stimulating rather than confusing, and facilitate further experimental clarification of the exact mechanism of action of the phospholipid mediator and the protective effect of its antagonists.

As mentioned in the Introduction, the basic concept of the molecular biochemical mode of action of PAF has been confirmed by recent studies providing additional evidence for the fundamental role of the phospholipid mediator in a variety of pathophysiological processes. In this context, the effect of PAF antagonists on cellular calcium metabolism deserves particular interest and may be the most important in various ischemic states. The recognition of the modulatory role for PAF in cell to cell interaction and the concept of PAF/cytokine interaction as a basic mechanism of cellular injury has shed more light on the significance of PAF in pathophysiological disorders, and the possible therapeutic application of PAF antagonists.

APPENDIX

The chemistry of PAF antagonists has recently been reviewed by Hosford and Braquet.[412] Here we intend to summarize briefly the classification and chemical structure of the most important PAF antagonists mentioned in this review without the special design of a detailed description of their chemistry.

CLASSIFICATION OF PAF ANTAGONISTS

The most important PAF antagonists can be divided into two groups: (1) synthetic and (2) natural compounds.

SYNTHETIC PAF ANTAGONISTS
The majority of these compounds are modified derivatives of the PAF framework.

Non-Constrained PAF Framework-Related Antagonists
These antagonists, such as CV-3988 (**1**), CV-6209 (**2**), SRI 63-119 (**3a**), ONO 6240 (**3b**), Ro 19-3704 (**3c**) and other Ro compounds (**4**) derive directly from the PAF structure and are open chain analogues of the mediator. Scheme 1 indicates the structure of such compounds.

Constrained PAF Framework-Related Antagonists
These compounds, like SRI 63-072 (**5**), SRI 63-441 (**6a**), SRI 63-675 (**6a**), BN 52111 (**7**) and BN 52115 (**8**) are produced by cyclization of parts of the PAF molecular backbone as indicated in Scheme 2.

Synthetic Antagonists Unrelated to the PAF Framework
Among these compounds 48470 RP (**9a**) and 52770 RP (**9b**) have a (3-pyridyl)-1*H*,3*H*-pyrrolo[1,2-*c*]thiazol framework, while other highly potent antagonists belong to various benzodiazepine-derived groups, such as alprazolam (**10a**), triazolam (**10b**), brotizolam (**11**), WEB 2086 (**12**), WEB 2170 (**13**), and BN 50739 (**14**) as indicated in Scheme 3.

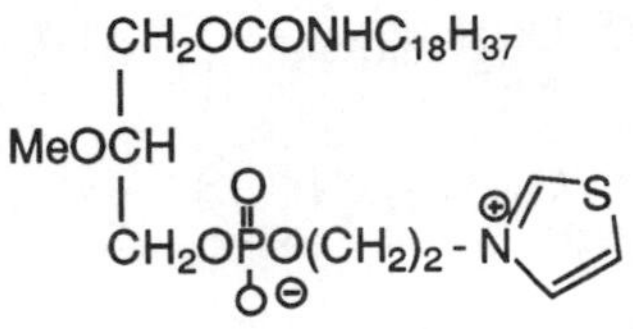
CH2OCONHC18H37
MeOCH
O
CH2OPO(CH2)2 - N
S
O⊖

(1) CV 3988

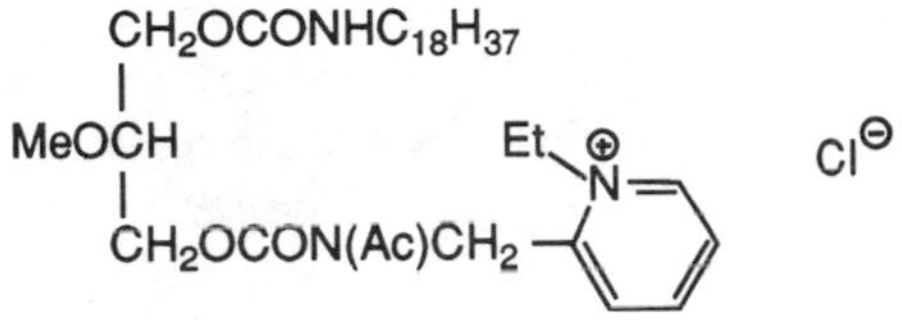
CH2OCONHC18H37
MeOCH
Et
N
CH2OCON(Ac)CH2
Cl⊖

(2) CV 6209

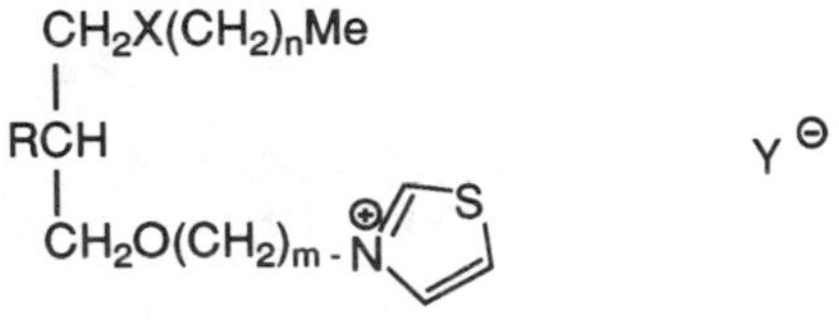
CH2X(CH2)nMe
RCH
CH2O(CH2)m - N
S
Y⊖

(2) CV 6209

(3a) SRI 63-119
n = 17, X = OCONH, R = OMe, m = 4, Y = I

(3b) ONO-6240
n = 15, X = O, R = OEt, m = 7, y = $MeSO_3$

(3c) Ro 19-3704
n = 17, X = OCONH, R = OCO_2Me, m = 4, Y = I
n = 17, X = OCONi-Pr, R = OCONHMe, m = 4

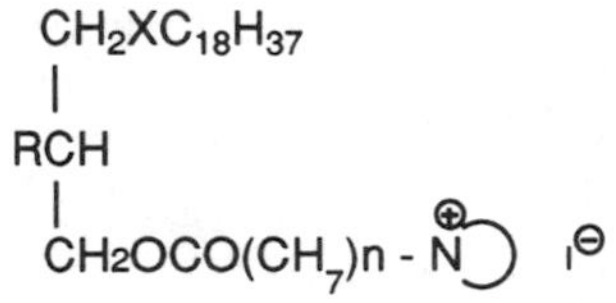
CH2XC18H37
RCH
CH2OCO(CH7)n - N
I⊖

(4a) Ro 18-7953
X = OCONH, R = OMe, n = 3

(4b) Ro 19-1400
X = OCONH, R = OCO_2Me, n = 3

(4c) Ro 18-8736
X = OCONH, R = $NHCO_2Me$, n = 3

(4d) RU 45,703
X = O, R = OEt, n = 4

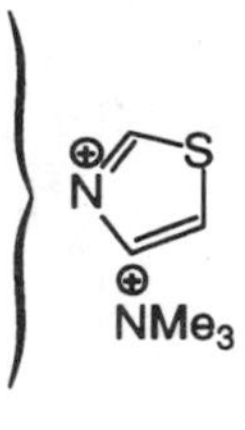
N
S
NMe3

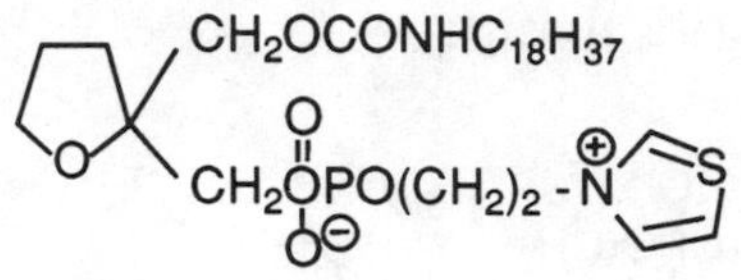

(5) SRI 63-072

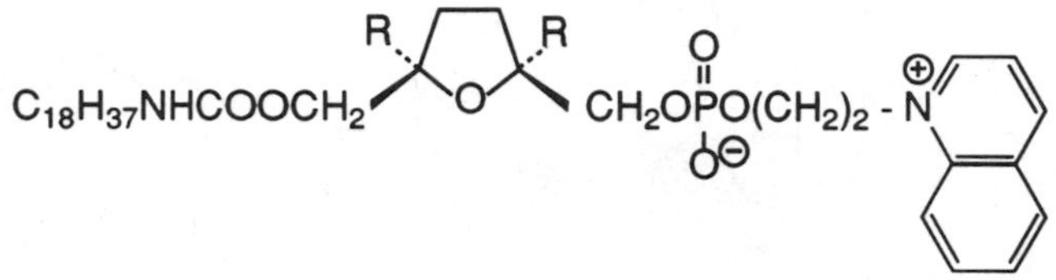

(6a) SRI 63-441

(6b) SRI 63-675

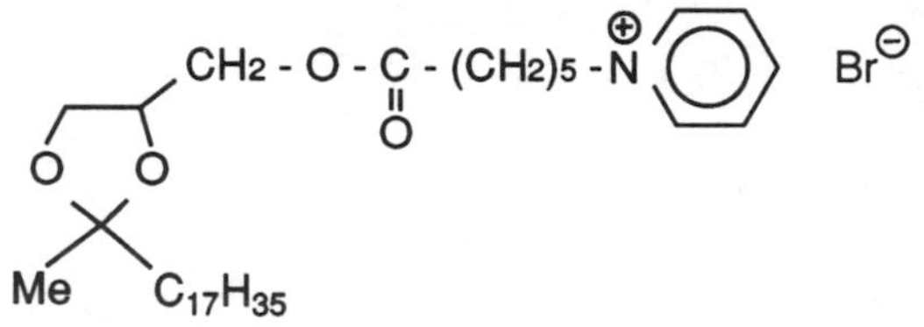

(7) BN 52111

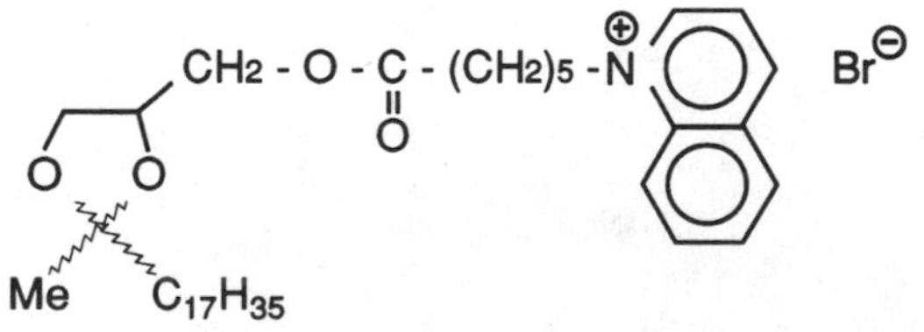

(8) BN 52115

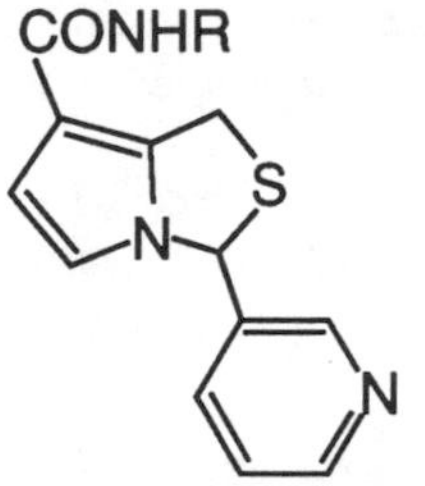

(9a) 48740 RP
(9c) 52770 RP

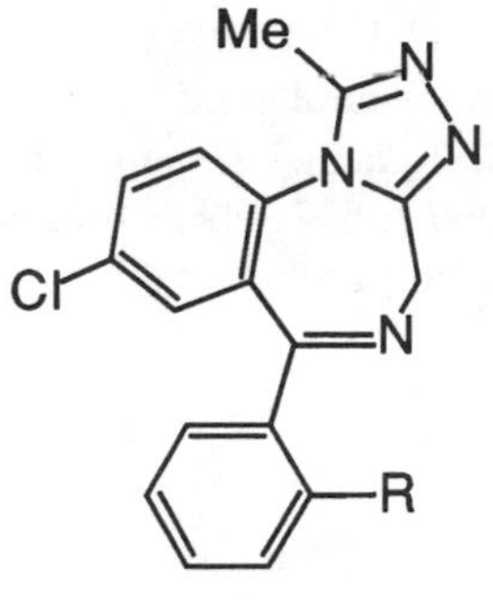

(10a) alprazolam   R = H
(10b) triazolam   R = Cl

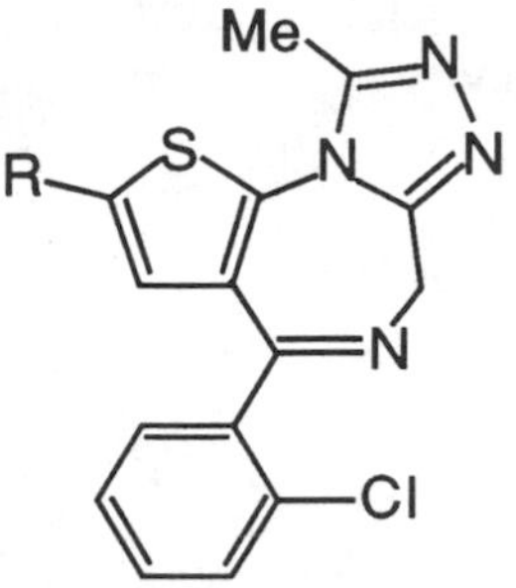

(11) brotizolam   r = Br

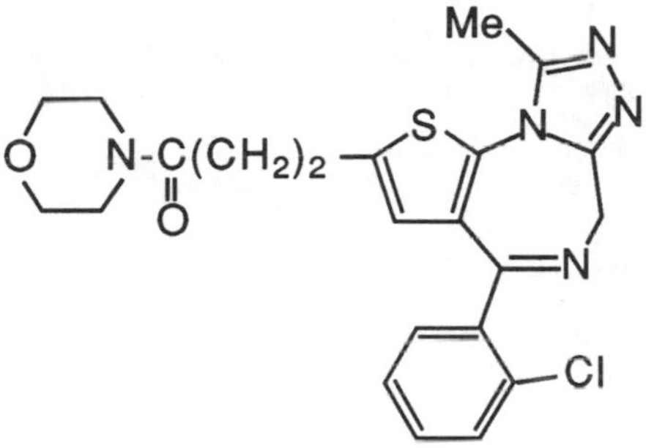

(12) WEB 2086

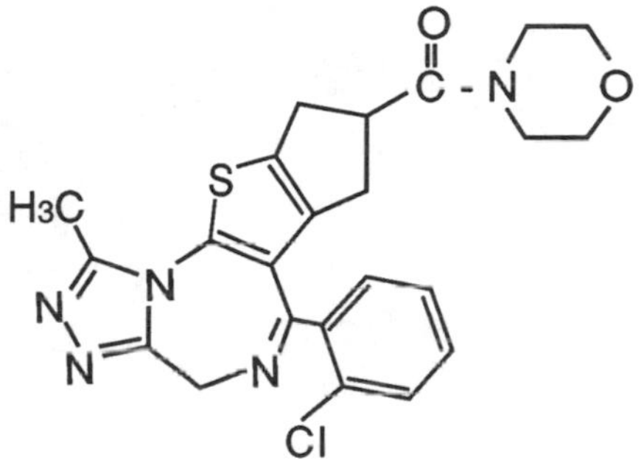

(13) WEB 2170

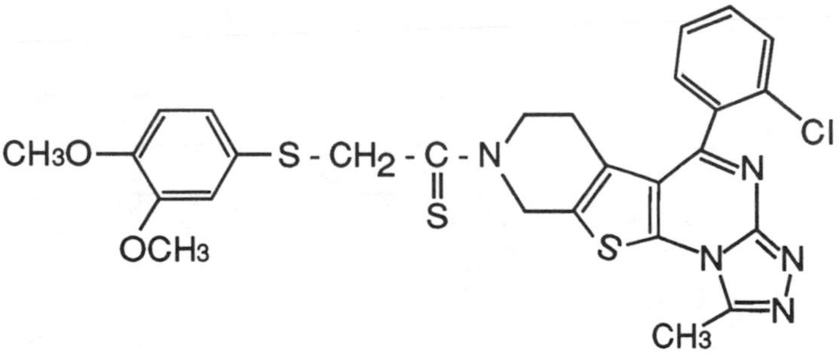

(14) BN 50739

NATURALLY OCCURRING PAF ANTAGONISTS

This relatively large group includes natural products represented by ginkgolides **(15)** and lignans, such as the benzofuranoid lignan, kadsurenone **(16)**, furthermore substituted furanoid lignans, like L-652,731 **(17)** and L-652,989 **(18)** as well as gliotoxin-related products, such as FR 900452 **(19)** as indicated in Scheme 4.

Ginkgolides (15)

Ginkgolide	IHB Nomenclature	R^1	R^2	R^3
A	BN 52020	OH	H	H
B	BN 52021	OH	OH	H
C	BN 52022	OH	OH	OH
J	BN 52024	OH	H	OH
M	BN 52023	H	OH	OH
synthetic	BN 50580	OH	OMe	H
synthetic	BN 50585	OH	OEt	H

(16) kadsurenone

Compound	R	R¹	R²	R³	R⁴	R⁵	R⁶	R⁷
(17) L-652,731	OMe	OMe	OMe	H	OMe	OMe	OMe	H
(18) L-652,989	H	OMe	OMe	OMe	H	SO_2Me	OPr	OMe

(19) FR 900452

REFERENCES

1. **Braquet, P., Touqui, L., Shen, T. S., et al.,** Perspectives in platelet-activating factor research, *Pharmacol. Rev.,* 39, 97, 1987.
2. **Braquet, P.,** The ginkgolides: potent platelet-activating factor antagonists isolated from Ginkgo biloba L.: chemistry, pharmacology and clinical applications, *Drugs Future,* 12, 643, 1987.
3. **Vargaftig, B. B. and Braquet, P.,** PAF-acether to day: relevance for acute experimental anaphylaxis, *Br. Med. Bull.,* 43, 312, 1987.
4. **Braquet, P., Chabrier, P. E., and Mencia-Huerta, J. M.,** The promise of PAF antagonists, *Adv. Inflammation Res.,* 16, 179, 1987.
5. **Hosford, D., Mencia-Huerta, J. M., Page, C., et al.,** Natural antagonists of platelet-activating factor, *Phytotherapy Res.,* 2, 1, 1988.
6. **Tahraoui, L., Floch, A., and Mondot, S.,** High affinity specific binding sites for tritiated platelet-activating factor in canine platelet membranes: counterparts of platelet-activating factor receptors mediating platelet aggregation, *Mol. Pharmacol.,* 34, 145, 1988.
7. **Chau, L. Y., Tsai, Y. M., and Cheng, J. R.,** Photoaffinity labeling of platelet activating factor binding sites in rabbit platelet membranes, *Biochem. Biophys. Res. Commun.,* 161, 1070, 1989.
8. **Morrison, W. J. and Shukla, S. D.,** Antagonism of platelet-activating factor receptor binding and stimulated phosphoinositide-specific phospholipase C in rabbit platelets, *J. Pharmacol. Exp. Ther.,* 250, 831, 1989.
9. **Dive, G., Godfroid, J. J., Lamotte-Brasseur, J., et al.,** PAF-receptor 1, "Cache-oreille" effect of selected high-potency platelet-activating factor (PAF) antagonists, *J. Lipid Med.,* 1, 201, 1989.
10. **Barone, D., Maggi, C. A., Baroldi, P., et al.,** Octylinium bromide interacts competitively with the PAF receptor, *Drugs Exp. Clin. Res.,* 15, 363, 1989.
11. **Schattner, M., Parini, A., Fouque, F., et al.,** Selective inhibition of adrenaline-induced human platelet aggregation by the structurally related PAF antagonist Ro 19-3704, *Br. J. Pharmacol.,* 96, 759, 1989.
12. **Selak, M. A. and Smith, J. B.,** Platelet-activating factor-induced calcium mobilization in human platelets and neutrophils: effects of PAF-acether antagonists, *J. Lipid Med.,* 1, 152, 1989.
13. **Shukla, S. D., Morrison, W. J., and Dhar, A.,** Desensitization of platelet-activating factor-stimulated protein phosphorylation in platelets, *Mol. Pharmacol.,* 35, 409, 1989.

14. **O'Donnel, S. R. and Barnett, C. J. K.,** pA$_2$ values for antagonists of platelet-activating factor on aggregation of rabbit platelets, *Br. J. Pharmacol.,* 94, 437, 1988.

15. **Yue, T. L., Robinovici, R., Farhat, M., et al.,** Pharmacologic profile of BN 50739 a new PAF antagonist *in vitro* and *in vivo, Prostaglandins,* 39, 469, 1990.

16. **Yue, T. L., Rabinovici, R., Farhat, M., et al.,** Inhibitory effect of novel PAF antagonists on PAF-induced rabbit platelet aggregation *in vitro* and *ex vivo, J. Lipid Med.,* submitted.

17. **Weichert, W. and Breddin, H. K.,** A PAF-acether antagonist (N 48740 RP/Rhone-Poulenc) and laser-induced thrombi in rat mesenteric vessels, *Haemostasis,* 19, 229, 1989.

18. **Hofmann, B., Meisgeier, Ud., Ostermann, G., et al.,** Effect of BN 52021 on PAF-induced release of tissue-type plasminogen activator, in *Ginkgolides: Chemistry, Biology, Pharmacology and Clinical Perspectives, Vol. 2,* Braquet, P., Ed., J. R. Prous, Barcelona, 1990, 291.

19. **Braquet, P. and Godfroid, J. J.,** Conformational properties of the PAF-acether receptor on platelets based on structure-activity studies, in *Platelet Activating Factor,* Snyder, F., Ed., Plenum Press, New York, 1987, 191.

20. **Stewart, A. G. and Dusting, G. J.,** Characterization of receptors for platelet-activating factor on platelets, polymorphonuclear leukocytes and macrophages, *Br. J. Pharmacol.,* 94, 1225, 1988.

21. **Dent, G., Ukena, D., Chanez, P., et al.,** Characterization of PAF receptors on human neutrophils using the specific antagonist, WEB 2086. Correlation between receptor binding and function, *FEBS Lett.,* 244, 365, 1989.

22. **Marquis, O., Robaut, C., and Cavero, I.,** Evidence for the existence and ionic modulation of platelet-activating factor receptors mediating degranulatory responses in human polymorphonuclear leukocytes, *J. Pharmacol. Exp. Ther.,* 250, 293, 1989.

23. **Gomez-Cambronero, J., Durstin, M., Molski, T. F., et al.,** Calcium is necessary for the platelet-activating factor release in human neutrophils stimulated by physiological stimuli. Role of G-proteins, *J. Biol. Chem.,* 264, 12699, 1989.

24. **Del Maschio, A., Albors, M., Evangelista, V., et al.,** Measurement of ionized cytoplasmic calcium mobilization with the photoprotein aequorin in human polymorphonuclear leukocytes activated by platelet-activating factor (PAF), *J. Lipid Med.,* 1, 25, 1989.

25. **Del Maschio, A., Chen, Z. M., Evangelista, V., et al.,** Increased platelet response to PAF by poly-morphonuclear leukocytes: inhibitory effect of BN 52021, in *Ginkgolides: Chemistry, Biology, Pharmacology and Clinical Perspectives, Vol. 2,* Braquet, P., Ed., J. R. Prous, Barcelona, 1990, 83.

26. **Tool, A. T., Verhoeven, A. J., Roos, D., et al.,** Platelet-activating factor (PAF) acts as an intercellular messenger in the changes of cytosolic free Ca^{2+} in human neutrophils induced by opsonized particles, *FEBS Lett.,* 259, 209, 1989.

27. **Bruijnzeel, P. L. B., Warringa, R. A. J., and Kok, P. T. M.,** Inhibition of platelet-activating factor and zymosan-activated serum-induced chemotaxis of human neutrophils by nedocromil sodium, BN 52021 and sodium cromoglycate, *Br. J. Pharmacol.,* 97, 1251, 1989.

28. **Pieper, G. M. and Gross, G. J.,** Priming by platelet-activating factor of neutrophil-induced impairment of endothelium-dependent relaxation, *J. Vasc. Med. Biol.,* in press.

29. **Rivero, A., Gomez-Guerrero, C., Egido, J., et al.,** Effect of BN 52021 on the superoxide anion release by human neutrophils and monocytes induced by tumor necrosis factor and gamma interferon, in *Ginkgolides: Chemistry, Biology, Pharmacology* and *Clinical Perspectives, Vol. 2.* Braquet, P., Ed., J. R. Prous, Barcelona, 1990, 65.

30. **Paubert-Braquet, M., Hosford, D., Klotz, P., et al.,** Tumor necrosis factor a "primes" the platelet-activating factor-induced superoxide production by human neutrophils: possible involvement of G proteins, *J. Lipid Med.,* 2, 51, 1990.

31. **McColl, S. R., Krump, R., Naccache, P. H., et al.,** Enhancement of platelet-activating factor-induced leukotriene synthesis in human neutrophils primed with granulocyte-macrophage colony-stimulating factor: effect of the ginkgolide BN 52021, in *Ginkgolides: Chemistry, Biology, Pharmacology and Clinical Perspectives, Vol. 2,* Braquet, P., Ed., J. R. Prous, Barcelona, 1990, 75.

32. **Rabier, M., Damon, M., Chanez, P., et al.,** Platelet-activating factor, neutrophil chemotaxis and gink-golides. in *Ginkgolides: Chemistry, Biology, Pharmacology and Clinical Perspectives, Vol. 2,* Braquet, P., Ed., J. R. Prous, Barcelona, 1990, 105.

33. **Sipka, S., Dinya, Z., Koltai, M., et al.,** Inhibition of neutrophil capillary migration by platelet-activating factor, in *Ginkgolides: Chemistry, Biology, Pharmacology and Clinical Perspectives, Vol. 2,* Braquet, P., Ed., J. R. Prous, Barcelona, 1990, 96.

34. **Hunyadi, J., Judak, R., Kenderessy, A. S., et al.,** Enhancing effect of whole-body ultraviolet light irradiation on *Candida albicans* activity of human polymorphonuclear leukocytes, *Dermatol. Monatsschr.,* 175, 326, 1989.

35. **Hayashi, H., Kudo, I., Kato, I., et al.,** A novel bioaction of PAF: induction of microbicidal activity in guinea-pig bone marrow cells, *Lipids,* 23, 1119, 1988.

36. **Bussolino, F., Turrini, F., Alessi, D., et al.,** BN 52021 inhibits (R)PAF-induced increase of CR_1-mediated erythrophagocytosis, in *Ginkgolides: Chemistry, Biology, Pharmacology and Clinical Perspectives, Vol. 2,* Braquet, P., Ed., J. R. Prous, Barcelona, 1990, 117.

37. **Valone, F. H.,** Identification of platelet-activating factor receptors in PS88D murine macrophages, *J. Immunol.,* 140, 2389, 1988.

38. **Parnham, M. J., Bittner, C., and Lambrecht, G.,** Antagonism of platelet-activating factor induced chemiluminescence in guinea-pig peritoneal macrophages in differing states of activation, *Br. J. Pharmacol.,* 98, 574, 1989.

39. **Elstad, M. R., Stafforini, D. M., McIntyre, T. M., et al.,** Platelet-activating factor acetylhydrolase increases during macrophage differentiation, *J. Biol. Chem.,* 264, 8467, 1989.

40. **Adolfs, M. J. P., Beusenberg, F. D., and Bonta, I. L.,** PAF-acether modifies human peritoneal macrophage cAMP levels in a biphasic fashion, *Agents Actions,* 26, 119, 1989.

41. **Ng, D. S. and Wong, K.,** Platelet-activating factor (PAF) stimulates phosphatidylinositol hydrolysis in human peripheral blood mononuclear leukocytes, *Res. Commun. Chem. Pathol. Pharmacol.,* 66, 219, 1989.

42. **Ward, S. G. and Westwick, J.,** Antagonism of the platelet-activating factor-induced rise of the intracellular calcium ion concentration of U 937 cells, *Br. J. Pharmacol.,* 93, 769, 1988.

43. **Barzaghi, G., Sarau, H. M., and Mong, S.,** Platelet-activating factor-induced phosphoinositide metabolism in differentiated U-937 cells in culture, *J. Pharmacol. Exp. Ther.,* 248, 559, 1989.

44. **Fitzgerald, M. F., Parente, L., and Whittle, B. J.,** Release of PAF-acether and eicosanoids from guinea-pig alveolar macrophages by FMLP: effect of cyclooxygenase and lipoxygenase inhibition, *Eur. J. Pharmacol.,* 164, 539, 1989.

45. **Stewart, A. G. and Phillips, W. A.,** Intracellular platelet-activating factor regulates eicosanoid generation in guinea-pig resident peritoneal macrophages, *Br. J. Pharmacol.,* 98, 141, 1989.

46. **Fauler, J., Sielhorst, G., and Frölich, J. C.,** Platelet-activating factor induces the production of leukotrienes by human monocytes, *Biochim. Biophys. Acta,* 1013, 80, 1989.

47. **Morris, D. D. and Moore, J. N.,** Equine peritoneal macrophage production of thromboxane and prostacyclin in response to platelet-activating factor and its receptor antagonist SRI 63-441, *Circ. Shock,* 28, 149, 1989.

48. **Dubois, C., Bissonnette, E., and Rola-Pleszczynski, M.,** Platelet-activating factor (PAF) enhances tumor necrosis factor production by alveolar macrophages. Prevention by PAF receptor antagonists and lipoxygenase inhibitors, *J. Immunol.,* 143, 964, 1989.

49. **Poubelle, P. and Rola-Pleszczynski, M.,** PAF enhances the production of tumor necrosis factor alpha by human monocytes: partial antagonism by BN 52021, in *Ginkgolides: Chemistry, Biology, Pharmacology and Clinical Perspectives,* Vol. 2, Braquet, P., Ed., J. R. Prous, Barcelona, 1990, 695.

50. **Bonivada, B., Mencia-Huerta, J. M., and Braquet, P.,** Effects of platelet-activating factor on peripheral blood monocytes: induction and priming for TNF secretion, *J. Lipid Med.,* 2, S65, 1990.

51. **Bonavida, B., Jewett, A., Mencia-Huerta, J. M., et al.,** Biology of platelet-activating factor (PAF) interaction with human peripheral blood monocytes and induction of tumor necrosis factor (TNF) secretion, in *Ginkgolides: Chemistry, Biology, Pharmacology and Clinical Perspectives, Vol. 2,* Braquet, P., Ed., J. R. Prous, Barcelona, 1990, 885.

52. **Pignol, B., Henane, S., Chaumeron, S., et al.,** Modulation of the priming effects of platelet-activating factor on the release of interleukin-1 from lipopolysaccharide-stimulated rat spleen macrophages, *J. Lipid Med.,* S93, 1990.

53. **Travers, J. B., Li, Q., Kniss, D. A., et al.,** Identification of functional platelet-activating factor receptors in Raji lymphoblasts, *J. Immunol.,* 143, 3708, 1989.

54. **Ukena, D., Krogel, C., Dent, G., et al.,** PAF-receptors on eosinophils: identification with a novel ligand, (3H)WEB 2086, *Biochem. Pharmacol.,* 38, 1702, 1989.

55. **Kroegel, C., Yukawa, T., Westwick, J., et al.,** Evidence for two platelet-activating factor receptors on eosinophils: dissociation between PAF-induced intracellular calcium mobilization degranulation and superoxides anion generation in eosinophils, *Biochem. Biophys. Res. Commun.,* 162, 511, 1989.

56. **Aoki, S., Boubekeur, K., Burrows, L., et al.,** Recruitment of eosinophils by platelet-activating factor (PAF) in guinea-pig lung, *J. Physiol.,* 394, 130P, 1988.

57. **Arnoux, B., Denjean, A., Page, C. P. et al.,** Accumulation of platelets and eosinophils in baboon lung following PAF-acether challenge: inhibition by ketotifen, *Am. Rev. Respir. Dis.,* 137, 855, 1988.

58. **Sanjar, S., Aoki, S., Boubekeur, K., et al.,** Inhibition of PAF-induced eosinophil accumulation in pulmonary airways of guinea-pigs by anti-asthma drugs, *Jpn. J. Pharmacol.,* 51, 167, 1989.

59. **Lellouch-Tubiana, A., Lefort, J., Simon, M. T., et al.,** Eosinophil recruitment into guinea-pig lungs after PAF-acether and allergen administration, *Am. Rev. Respir. Dis.,* 137, 948, 1988.

60. **Page, C. P. and Coyle, A. J.,** The interaction between PAF, platelets and eosinophils in bronchial asthma, *Eur. Respir. J.,* Suppl. 2, 483s, 1989.

61. **Sanjar, S., Aoki, S., Boubekeur, K., et al.,** Eosinophil accumulation in pulmonary airways of guinea-pigs induced by exposure to an aerosol of platelet-activating factor: effect of anti-asthma drugs, *Br. J. Pharmacol.,* 99, 267, 1990.

62. **Chihara, J. and Nakajima, S.,** Induction of hypodense eosinophils and nuclear hypersegmentation of eosinophils by various chemotactic factors and lymphokines *in vitro, Allergy Proc.,* 1, 27, 1989.

63. **Kloprogge, E., de Leuw, A. J., de Monchy, J. G., et al.,** Hypodense eosinophilic granulocytes in normal individuals and patients with asthma: generation of hypodense cell populations *in vitro, J. Allergy Clin. Immunol.,* 83, 393, 1989.

64. **Yukawa, T., Kroegel, C., Evans, P., et al.,** Density heterogeneity of eosinophil leucocytes: induction of hypodense eosinophils by platelet-activating factor, *Immunology,* 68, 140, 1989.

65. **Ebisawa, M., Saito, H., Reason, D. C., et al.,** Effects of human recombinant interleukin 5 and 3 on the differentiation of cord blood-derived eosinophils and basophils, *Arerugi,* 38, 442, 1989.

66. **Popper, H., Knipping, G., Czarnetski, B. M., et al.,** Activation and release of enzymes and major basic protein from guinea-pig eosinophil granulocytes induced by different inflammatory stimuli and other substances. A histochemical, biochemical, and electron microscopic study, *Inflammation,* 13, 147, 1989.

67. **Koenderman, L., and Bruijnzeel, P. L.,** Increased sensitivity of the chemoattractant-induced chemiluminiscence in eosinophils isolated from atopic individuals, *Immunology,* 67, 534, 1989.

68. **Kroegel, C., Pleass, R., Yukawa, T., et al.,** Characterization of platelet-activating factor-induced elevation of cytosolic free calcium concentration in eosinophils, *FEBS Lett.,* 243, 41, 1989.

69. **Moqbel, R., Cromwell, O., and Kay, A. B.,** The effect of nedocromil sodium on human eosinophil activation, *Drugs 37* suppl. 1, 19, 1989.

70. **Moqbel, R., Kurihara, K., Wardlaw, A. J., et al.,** BN 52021 inhibits PAF-induced eosinophil chemotaxis and cytotoxicity, in *Ginkgolides: Chemistry, Biology, Pharmacology and Clinical Perspectives, Vol. 2,* Braquet, P., Ed., J. R. Prous, Barcelona, 1990, 143.

71. **Kurihara, K., Wardlaw, A. J., Moqbel, R., et al.,** Inhibition of platelet-activating factor (PAF)-induced chemotaxis, and PAF binding to human eosinophils and neutrophils, by the specific gingkolide-derived PAF antagonist, BN 52021, *Arch. Allergy Appl. Immunol.,* in press.

72. **Bruijnzell, P. L. B., Burgers, J. A., Kok, P. T. M., et al.,** BN 52021 and leukotriene C$_4$ formation by human eosinophils, in *Ginkgolides: Chemistry, Biology, Pharmacology and Clinical Perspectives, Vol. 2,* Braquet, P., Ed., J. R. Prous, Barcelona, 1990, 125.

73. **Thomson, A. W., Milton, J. I., Aldridge, R. D., et al.,** Inhibition by cyclosporine of eosinophilia induced by high-dose cyclophosphamide prior to immunization, *Transplant. Proc.,* 18, 895, 1986.

74. **Etienne, A., Soulard, C., Thonier, F., et al.,** Modulation of eosinophil recruitment in the rat by the platelet-activating factor (PAF) antagonist, BN 52021, the somatostatin analog, BIM 23014, and by cyclosporin A, *Prostaglandins,* 37, 345, 1989.

75. **Morita, E., Schroder, J. M., and Christophers, E.,** Chemotactic responsiveness of eosinophils isolated from patients with inflammatory skin diseases, *J. Dermatol.,* 16, 348, 1989.

76. **Thiermermann, C., May, G. R., Page, C. P., et al.,** Endothelin-1 inhibits platelet aggregation *in vivo:* a study with [111]indium-labeled platelets, *Br. J. Pharmacol.,* 99, 303, 1990.

77. **Whatley, R. E., Zimmermann, G. A., McIntyre, T. M., et al.,** Endothelium from diverse vascular sources synthesizes platelet-activating factor, *Arteriosclerosis,* 8, 321, 1988.

78. **Lewis, M. S., Whatley, R. E., Cain, P., et al.,** Hydrogen peroxide stimulates the synthesis of platelet-activating factor by endothelium and induces endothelial cell-dependent neutrophil adhesion, *J. Clin. Invest.,* 82, 2045, 1988.

79. **Hirafuji, M., Maeyama, K., Watanabe, T., et al.,** Transient increase of cytosolic free calcium in cultured human vascular endothelial cells by platelet-activating factor, *Biochem. Biophys. Res. Commun.,* 154, 910, 1988.

80. **Vercellotti, G. M., Yin, H. Q., Gustafson, K. S., et al.,** Platelet-activating factor primes neutrophil responses to agonist role in promoting netrophil-mediated endothelial damage, *Blood* 71, 1100, 1988.

81. **Vercellotti, G. M., Wickham, N. W., Gustafson, K. S., et al.,** Thrombin-treated endothelium primes neutrophil functions: inhibition by platelet-activating factor receptor antagonists, *J. Leukocyte Biol.,* 45, 483, 1989.

82. **Stewart, A. G. and Harris, T.,** Effects of BN 52021 on receptor-mediated activation of leukocytes and endothelial cells, in *Ginkgolides: Chemistry, Biology, Pharmacology and Clinical Perspectives, Vol. 2,* Braquet, P., Ed., J. R. Prous, Barcelona, 1990, 155.

83. **Northover, A. M.,** Effects of PAF and PAF antagonists on the shape of venous endothelial cells *in vitro, Agents Actions,* 28, 142, 1989.

84. **Northover, A. M.,** Effects of platelet-activating factor on vascular endothelial cell shape *in vitro,* in *Ginkgolides: Chemistry, Biology, Pharmacology and Clinical Perspectives, Vol. 2,* Braquet, P., Ed., J. R. Prous, Barcelona, 1990, 143.

85. **Korth, R., Hirafuji, M., Keraly, C. L., et al.,** Interaction of the PAF antagonist WEB 2086 and its hetrazepine analogues with human platelets and endothelial cells, *Br. J. Pharmacol.,* 98, 653, 1989.

86. **Koltai, M., Tosaki, A., Guillon, J. M., et al.,** PAF-antagonists as potential therapeutic agents in cardiac anaphylaxis and myocardial ischemia, *Cardiovasc. Drug Rev.*, 7, 177, 1989.

87. **Levi, R., Genovese, A., and Pinckard, R. N.,** Alkyl chain homologs of platelet-activating factor and their effects on the mammalian heart, *Biochem. Biophys. Res. Commun.*, 161, 1341, 1989.

88. **Vornovitskii, E. G., Ignateva, V. B., Gollash, M., et al.,** Cardiodepressive effect of platelet activating factor, *Biull. Eksp. Biol. Med.*, 107, 27, 1989.

89. **Vornovitskii, E. G., Ignateva, V. B., Gollash, M., et al.,** Interactions of PAF and its antagonists in the guinea pig atrial myocardium, *Biull. Eksp. Biol. Med.*, 108, 137, 1989.

90. **Lagente, V., Simonetti, M. P., Fortez, Z. B., et al.,** Protective effect of a specific platelet-activating factor antagonist, BN 52021, on bupivacaine-induced cardiovascular impairments in rats, *Pharmacol. Res.*, 21, 577, 1989.

91. **Simonetti, M. P., and Lagente, V.,** Effect of BN 52021 on bupivacaine-induced cardiovascular impairments, in *Ginkgolides: Chemistry, Biology, Pharmacology and Clinical Perspectives, Vol. 2*, Braquet, P., Ed., J. R. Prous, Barcelona, 1990, 445.

92. **Riedel, A., Meyer, E., Heinroth-Hoffmann, I., et al.,** BN 52021 abolishes PAF-induced cardiac rhythm disturbances, in *Ginkgolides: Chemistry, Biology, Pharmacology and Clinical Perspectives, Vol. 2*, Braquet, P., Ed., J. R. Prous, Barcelona, 1990, 275.

93. **Soloviev, A. I. and Braquet, P.,** The role of PAF-acether in the mechanisms of isolated coronary arteries spasm under hypoxia and its inhibition by BN 52021, in *Ginkgolides: Chemistry, Biology, Pharmacology and Clinical Perspectives, Vol. 2*, Braquet, P., Ed., J. R. Prous, Barcelona, 1990, 353.

94. **Tosaki, A., Koltai, M., Braquet, P., et al.,** Possible involvement of platelet activating factor in anaphylaxis of passively sensitized, isolated guinea pig hearts, *Cardiovasc., Res.*, 23, 715, 1989.

95. **Joseph, R. and Welch, K. M.,** Granulocytes, platelet-activating factor and myocardial injury (letter), *Circulation*, 79, 140, 1989.

96. **Lefer, A. M.,** Platelet-activating factor (PAF) and its role in cardiac injury, *Prog. Clin. Biol. Res.*, 301, 53, 1989.

97. **Mickelson, J. K., Simpson, P. J., and Lucchesi, B. R.,** Myocardial dysfunction and coronary vasoconstriction induced by platelet-activating factor in the post-infarcted rabbit isolated heart, *J. Mol. Cell. Cardiol.*, 20, 547, 1988.

98. **Montrucchio, G., Alloatti, G., Tetta, C., et al.,** Release of platelet-activating factor from ischemic-reperfused rabbit heart, *Am. J. Physiol.*, 25, H1236, 1989.

99. **Nidorf, S. M., Sturm, M., Strophair, J., et al.,** Whole blood aggregation, thromboxane release and the lyso derivative of platelet-activating factor in myocardial infarction and unstable angina, *Cardiovasc. Res.*, 23, 273, 1989.

100. **Leonelli, F. M., Leon, L. L., Sturm, M. J., et al.,** Plasma levels of the lyso-derivative of platelet-activating factor in acute severe systemic illness, *Clin. Sci.*, 77, 561, 1989.

101. **Taylor, R. R., Sturm, M., Kendrew, P. J., et al.,** Plasma levels of the lyso-derivative of platelet-activating factor are related to age, *Clin. Sci.*, 76, 195, 1989.

102. **Koltai, M., Tosaki, A., Hosford, D., et al.,** BN 52021, a PAF receptor antagonist, protects isolated working rat hearts against arrhythmias induced by ischemia but not reperfusion, *Eur. J. Pharmacol.*, 164, 293, 1989.

103. **Tosaki, A., Hosford, D., and Koltai, M.,** Effect of Ginkgolide B (BN 52021) on ischemia/reperfusion-induced arrhythmias in isolated working rat hearts, in *Ginkgolides: Chemistry, Biology, Pharmacology and Clinical Perspectives, Vol. 2*, Braquet, P., Ed., J. R. Prous, Barcelona, 1990, 427.

104. **Berti, F., Rossoni, G., Puglisi, L., et al.,** The Ginkgolide BN 52021 prevents myocardial contracture and arrhythmia in ischemic rabbit heart, in *Ginkgolides: Chemistry, Biology, Pharmacology and Clinical Perspectives, Vol. 2*, Braquet, P., Ed., J. R. Prous, Barcelona, 1990, 381.

105. **Felix, S. B., Steger, A., Baumann, G., et al.,** Platelet-activating factor-induced coronary constriction in the isolated perfused guinea-pig heart and antagonistic effects of the PAF antagonist WEB 2086, *J. Lipid Med.*, 2, 9, 1990.

106. **Guillon, J. M., Rochette, L., and Baranès, J.,** Effects of *Ginkgo biloba* extract on two models of experimental myocardial ischemia, in Rökan *(Ginkgo biloba). Recent Results in Pharmacology and Clinic*, Fünfgeld, E. W., Ed., Springer-Verlag, Berlin, 1988, 153.

107. **Guillon, J. M. and Koltai, M.,** Effect of BN 52021 (Ginkgolide B) on arrhythmias evoked by coronary artery ligation in the zucker rat, in *Ginkgolides: Chemistry, Biology, Pharmacology and Clinical Perspectives, Vol. 2*, Braquet, P., Ed., J. R. Prous, Barcelona, 1990, 427.

108. **Stahl, G. L., Terashita, Z. I., and Lefer, A. M.,** Role of platelet-activating factor in propagation of cardiac damage during myocardial ischemia, *J. Pharmacol. Exp. Ther.*, 244, 898, 1988.

109. **Stahl, G. L. and Lefer, A. M.,** Mechanisms of platelet-activating factor-induced cardiac depression in the isolated perfused rat heart, *Circ. Shock*, 23, 165, 1987.

110. **Wainwright, C. L., Parratt, J. R., and Bigaud, M.,** The effects of PAF antagonists on arrhythmias and platelets during acute myocardial ischaemia and reperfusion, *Eur. Heart J.*, 10, 235, 1989.

111. **Wainwright, C. L. and Parratt, J. R.,** Effect of BN 52021 on platelet behavior and arrhythmias during myocardial ischemia and reperfusion, in *Ginkgolides: Chemistry, Biology, Pharmacology and Clinical Perspectives, Vol. 2,* Braquet, P., Ed., J. R. Prous, Barcelona, 1990, 391.

112. **Jouve, R., Puddu, P. E., Langlet, F., et al.,** Anti-arrhythmic effects of BN 52021 after circumflex coronary artery occlusion-reperfusion in dogs: analysis of 87 experiments using the proportional hazards cox's model, in *Ginkgolides: Chemistry, Biology, Pharmacology and Clinical Perspectives, Vol. 2,* Braquet, P., Ed., J. R. Prous, Barcelona, 1990, 437.

113. **Thiévant, P., Guillon, J. M., and Koltai, M.,** Effect of Ginkgolide B (BN 52021) on ischemia/reperfusion-induced arrhythmias in mongrel dogs, in *Ginkgolides: Chemistry, Biology, Pharmacology and Clinical Perspectives, Vol. 2,* Braquet, P., Ed., J. R. Prous, Barcelona, 1990, 413.

114. **Fontaliran, F., Guillon, J. M., Koltai, M., et al.,** Reduction of infarct size by Ginkgolide B (BN 52021) in coronary artery ligated rats, in *Ginkgolides: Chemistry, Biology, Pharmacology and Clinical Perspectives, Vol. 2,* Braquet, P., Ed., J. R. Prous, Barcelona, 1990, 405.

115. **Gross, G. J., Maruyama, M., Vercellotti, G. M., et al.,** Effect of the PAF antagonist, BN 52021, on myocardial infarct size in dogs, in *Ginkgolides: Chemistry, Biology, Pharmacology and Clinical Perspectives, Vol. 2,* Braquet, P., Ed., J. R. Prous, Barcelona, 1990, 421.

116. **Maruyama, M., Farber, N. E., Vercellotti, G. M., et al.,** Evidence for a role of platelet activating factor in the pathogenesis of irreversible but not reversible myocardial injury after reperfusion in dogs, *Am. Heart J.,* 120, 510, 1990.

117. **Braquet, P., Paubert-Braquet, M., Koltai, M., et al.,** Is there a case for PAF antagonists in the treatment of ischemic states?, *Trends Pharmacol. Sci.,* 10, 23, 1989.

118. **Braquet, P. and Hosford, D.,** The potential role of platelet-activating factor (PAF) in shock, sepsis and adult respiratory distress syndrome (ARDS), *Prog. Clin. Biol. Res.,* 308, 425, 1989.

119. **Hosford, D. and Braquet, P.,** Potential role for platelet activating factor and tumor necrosis factor in the immune impairments in shock and trauma, in *Immune Consequences of Trauma, Shock and Sepsis,* 1989, 311.

120. **Laurindo, F. R., Goldstein, R. E., Davenport, N. J., et al.,** Mechanisms of hypotension produced by platelet-activating factor, *J. Appl. Physiol.,* 66, 2681, 1989.

121. **Filep, J., Herman, F., Braquet, P., et al.,** Increased levels of platelet-activating factor in blood following intestinal ischemia in the dog, *Biochem. Biophys. Res. Commun.,* 158, 353, 1989.

122. **Mozes, T., Braquet, P., and Filep, J.,** Platelet-activating factor: an endogenous mediator of mesenteric ischemia-reperfusion-induced shock, *Am. J. Physiol.,* 257, R872, 1989.

123. **Mozes, T. and Filep, J.,** Protective effect of BN 52021 in mesenteric ischemia/reperfusion-induced shock in anesthetized dogs, in *Ginkgolides: Chemistry, Biology, Pharmacology and Clinical Perspectives, Vol. 2,* Braquet, P., Ed., J. R. Prous, Barcelona, 1990, 331.

124. **Stahl, G. L., Craft, D. V., Lento, P. H., et al.,** Detection of platelet-activating factor during traumatic shock, *Circ. Shock,* 26, 237, 1988.

125. **Siren, A. L. and Feuerstein, G.,** Effects of PAF and BN 52021 on cardiac function and regional blood flow in conscious rats, *Am. J. Physiol.,* 257, H25, 1989.

126. **Gerkens, J. F.,** Inhibition of vasoconstriction by platelet-activating factor in the in situ blood perfused rat mesentery, *Clin. Exp. Pharmacol. Physiol.,* 16, 161, 1989.

127. **Lagente, V., Fortes, Z. B., and Garcia-Leme, J.,** Effect of BN 52021 on PAF-induced changes of the mesenteric microvasculature, in *Ginkgolides: Chemistry, Biology, Pharmacology and Clinical Perspectives, Vol. 2,* Braquet, P., Ed., J. R. Prous, Barcelona, 1990, 267.

128. **Bahr, T., Schaper, U., Becker, K., et al.,** Influence of inhibitors of the eicosanoid metabolism, and of eicosanoids- and PAF-acether antagonists on mortality and some biochemical parameters of three shock models, *Prog. Clin. Biol. Res.,* 301, 229, 1989.

129. **Sagach, V. F., Dmitrieva, A. V., and Braquet, P.,** Influence of BN 52021 on cardiac and hemodynamic changes during the development of post-ischemic shock reaction, in *Ginkgolides: Chemistry, Biology, Pharmacology and Clinical Perspectives, Vol. 2,* Braquet, P., Ed., J. R. Prous, Barcelona, 1990, 341.

130. **Stanton, A. W. B., Izumi, T., Antoniw, J. W., et al.,** Platelet-activating factor (PAF) antagonist, WEB 2086, protects against PAF-induced hypotension in *Macaca fascicularis, Br. J. Pharmacol.,* 97, 643, 1989.

131. **Bauer, J. A., Wuster, K., Conzen, P., et al.,** Modulation of re-synthesis of 1-alkyl-2-arachidonyl-glycero-3-phosphocholine and phosphatidylinositols for interception in vivo of free arachidonic acid, lyso-PAF, diacyl-glycero-, and phospho-inositides, *Prog. Clin. Biol. Res.,* 308, 455, 1989.

132. **Lavaud, P., Mathieu, J., Bienvenu, P., et al.,** Modulation of leucocyte activation in the early phase of the rabbit burn injury, *Burns,* 14, 15, 1988.

133. **Terashita, Z., Shibouta, Y., Imura, Y., et al.,** Endothelin-induced sudden death and the possible involvement of platelet-activating factor (PAF), *Life Sci.,* 45, 1911, 1989.

134. **Lang, C. and Dobrescu, C.,** Attenuation of burn-induced changes in hemodynamics and glucose metabolism by the PAF antagonist SRI 63-675, *Eur. J. Pharmacol.,* 156, 207, 1988.

135. **Bradley, L. M., Goldstein, R. E., Feuerstein, G., et al.,** Circulatory effects of PAF-acether in newborn piglets, *Am. J. Physiol.,* 256, H205, 1989.

136. **Bradley, L. M., Stambouly, J. J., Czaja, J. F., et al.,** Influence of thromboxane A_2 receptor antagonism on pulmonary vasoconstrictor responses, *Pediatr. Res.,* 26, 175, 1989.

137. **Aguggini, G., Berti, F., Clement, M. G., et al.,** The Ginkoglide BN 52021 antagonizes the increase in pulmonary pressure induced by platelet-activating factor in pig: a link to TXA_2 generation, in *Ginkgolides: Chemistry, Biology, Pharmacology and Clinical Perspectives, Vol. 2,* Braquet, P., Ed., J. R. Prous, Barcelona, 1990, 241.

138. **Imai, T., Vercellotti, G. M., Moldowyn, C. F., et al.,** The pulmonary hypertension and edema induced by platelet-activating factor in isolated, perfused rat lungs is blocked by BN 52021, *J. Lab. Clin. Med.,* in press.

139. **Pinheiro, J. M., Pitt, B. R., and Gillis, C. N.,** Roles of platelet-activating factor and thromboxane in group B Streptococcus-induced pulmonary hypertension in piglets *Pediatr. Res.,* 26, 420, 1989.

140. **McCormack, D. G., Barnes, P. G., and Evans, T. W.,** Evidence against a role for platelet-activating factor in hypoxic pulmonary vasoconstriction in the rat, *Clin. Sci.,* 77, 439, 1989.

141. **Ibbotson, G. C. and Wallace, J. L.,** Beneficial effects of prostaglandin E_2 in endotoxic shock are unrelated to effects on PAF-acether synthesis, *Prostaglandins,* 37, 237, 1989.

142. **Fletcher, J. R., DiSimone, A. G., and Earnest, M.,** The effects of BN 52021 on PAF induced hypotension or endotoxin induced hypotension in the conscious rat, in *Ginkgolides: Chemistry, Biology, Pharmacology and Clinical Perspectives, Vol. 1,* Braquet, P., Ed., J.R. Prous, Barcelona, 1988, 457.

143. **Lagente, V., Fortes, Z. B., Garcia-Leme, J., et al.,** PAF-acether and endotoxin display similar effects on rat mesenteric microvessels: inhibition by specific antagonists, *J. Pharmacol. Exp. Ther.,* 247, 254, 1988.

144. **Earnest, M. A., DiSimone, A. G., and Fletcher, J. R.,** The effects of BN 52021, a PAF receptor antagonist, in canine endotoxemia, in *Ginkgolides: Chemistry, Biology, Pharmacology and Clinical Perspectives, Vol. 2,* Braquet, P., Ed., J. R. Prous, Barcelona, 1990, 463.

145. **Damas, J., Remacle-Volon, G., Adma, A., et al.,** Endotoxin shock, kinin system and PAF-acether in the rat, in *Kinins V, Part B,* Abe, K., Moriya, H., and Fujii, S., Eds., Plenum Press, New York, 1989, 547.

146. **Lomazova, K. D., Poliakova, A. M., Astrina, O. S., et al.,** The thrombocyte activation factor and endotoxin-induced thrombocyte activation, *Biull. Eksp. Biol. Med.,* 107, 538, 1989.

147. **Beijer, L., Botting, J., Crook, P., et al.,** The involvement of platelet-activating factor in endotoxin-induced pulmonary platelet recruitment in the guinea-pig, *Br. J. Pharmacol.,* 92, 803, 1987.

148. **Rylander, R. and Beijer, L.,** PAF antagonist BN 52021 modifies lung wall and airway cell responses to endotoxin inhalation, in *Ginkgolides: Chemistry, Biology, Pharmacology and Clinical Perspectives, Vol. 2,* Braquet, P., Ed., J. R. Prous, Barcelona, 1990, 219.

149. **Pons, L., Droay-Lefay, M. T., Braquet, P., et al.,** Involvement of platelet-activating factor (PAF) in endotoxin-induced intestinal motor disturbances in rats, *Life Sci.,* 45, 533, 1989.

150. **Boughton-Smith, N. K., Hutcheson, I., and Whittle, B. J.,** Relationship between PAF-acether and thromboxane A_2 biosynthesis in endotoxin-induced intestinal damage in the rat, *Prostaglandins,* 38, 319, 1989.

151. **Redl, H., Gasser, H., Bahrami, S., et al.,** The role of PAF in an ovine model of endotoxin shock, in *Ginkgolides: Chemistry, Biology, Pharmacology and Clinical Perspectives, Vol. 2,* Braquet, P., Ed., J. R. Prous, Barcelona, 1990, 471.

152. **Nijkamp, F. P. and van Heuven-Nolsen, D.,** The PAF antagonist BN 52021 inhibits endotoxin-induced hyperreactivity to histamine in guinea-pig airways but not in coronary vessels, in *Ginkgolides: Chemistry, Biology, Pharmacology and Clinical Perspectives, Vol. 2,* Braquet, P., Ed., J. R. Prous, Barcelona, 1990, 197.

153. **Nijkamp, F. P., Braquet, P., and van Heuven-Nolsen, D.,** BN 52021 inhibits the endotoxin-induced tracheal hyperreactivity to histamine in the guinea-pig but not the increased response to histamine in the coronary vessels, in *Immune Consequence of Trauma,* Springer-Verlag, Berlin, in press.

154. **Tolins, J. P.,** The role of PAF in endotoxemic acute renal failure in the rat: protection by BN 52021, in *Ginkgolides: Chemistry, Biology, Pharmacology and Clinical Perspectives, Vol. 2,* Braquet, P., Ed., J. R. Prous, Barcelona, 1990, 455.

155. **Floch, A., Bousseau, A., Hetier, E., et al.,** RP 55778, a PAF receptor antagonist, prevents and reverses LPS-induced hemoconcentration and TNF release, *J. Lipid Med.,* 1, 349, 1989.

156. **Yue, T. L., Farhat, M., Rabinovici, R., et al.,** Protective effect of BN 50739, a new PAF antagonist, in endotoxin-treated rabbits, *J. Pharmacol. Exp. Ther.,* 254, 976, 1990.

157. **Rabinovici, R., Yue, T. L., Farhat, M., et al.,** Platelet-activating factor (PAF) and tumor necrosis factor (TNF) interactions in endotoxemic shock, *J. Pharmacol. Exp. Ther.,* 255, 256, 1990.

158. **Satoh, K., Imaizumi, T., Kawamura, Y., et al.,** Increased activity of the platelet-activating factor acetylhydrolase in plasma low density lipoprotein from patients with essential hypertension, *Prostaglandins,* 37, 673, 1989.
159. **Bodzenta-Lukaszyk, A., Krupinski, K., Dabrowski, S., et al.,** Blood platelet function in patients with obliterative arteriosclerosis of the lower limbs, *Folia Haematol.,* 115, 470, 1988.
160. **Ostermann, G., Lans, A., Holtz, H., et al.,** The degradation of platelet-activating factor in serum and its discriminative value in atherosclerotic patients, *Thromb. Res.,* 52, 529, 1988.
161. **Masugi, F., Sakaguchi, K., Saeki, S., et al.,** Dietary salt, blood pressure and circulating levels of 1-O-hexadecyl-2-acetyl-sn-glycero-3-phosphocholine in patients with essential hypertension, *J. Lipid Med.,* 1, 341, 1989.
162. **Kawaguchi, H., Sawa, H., Izuka, K., et al.,** Platelet-activating factor stimulates angiotensin converting enzyme activity, *J. Hypertens.,* 8, 173, 1990.
163. **Sturm, M. J., Strophair, J. M., Kendrew, P. J., et al.,** Whole blood aggregation and plasma lyso-PAF related to smoking and atherosclerosis, *Clin. Exp. Pharmacol. Physiol.,* 16, 597, 1989.
164. **Feliste, R., Perret, B., Braquet, P., et al.,** Protective effect of BN 52021, a specific antagonist of platelet-activating factor (PAF-acether) against diet-induced cholesteryl ester deposition in rabbit aorta, *Atherosclerosis,* 78, 151, 1989.
165. **Lopez, J. A., Armstrong, M. L., Harrison, D. G., et al.,** Vascular responses to leukocyte products in atherosclerotic primates, *Circ. Res.,* 65, 1078, 1989.
166. **Hellegouarch, A. and Pirotzky,** Effects of ANF and BN 52021 on PAF-induced modulation of venal tone, in *Ginkgolides: Chemistry, Biology, Pharmacology and Clinical Perspectives, Vol. 2,* Braquet, P., Ed., J. R. Prous, Barcelona, 1990, 305.
167. **Hellegouarch, A., Auguet, M., Guillon, J. M., et al.,** Lack of effect of atrial natriuretic factor on the tone induced in rat portal vein by platelet-activating factor, *Eur. J. Pharmacol.,* 145, 345, 1988.
168. **Hellegouarch, A., Auguet, M., Clostre, F., et al.,** Effects of BN 52063 and other agents inhibiting platelet-activating factor-induced contractile responses in rat portal vein, *J. Pharm. Pharmacol.,* 49, 589, 1988.
169. **Kumar, R., Harvey, S. A., Kester, M., et al.,** Production and effects of platelet-activating factor in the rat brain, *Biochim. Biophys. Acta,* 963, 375, 1988.
170. **Yue, T. L., Lysko, P. G., and Feuerstein, G.,** Production of platelet-activating factor from rat cerebellar granule cells in culture, *J. Neurochem.,* 54, 1809, 1990.
171. **Francescangeli, E. and Goracci, G.,** The de novo biosynthesis of platelet-activating factor in rat brain, *Biochem. Biophys. Res. Commun.,* 16, 107, 1989.
172. **Kornecki, E. and Ehrlich, Y. H.,** Neuroregulatory and neuropathological actions of the ether-phospholipid platelet-activating factor, *Science,* 240, 92, 1988.
173. **Dray, F., Wisner, A., Bommelaer-Bayet, M. C., et al.,** Prostaglandin E2, leukotriene C4, and platelet-activating factor receptor sites in the brain. Binding parameters and pharmacological studies, *Ann. N.Y. Acad. Sci.,* 559, 100, 1989.
174. **Domingo, M. T., Spinnewyn, B., Chabrier, P. E., et al.,** Specific binding site for PAF in the brain and inhibition by BN 52021, in *Ginkgolides: Chemistry, Biology, Pharmacology and Clinical Perspectives, Vol. 2,* Braquet, P., Ed., J. R. Prous, Barcelona, 1990, 613.
175. **Murphy, S. and Welk, S.,** Arachidonic acid evokes inositol phospholipid hydrolysis in astrocytes, *FEBS-Lett.,* 257, 68, 1989.
176. **Miller, L. G., Roy, R. B., Gaver, A., et al.,** Platelet-activating factor antagonists augment benzodiazepine receptor binding and GABA$_A$ receptor function, *J. Pharmacol. Exp. Therap.,* submitted.
177. **Junier, M. P., Tiberghien, C., Rougeat, C., et al.,** Inhibitory effect of platelet-activating factor (PAF) on luteinizing hormone-releasing hormone and somatostatin release from rat median eminence in vitro correlated with the characterization of specific PAF receptor sites in rat hypothalamus, *Endocrinology,* 123, 72, 1988.
178. **Tiberghien, C., Junier, M. P., Rougeot, C., et al.,** Effect of BN 52021, kadsurenone and L-652,731 on neuropeptide release in vitro, relation with PAF binding site receptor in rat brain, in *Ginkgolides: Chemistry, Biology, Pharmacology and Clinical Perspectives, Vol. 2,* Braquet, P., Ed., J. R. Prous, Barcelona, 1990, 639.
179. **Bernardini, R., Calogero, A. E., Ehrlich, Y. H., et al.,** The alkyl-ether phospholipid platelet-activating factor is a stimulator of the hypothalamic-pituitary-adrenal axis in the rat, *Endocrinology,* 125, 1067, 1989.
180. **Camoratto, A. M. and Grandison, L.,** Platelet-activating factor stimulates prolactin release from dispersed rat anterior pituitary cells *in vitro, Endocrinology,* 124, 1502, 1989.
181. **Blasquez, C., Jégou, S., Delarue, C., et al.,** Effects of platelet-activating factor (PAF) and ginkgolide BN 52021 on hypothalamic neutropeptides and pituitary hormones, in *Ginkgolides: Chemistry, Biology, Pharmacology and Clinical Perspectives, Vol. 2,* Braquet, P., Ed., J. R. Prous, Barcelona, 1990, 657.
182. **Squinto, S. P., Block, A. L., Braquet, P., et al.,** Platelet-activating factor stimulates a fox/jun/AP-1 transcriptional signaling system in human neuroblastoma cells, *J. Neurosci. Res.,* 24, 558, 1989.

183. **Ernst, A., Syka, J., Riedel, A., et al.,** The effect of PAF in the cochlea of guinea-pigs, *Prostaglandins,* 38, 523, 1989.

184. **Ernst, A., Syka, J., and Mest, H. J.,** Arachidonate metabolites change furosemide-induced cochlear potentials, *Hearing Res.,* 40, 39, 1989.

185. **Ernst, A., Syka, J., Riedel, A., et al.,** The effect of PAF and BN 52021 on inner ear potentials, in *Ginkgolides: Chemistry, Biology, Pharmacology and Clinical Perspectives, Vol. 2,* Braquet, P., Ed., J. R. Prous, Barcelona, 1990, 797.

186. **Ernst, A, Syka, J., Riedel, A., et al.,** Local effects of PAF in guinea-pig inner ear, *J. Lipid Med.,* 1, 297, 1989.

187. **Ernst, A., Syka, J., Riedel, A., et al.,** The effect of PAF in the cochlea of guinea-pigs, *Prostaglandins,* 38, 523, 1989.

188. **Woodward, D. F., Spada, C. S., Nieves, A. L., et al.,** Platelet-activating factor causes goblet cell depletion in the conjunctiva, *Eur. J. Pharmacol.,* 168, 23, 1989.

189. **Bazan, H. E., Braquet, P., Raddy, S. T., et al.,** Inhibition of the alkali burn-induced lipoxygenation of arachidonic acid in the rabbit cornea in vivo by a platelet-activating factor antagonist, *J. Ocular Pharmacol.,* 2, 237, 1987.

190. **Domingo, M. T., Chabrier, P. E., van Delft, J. L., et al.,** Effect of BN 52021 on PAF specific binding site in the eye. in *Ginkgolides: Chemistry, Biology, Pharmacology and Clinical Perspectives, Vol. 2,* Braquet, P., Ed., J. R. Prous, Barcelona, 1990, 739.

191. **Verbey, N. L., van Delft, J. L., van Haeringen, N. J., et al.,** Platelet-activating factor and laser trauma of the iris, *Invest. Ophthalmol. Vis. Sci.,* 30, 1101, 1989.

192. **Verbey, N. L., van Delft, J. L., Haeringen, N. J., et al.,** Interference of Ginkgolides with the rise in intraocular pressure after laser irradiation of the iris in the rabbit eye, in *Ginkgolides: Chemistry, Biology, Pharmacology and Clinical Perspectives, Vol. 2,* Braquet, P., Ed., J. R. Prous, Barcelona, 1990, 757.

193. **Thierry, A., Doly, M., Braquet, P., et al.,** Presence of specific platelet-activating factor binding sites in the rat retina, *Eur. J. Pharmacol.,* 163, 97, 1989.

194. **Bussolino, F., Torelli, S., Stefanini, E., et al.,** Platelet-activating factor production occurs through stimulation of cholinergic and dopaminergic receptors in the chick retina, *J. Lipid Med.,* 1, 283, 1989.

195. **Doly, M., Hosford, D., Gaillard, G., et al.,** Electrophysiological demonstration of transducin inhibition by lithium, in *Ginkgolides: Chemistry, Biology, Pharmacology and Clinical Perspectives, Vol. 2,* Braquet, P., Ed., J. R. Prous, Barcelona, 1990, 745.

196. **Uski, T. K. and Reinstrup, P.,** Actions of platelet-activating factor on isolated feline and human cerebral arteries, *J. Cereb. Blood Flow Metab.,* submitted.

197. **Armstead, W. M., Pourcyrous, M., Mirro, R., et al.,** Platelet-activating factor: a potent constrictor of cerebral arterioles in newborn pigs, *Circ. Res.,* 62, 1, 1088.

198. **Armstead, W. M., Mirro, R., Busija, D. W., et al.,** Permissive role of prostanoids in acetylcholine-induced cerebral vasoconstriction, *J. Pharmacol. Exp. Ther.,* 251, 1012, 1989.

199. **Herman, F., Magyar, K., Kovacs, K., et al.,** Decreased sensitivity of platelets to platelet-activating factor in migraine patients during the headache-free interval (letter), *Thromb. Haemost.,* 62, 818, 1989.

200. **Panetta, T., Marcheselli, V. L., Braquet, P., et al.,** Effects of a platelet-activating factor antagonist (BN 52021) on free fatty acids, diacylglycerols, polyphospho-inositides and blood flow in the gerbil brain: inhibition of ischemia-reperfusion induced cerebral injury, *Biochem. Biophys. Res. Commun.,* 149, 580, 1987.

201. **Spinnewyn, B., Blavet, N., Clostre, F., et al.,** Involvement of platelet-activating factor (PAF) in cerebral post-ischemic phase in mongolian gerbils, *Prostaglandins,* 34, 337, 1987.

202. **Kochanek, P. M., Dutka, A. J., Kumaroo, K. K., et al.,** Platelet-activating factor receptor blockade enhances early neuronal recovery after multifocal brain ischemia in dogs, *Life Sci.,* 41, 2639, 1987.

203. **Kochenek, P. M., Nemoto, E. M., and Schoettle, R.,** Cerebrovascular effects of platelet-activating factor receptor antagonism in the rat : effects on normal cerebral blood flow and posttraumatic edema, in *Ginkgolides: Chemistry, Biology, Pharmacology and Clinical Perspectives, Vol. 2,* Braquet, P., Ed., J. R. Prous, Barcelona, 1990, 619.

204. **Braquet, P., Spinnewyn, B., Demerle, C., et al.,** The role of platelet-activating factor in cerebral ischemia and related disorders, *Ann. N.Y. Acad. Sci.,* 559, 296, 1989.

205. **Panetta, T., Marcheselli, V. L., Braquet, P., et al.,** Arachidonic acid metabolism and cerebral blood flow in the normal, ischemic, and reperfused gerbil brain. Inhibition of ischemia-reperfusion-induced cerebral injury by a platelet-activating factor antagonist (BN 52021), *Ann. N.Y. Acad. Sci.,* 559, 340, 1989.

206. **Birkle, S. L., Kuran, P., Braquet, P., et al.,** Platelet-activating factor antagonist BN 52021 decreases accumulation of free polyunsaturated fatty acid in mouse brain during ischemia and electroconvulsive shock, *J. Neurochem.,* 31, 1900, 1988.

207. **Gilboe, D. D., Kintner, D., Fitzpatrick, J. H., et al.,** Recovery of postichemic brain metabolism and function following treatment of a free radical scavenger and platelet-activating factor antagonists, *J. Neurochem.,* 56, 113, 1991.

208. **Frerichs, K. U., Lindsberg, P. J., Hallengeck, J. M., et al.,** Platelet-activating factor and progressive brain damage following focal brain injury, *J. Neurosurg.,* 73, 223, 1990.

209. **Howat, D. W., Chand, N., Braquet, P., et al.,** An investigation into the possible involvement of platelet-activating factor in experimental allergic encephalomyelitis in rats, *Agents Actions,* 27, 473, 1989.

210. **Howat, D. W. and Willoughby, D. A.,** BN 52021 and immune encephalomyelitis in the rat, in *Ginkgolides: Chemistry, Biology, Pharmacology and Clinical Perspectives, Vol. 2,* Braquet, P., Ed., J. R. Prous, Barcelona, 1990, 649.

211. **Barnes, P. J.,** New concepts in the pathogenesis of bronchial hyperresponsiveness and asthma, *J. Allergy Clin. Immunol.,* 83, 1013, 1989.

212. **Larsen, G. L.,** New concepts in the pathogenesis of asthma, *Clin. Immunol. Immunopathol.,* 53, 107, 1989.

213. **Mencia-Huerta, J. M., Hosford, D., and Braquet, P.,** Acute and long-term pulmonary effects of platelet-activating factor, *Clin. Exp. Allergy,* 19, 125, 1990.

214. **Hosford, D., Mencia-Huerta, J. M., and Braquet, P.,** Platelet-activating factor (PAF) and PAF antagonists in asthma, in *Critical Reviews in Vasoactive Lipids,* Feuerstein, G., Ed., CRC Press, London, in press.

215. **Page, C. P.,** The role of platelet activating factor in asthma, *J. Allergy Clin. Immunol.,* 81, 144, 1988.

216. **Desquand, S., Lefort, J., Liu, F. T., et al.,** Antigen-induced bronchopulmonary alterations in the guinea-pig: a new model of passive sensitization mediated by mouse IgE antibodies, *Int. Arch. Allergy Appl. Immunol.,* 89, 71, 1989.

217. **Heuer, H. O.,** Effect of the hetrazepinoic PAF-antagonist WEB 2170 in several models of anaphylaxis in mice and guinea-pigs, *Lipids,* in press.

218. **Iwama, T., Shikada, K., and Tanaka, S.,** Pharmacological modulation of platelet-activating factor (PAF)-induced bronchoconstriction and hypertension in anaesthetized guinea-pigs, *J. Pharm. Pharmacol.,* 40, 544, 1988.

219. **Underwood, D. C. and Kadowitz, P. J.,** Analysis of bronchoconstrictor responses to platelet-activating factor in the cat, *J. Appl. Physiol.,* 67, 377, 1989.

220. **Stengel, P. M. and Silbaugh, S. A.,** Reversal of A23187-induced airway constriction in the guinea-pig, *J. Pharmacol. Exp. Ther.,* 248, 1084, 1989.

221. **Abraham, W. M., Stevenson, J. S., and Garrido, R.,** A possible role for PAF in allergen-induced late responses: modification by a selective antagonist, *J. Appl. Physiol.,* 66, 2351, 1989.

222. **Pons, F., Touvay, C., Lejeune, V., et al.,** Action of platelet-activating factor (PAF) antagonists on the bronchopulmonary effects of PAF in the guinea-pig, *J. Lipid Med.,* 1, 329, 1989.

223. **Soler, M., Sielczak, M. W., and Abraham, W. M.,** A PAF antagonist blocks antigen-induced airway hyperresponsiveness and inflammation in sheep, *J. Appl. Physiol.,* 67, 406, 1989.

224. **Chang, S. W., Ohara, N., Juo, G., et al.,** Tumor necrosis factor-induced lung injury is not mediated by platelet-activating factor, *Am. J. Physiol.,* 257, C232, 1989.

225. **Touvay, C., Vilain, B., Lejeune, V., et al.,** Effect of cyclosporin A and platelet-activating factor (PAF) antagonist, BN 52021, on PAF, and antigen-induced bronchoconstriction in the guinea-pig, *Biochem. Biophys. Res. Commun.,* 163, 118, 1989.

226. **Touvay, C., Vilain, B., Lejeune, V., et al.,** Effect of cyclosporin A and the platelet-activating factor (PAF) antagonist BN 52021 on PAF- and antigen-induced bronchoconstriction in the guinea-pig, in *Ginkgolides: Chemistry, Biology, Pharmacology and Clinical Perspectives, Vol. 2,* Braquet, P., Ed., J. R. Prous, Barcelona, 1990, 207.

227. **Dixon, E. J. A., Wilsoncroft, P., Robertson, D. N., et al.,** The effect of PAF antagonists on bronchial hyperresponsiveness induced by PAF, propranolol or indomethacin, *Br. J. Pharmacol.,* 97, 717, 1989.

228. **Desquand, S., Lefort, J., Dumarey, C., et al.,** Interference of BN 52021, an antagonist of PAF with different forms of active anaphylaxis in the guinea-pig; importance of the booster injection, *Br. J. Pharmacol.,* in press.

229. **Desquand, S. and Vargaftig, B. B.,** Interference of the PAF-antagonist BN 52021 with different forms of active anaphylaxis in the guinea-pig: modulation of its activity by the booster injection of antigen during sensitization, in *Ginkgolides: Chemistry, Biology, Pharmacology and Clinical Perspectives, Vol. 2,* Braquet, P., Ed., J. R. Prous, Barcelona, 1990, 227.

230. **Chand, N., Diamanti, W., and Sofia, R. D.,** Effect of PAF-acether on isoprenaline-induced relaxation in isolated tracheal segments of rats and guinea-pigs, *Eur. J. Pharmacol.,* 158, 135, 1988.

231. **Bethel, R. A., Curtis, S. P., Lien, D. C., et al.,** Effect of PAF on parasympathetic contraction of canine airways, *J. Appl. Physiol.,* 66, 2629, 1989.

232. **Inoue, T. and Kannan, R. S.,** Platelet-activating factor-induced functional changes in the guinea-pig trachea *in vitro, Respir. Physiol.,* 77, 157, 1989.

233. **Burka, J. F., Briand, H., Scott-Savage, P., et al.,** Leukotriene D4 and platelet-activating factor-acether antagonists on allergic and arachidonic acid-induced reactions in guinea-pig airways, *Can. J. Physiol. Pharmacol.,* 67, 483, 1989.

234. **Jancar, S., Theriault, P., Procenccal, B., et al.,** Mechanisms of action of platelet-activating factor on guinea-pig lung parenchyma strips, *Can. J. Physiol. Pharmacol.,* 66, 1187, 1988.

235. **Jancar, S., Theriault, P., Lauziere, M., et al.,** PAF-induced release of spasmogens from guinea-pig lungs, *Br. J. Pharmacol.,* 96, 153, 1989.

236. **Pretolani, M., Lefort, J., and Vargaftig, B. B.,** Limited interference of specific PAF antagonists with hyperresponsiveness to PAF itself of lungs from actively sensitized guinea-pigs, *Br. J. Pharmacol.,* 97, 433, 1989.

237. **Yaghi, A., Hamilton, J. T., and Paterson, N. A.,** Influence of platelet-activating factor on leukotriene D_4-induced contractions of the guinea-pig parenchymal strip, *Can. J. Physiol. Pharmacol.,* 67, 315, 1989.

238. **Brunelleshi, S., Ledda, F., Giotti, A., et al.,** Interference of WEB 2086 and BN 52021 with PAF-induced effects on guinea-pig trachea, *Br. J. Pharmacol.,* 97, 469, 1989.

239. **Goswami, S. K., Ohashi, M., Stathas, P., et al.,** Platelet-activating factor stimulates secretion of respiratory glycoconjugate from human airways in culture, *J. Allergy Clin. Immunol.,* 84, 726, 1989.

240. **Dent, G., Ukena, D., Sybrech, G. W., et al.,** (3H)WEB 2086 labels platelet-activating factor receptors in guinea-pig and human lung, *Eur. J. Pharmacol.,* 169, 313, 1989.

241. **Feogh, M. L.,** Eicosanoids and platelet-activating factor mechanisms in organ rejection, *Transplant. Proc.,* 20, 1260, 1988.

242. **Feogh, M. L., Chambers, E., Khirabadi, B. S., et al.,** Platelet-activating factor in organ transplant rejection, *Adv. Prostaglandin Thromboxane Leukotriene Res.,* 19, 377, 1989.

243. **Becker, K., Lueddeckens, G., and Förster, W.,** Influence of BN 52021 on the rejection of murine tail skin allografts and mortality in mice, in *Ginkgolides: Chemistry, Biology, Pharmacology and Clinical Perspectives, Vol. 2,* Braquet, P., Ed., J. R. Prous, Barcelona, 1990, 715.

244. **Kagawa, K., Kasahara, K., Sakurai, Y., et al.,** Prolongation of rat cardiac allograft survival with arachidonic acid metabolism inhibitor, *Transplant. Proc.,* 19, 1308, 1987.

245. **Becker, K., Lueddeckens, G., and Förster, W.,** Protective effect of BN 52021 compared with prostaglandin-related drugs versus skin graft rejection, significance of thromboxane, in *Ginkgolides: Chemistry, Biology, Pharmacology and Clinical Perspectives, Vol. 2,* Braquet, P., Ed., J. R. Prous, Barcelona, 1990, 725.

246. **Filipponi, F., Michel, A., van de Stadt, J., et al.,** Protection effect of BN 52063 on xenograft rejection, in *Ginkgolides: Chemistry, Biology, Pharmacology and Clinical Perspectives, Vol. 2,* Braquet, P., Ed., J. R. Prous, Barcelona, 1990, 707.

247. **Foegh, M. L., Conte, J. V., Jacobsson, J., et al.,** Organ preservation and BN 52021, in *Ginkgolides: Chemistry, Biology, Pharmacology and Clinical Perspectives, Vol. 2,* Braquet, P., Ed., J. R. Prous, Barcelona, 1990, 719.

248. **Mencia-Huerta, J. M., Pignol, B., Paubert-Braquet, M., et al.,** The role of platelet-activating factor (PAF) in immune and cytotoxic processes, *Prog. Clin. Biol. Res.,* 308, 441, 1989.

249. **Fernandez-Gallardo, S., Cano, E., Braquet, P., et al.,** Role of PAF-acether in the mediation of pathophysiological responses to aggregated immunoglobulins. Studies with the platelet-activating factor receptor antagonist BN 52021, *Int. J. Immunopharmacol.,* 10, 353, 1988.

250. **Tavares de Lima, W., Taixeira, C. F. P., Sirois, P., et al.,** Involvement of eicosanoids and PAF in immune-complex alveolitis, *Brazilian J. Med. Biol. Res.,* 22, 745, 1989.

251. **Pignol, B., Henane, S., Pirotzky, E., et al.,** Effect of platelet-activating factor antagonists on the immunosuppressive action of cyclosporine A, in *Ginkgolides: Chemistry, Biology, Pharmacology and Clinical Perspectives, Vol. 2,* Braquet, P., Ed., J. R. Prous, Barcelona, 1990, 773.

252. **Mandi, Y., Farkas, G., Koltai, M., et al.,** The effect of the platelet-activating factor antagonist, BN 52021, on human natural killer cell-mediated cytotoxicity, *Immunology,* 67, 370, 1989.

253. **Silva, P. M., Martins, M. A., Castro-Faria-Neto, H. C., et al.,** Adrenalectomy exacerbates paw edema without interfering with desensitization induced by PAF-acether in rats, *Brazilian J. Med. Biol. Res.,* 21, 855, 1988.

254. **Trebien, H. A. and Calixto, J. B.,** Pharmacological evaluation of rat paw oedema induced by Bothrops jaracaca venom, *Agents Actions,* 26, 292, 1989.

255. **Marshall, L. A., Chang, J. V., Calhoun, W., et al.,** Preliminary studies on phospholipase A_2-induced mouse paw edema as a model to evaluate antiinflammatory agents, *J. Cell. Biochem.,* 40, 147, 1989.

256. **Bekker, A. Y., Dillon, P. K., Paul, J., et al.,** Dose-response relationships between platelet-activating factor and permeability surface area product of FITC-dextran 150 in the hamster cheek pouch, *Microcirc. Endothelium-Lymphatics,* 4, 433, 1988.

257. **Sirois, M. G., Jancar, S., Braquet, P., et al.,** PAF increases vascular permeability in selected tissues: effect of BN 52021 and L-655,240, *Prostaglandins,* 36, 631, 1988.

258. **Sirois, M. G., Jancar, S., Braquet, P., et al.,** PAF increases protein extravasation in selected rat tissues, in *Ginkgolides: Chemistry, Biology, Pharmacology and Clinical Perspectives, Vol. 2,* Braquet, P., Ed., J. R. Prous, Barcelona, 1990, 255.

259. **Martins, M. A., Silva, P. M., Faria-Neto, H. C., et al.,** Pharmacological modulation of PAF-induced rat pleurisy and its role in inflammation by zymosan, *Br. J. Pharmacol.,* 96, 363, 1989.

260. **Martins, M. A., Machado Rodrigues e Silva, P., Castro-Faria-Neto, H. C., et al.,** Effect of BN 52021 on pleurisy induced by zymosan in rats, in *Ginkgolides: Chemistry, Biology, Pharmacology and Clinical Perspectives, Vol. 2,* Braquet, P., Ed., J. R. Prous, Barcelona, 1990, 187.

261. **Oh Ishi, S., Hayashi, I., Hayashi, M., et al.,** Pharmacological demonstration of inflammatory mediators using experimental inflammatory models: rat pleurisy induced by carrageenin and phorbol myristate acetate, *Dermatologica,* 179 *(Suppl.* 1), 68, 1989.

262. **Jancar, S., Braquet, P., and Sirois, P.,** Release of eicosanoids in rat peritoneal cavity during the Arthus reaction. Effect of the PAF-antagonist BN 52021 and indomethacin, *Int. J. Immunopharmacol.,* 11, 129, 1989.

263. **Jancar, S., Braquet, P., and Sirois, P.,** Release of eicosanoids in rat peritoneal cavity stimulated with platelet-activating factor (PAF). Effect of the PAF-antagonist BN 52021, *Prostaglandins Leukot. Essent. Fatty Acids,* 37, 23, 1989.

264. **Noguchi, K., Morita, I., and Murota, S.,** The detection of platelet-activating factor in inflammed human gingival tissue, *Arch. Oral Biol.,* 34, 37, 1989.

265. **Beck, J. C., Goodner, J., Wilson, C., et al.,** The platelet-activating factor inhibitor, BN 52021, attenuates insulitis in the BB rat, *Gastroenterology,* in press.

266. **Maestre, C., Zarco, P., Egido, J., et al.,** Possible role of platelet-activating factor in experimental and human arthritis. Studies with PAF receptor antagonists, in *Ginkgolides: Chemistry, Biology, Pharmacology and Clinical Perspectives, Vol. 2,* Braquet, P., Ed., J. R. Prous, Barcelona, 1990, 165.

267. **Howat, D. W., Desa, F. M., Chander, C. L., et al.,** Platelet-activating factor and the arthropathies: synergism with interleukin 1, in *Ginkgolides: Chemistry, Biology, Pharmacology and Clinical Perspectives, Vol. 2,* Braquet, P., Ed., J. R. Prous, Barcelona, 1990, 177.

268. **Montrucchio, G., Mariano, F., Cavalli, P. L., et al.,** Platelet-activating factor is produced during infectious peritonitis in CAPD patients, *Kidney Int.,* 36, 1029, 1989.

269. **Michel, L., Denizot, Y., Thomas, Y., et al.,** Release of PAF-acether and precursors during allergic cutaneous reactions, *Lancet,* 2, 404, 1988.

270. **Fisher, G. J., Talwar, H. S., Ryder, N. S., et al.,** Differential activation of human skin cells by platelet-activating factor: stimulation of phosphoinositide turnover and arachidonic acid mobilization in keratinocytes but not in fibroblasts, *Biochem. Biophys. Res. Commun.,* 163, 1344, 1989.

271. **Hellewell, P. G. and Williams, T. J.,** Antagonism of PAF-induced oedema formation in rabbit skin: a comparison of different antagonists, *Br. J. Pharmacol.,* 97, 171, 1989.

272. **Kemeny, L., Csato, M., and Dobozy, A.,** Pharmacological studies on dithranol-induced irritative dermatitis in mice, *Arch. Dermatol. Res.,* 281, 362, 1989.

273. **Kemény, L., Csato, M., and Dobozy, A.,** Effect of BN 52021 on dithranol-induced dermatitis, in *Ginkgolides: Chemistry, Biology, Pharmacology and Clinical Perspectives, Vol. 2,* Braquet, P., Ed., J. R. Prous, Barcelona, 1990, 775.

274. **Lavaud, P., Rodrigue, F., Carré, C., et al.,** Effect of the platelet-activating factor antagonist, BN 52063, on contact dermatitis in the mouse, in *Ginkgolides: Chemistry, Biology, Pharmacology and Clinical Perspectives, Vol. 2,* Braquet, P., Ed., J. R. Prous, Barcelona, 1990, 787.

275. **Pignol, P., Lonchampt, M. O., Chabrier, P. E., et al.,** Platelet-activating factor potentiates interleukin-1/epidermal cell-derived thymocyte-activating factor release by guinea-pig keratinocytes stimulated with lipopoly-saccharide, *J. Lipid Med.,* 2, S93, 1990.

276. **Csato, M., Pignol, B., Hunyadi, J., et al.,** Effect of BN 52021 on interleukin 1 production by UV-irradiated human keratinocytes, in *Ginkgolides: Chemistry, Biology, Pharmacology and Clinical Perspectives, Vol. 2,* Braquet, P., Ed., J. R. Prous, Barcelona, 1990, 767.

277. **Whittle, B. J.,** The defensive role played by the gastric microcirculation, *Meth. Find. Exp. Clin. Pharmacol.,* 11, (Suppl. 1), 25, 1989.

278. **Esplugues, J. V. and Whittle, B. J.,** Gastric effects of PAF, *Meth. Find. Exp. Clin. Pharmacol.,* 11 (Suppl. 1), 61, 1989.

279. **Binnaka, T., Yamaguchi, T., Hirohara, J., et al.,** Gastric mucosal damage induced in rats by intravenous administration of platelet-activating factor, *Scand. J. Gastroenterol. (Suppl.)* 162, 67, 1989.

280. **Yoshida, N., Yoshikawa, T., Ando, T., et al.,** Pathogenesis of platelet-activating factor-induced gastric mucosal damage in rats, *Scand. J. Gastroenterol. (Suppl.),* 162, 210, 1989.

281. **Fujimura, K., Sugatani, J., Miwa, M., et al.,** Serum platelet-activating factor acetylhydrolase activity in rats with gastric ulcers induced by water-immersion stress, *Scand. J. Gastroenterol. (Suppl.),* 162, 59, 1989.

282. **Hatakeyama, K., Yano, S., and Watanabe, K.,** Platelet-activating factor induced gastric damage in rats: participation of increased gastric vascular permeability, *Scand. J. Gastroenterol. (Suppl.),* 162, 71, 1989.

283. **Hanglow, A. C., Bienenstock, J., and Perdue, M. H.,** Effects of platelet-activating factor on ion transport in isolated rat jejunum, *Am. J. Physiol.,* 257, G845, 1989.

284. **Braquet, P., Etienne, A., Mencia-Huerta, J. M., et al.,** Effects of the specific platelet-activating factor antagonists, BN 52021 and BN 52063, on various experimental gastrointestinal ulcerations, *Eur. J. Pharmacol.*, 150, 269, 1988.

285. **Etienne, A., Thonier, F., and Braquet, P.,** Protective effect of the PAF-antagonist BN 52021 on several models of gastro-intestinal mucosal damage in rats, *Int. J. Tissue React.*, 11, 59, 1989.

286. **Esplugues, J. V., Whittle, B. J., and Moncada, S.,** Local opioid-sensitive afferent sensory neurones in the modulation of gastric damage induced by PAF, *Br. J. Pharmacol.*, 97, 579, 1989.

287. **Esplugues, J. V. and Whittle, B. J.,** Mechanisms contributing to gastric motility changes induced by PAF-acether and endotoxin in rats, *Am. J. Physiol.*, 256, G275, 1989.

288. **Konturek, S. J., Brzozowski, T., Drozdowicz, D., et al.,** Role of leukotrienes and platelet-activating factor in acute gastric mucosal lesions in rats, *Eur. J. Pharmacol.*, 164, 285, 1989.

289. **Dembinska-Kiec, A., Peskar, B. A., Müller, M. K., et al.,** The effects of platelet-activating factor on flow rate and eicosanoid release in the isolated perfused rat gastric vascular bed, *Prostaglandins*, 37, 69, 1989.

290. **Peskar, B. M.,** Cyteinyl leukotrienes in experimental ulcers in rats, in *New Trends in Lipid Mediators Research, Vol. 3-4*, Braquet, P., Ed., 451, 1988.

291. **Droy-Lefaix, M. T., Drouet, Y., Garaud, G., et al.,** The amplification role of PAF-acether in the oxidative stress following reperfusion of ischemic stomach, *Basic Life Sci.*, 49, 887, 1988.

292. **Filep, J., Herman, F., Schneider, F., et al.,** Involvement of platelet-activating factor in dexamethasone-induced gastric mucosal damage in the rat: studies with PAF receptor antagonist BN 52021, in *Ginkgolides: Chemistry, Biology, Pharmacology and Clinical Perspectives, Vol. 2*, Braquet, P., Ed., J. R. Prous, Barcelona, 1990, 503.

293. **Eliakim, R., Karmeli, F., Razin, E., et al.,** Role of platelet-activating factor in ulcerative colitis. Enhanced production during active disease and inhibition by sulfasalazine and prednisolone, *Gastroenterology*, 95, 1167, 1988.

294. **Ibbotson, G. C. and Wallace, J. L.,** Inhibitory effects of dexamethasone in endotoxic shock and its relation to PAF-acether synthesis in the gastrointestinal tract and lung, *J. Lipid Med.*, 1, 273, 1989.

295. **Cucala, M., Wallace, J. L., Salas, A., et al.,** Central regulation of gastric acid secretion by platelet-activating factor in anesthesized rats, *Prostaglandins*, 37, 275, 1989.

296. **Cucala, M., Wallace, J. L., Salas, A., et al.,** CNS effects of platelet-activating factor on the rat stomach, *Meth. Find. Exp. Clin. Pharmacol.*, 11, suppl. 1, 67, 1989.

297. **Filep, J., Herman, F., Braquet, et al.,** Increased levels of platelet-activating factor in blood following intestinal ischemia in the dog, *Biochem. Biophys. Res. Commun.*, 158, 353, 1989.

298. **Otamiri, T., Lindahl, M., and Tagesson, C.,** Phospholipase A₂ inhibition prevents mucosal damage associated with small intestinal ischaemia in rats, *Gut*, 29, 489, 1988.

299. **Iwai, A., Itoh, M., Yokoyama, Y., et al.,** Role of PAF in ischemia-reperfusion in injury in the rat stomach, *Scand. J. Gastroenterol. Suppl.*, 162, 63, 1989.

300. **Buckley, T. L. and Hoult, J. R.,** Platelet-activating factor is a potent colonic secretagogue with actions independent of specific PAF receptors, *Eur. J. Pharmacol.*, 163, 275, 1989.

301. **Sun, X. M. and Hsueh, W.,** Bowel necrosis induced by tumor necrosis factor in rats is mediated by platelet-activating factor, *J. Clin. Invest.*, 81, 1328, 1988.

302. **Hsueh, W. and Sun, X. M.,** Tumor necrosis factor-induced bowel necrosis: the role of platelet-activating factor, *Adv. Prostaglandin Thromboxane Leukotriene Res.*, 19, 363, 1989.

303. **Cueva, J. P. and Hsueh, W.,** Role of oxygen derived free radicals in platelet-activating factor induced bowel necrosis, *Gut*, 29, 1207, 1988.

304. **Rautureau, M., Bisalli, A., Heyman, M., et al.,** Effects of platelet-activating factor and BN 52021 on intestinal HRT-18 epithelial cells, in *Ginkgolides: Chemistry, Biology, Pharmacology and Clinical Perspectives, Vol. 2*, Braquet, P., Ed., J. R. Prous, Barcelona, 1990, 513.

305. **Wallace, J. L., Ibbotson, G. C., and Keenan, C. M.,** Mediatory role of platelet-activating factor in intestinal inflammation and ulceration, in *Ginkgolides: Chemistry, Biology, Pharmacology and Clinical Perspectives, Vol. 2*, Braquet, P., Ed., J. R. Prous, Barcelona, 1990, 481.

306. **Wallace, J. L.,** Release of platelet-activating factor (PAF) and accelerated healing induced by a PAF antagonist in an animal model of chronic colitis, *Can. J. Physiol. Pharmacol.*, 66, 422, 1988.

307. **Wallace, J. L., Braquet, P., Ibbotson, G. C., et al.,** Assessment of the role of platelet-activating factor in an animal model of inflammatory bowel disease, *J. Lipid Med.*, 1, 13, 1989.

308. **Wallace, J. L., MacNaughton, W. K., Morris, G. P., et al.,** Inhibition of leukotriene synthesis markedly accelerates healing in a rat model of inflammatory bowel disease, *Gastroenterology*, 76, 24, 1989.

309. **Emanuelli, G., Montrucchio, G., Gaia, E., et al.,** Experimental acute pancreatitis induced by platelet-activating factor in rabbits, *Am. J. Pathol.*, 134, 315, 1989.

310. **Dabrowski, A., Gabryelewicz, A., and Chyczewski, L.,** Oxygen radicals in cerulein-induced acute pancreatitis with reference to treatment with a platelet-activating factor antagonist, in *Ginkgolides: Chemistry, Biology, Pharmacology and Clinical Perspectives, Vol. 2*, Braquet, P., Ed., J. R. Prous, Barcelona, 1990, 493.

311. **Altin, J. G. and Bygrave, F. L.,** Non-parenchymal cells as mediators of physiological responses in liver, *Mol. Cell. Biochem.*, 83, 3, 1988.

312. **Chao, W., Liu, H., Hanahan, D. J., et al.,** Regulation of platelet-activating factor receptors in rat Kupffer cells, *J. Biol. Chem.*, 264, 20448, 1989.

313. **Chao, W., Siafaka-Karadai, A., Olson, M. S., et al.,** Biosynthesis of platelet-activating factor by cultured rat Kupffer cells stimulated with calcium ionophore A23187, *Biochem. J.*, 257, 823, 1989.

314. **Levine, L.,** Platelet-activating factor stimulates arachidonic acid metabolism in rat liver cells (C-9 cell line) by a receptor-mediated mechanism, *Mol. Pharmacol.*, 34, 793, 1988.

315. **Lapointe, D. S. and Olson, M. S.,** Platelet-activating factor-stimulated hepatic glycogenolysis is not mediated through cyclooxygenase-derived metabolites of arachidonic acid, *J. Biol. Chem.*, 264, 12130, 1989.

316. **Fisher, R. A., Sharma, R. V., and Bhalla, R. C.,** Platelet-activating factor increases inositol phosphate and cytosolic free CA^{2+} concentrations in cultured rat Kupffer cells, *FEBS Lett.*, 251, 22, 1989.

317. **Levine, L.,** Inhibition by antagonists of PAF-stimulated PGI_2 production in rat liver cells, in *Ginkgolides: Chemistry, Biology, Pharmacology and Clinical Perspectives, Vol. 2*, Braquet, P., Ed., J. R. Prous, Barcelona, 1990, 321.

318. **Sekiyama, T., Gaudin, C., Roulot, D., et al.,** Evidence for platelet-activating factor as a mediator for hyperdynamic circulation in conscious cirrhotic rats, in *Ginkgolides: Chemistry, Biology, Pharmacology and Clinical Perspectives, Vol. 2*, Braquet, P., Ed., J. R. Prous, Barcelona, 1990, 321.

319. **Guarner, F., Wallace, J. L., MacNaughton, W. K., et al.,** Endotoxin-induced ascites formation in the rat: partial mediation by platelet-activating factor, *Hepatology*, 10, 788, 1989.

320. **Schirmer, W. J., Schirmer, J. M., Galat, J. A., et al.,** Systemic and renal hemodynamic response to platelet-activating factor, *Prog. Clin. Biol. Res.*, 299, 227, 1989.

321. **Santos, O. F., Bregman, R., Boim, M. A., et al.,** Platelet-activating factor in nephrology: physiopathologic and therapeutic perspectives, *Rev. Paul Med.*, 106, 231, 1988.

322. **de Arriba, G., Bario, V., Hernando, L., et al.,** Changes in glomerular cross-sectional area induced by platelet-activating factor, *Nephrol. Dial. Transplant.*, 2, 224, 1987.

323. **Neuwirth, R., Satriano, J. A., DeCandido, S., et al.,** Angiotensin II causes formation of platelet-activating factor in cultured rat mesangial cells, *Circ. Res.*, 64, 1124, 1989.

324. **Hebert, R. L., Sirois, P., and Plante, G. E.,** Inhibition of platelet-activating factor induced renal hemodynamic and tubular dysfunctions with L-655-240, a new thromboxane-prostaglandin endoperoxide antagonist, *Can. J. Physiol. Pharmacol.*, 67, 304, 1989.

325. **Fonteles, M. C. and Ferreira, M. G.,** Effects of BN 52021 (PAF antagonist) on renal vascular escape and tachphylaxis in the perfused rabbit kidney, in *Ginkgolides: Chemistry, Biology, Pharmacology and Clinical Perspectives, Vol. 2*, Braquet, P., Ed., J. R. Prous, Barcelona, 1990, 605.

326. **Pirotzky, E., Colliez, P., Guilmard, C., et al.,** Renal diseases and platelet-activating factor, *Pediatrie*, 44, 163, 1989.

327. **Lopez-Farré, A., y Cajal, S. R., Braquet, P., et al.,** Ginkgolide BN 52021 protects against glycerol-induced acute renal failure, in *Ginkgolides: Chemistry, Biology, Pharmacology and Clinical Perspectives, Vol. 2*, Braquet, P., Ed., J. R. Prous, Barcelona, 1990, 591.

328. **Plante, G. E., Sirois, P., and Braquet, P.,** Platelet-activating factor antagonism with BN 52021 protects the kidney against acute ischemic injury, *Prostaglandins Leukot. Essent. Fatty Acids*, 34, 53, 1989.

329. **Tolins, J. P., Vercellotti, G. M., Wilkowske, M., et al.,** Role of platelet-activating factor in endotoxemic acute renal failure in the male rat, *J. Lab. Clin. Med.*, 113, 316, 1989.

330. **Lee, T. C., Malone, B., Woodard, D., et al.,** Renal necrosis and the involvement of a single enzyme of the de novo pathway for the biosynthesis of platelet-activating factor in the rat kidney inner medulla, *Biochem. Biophys. Res. Commun.*, 163, 1002, 1989.

331. **Yeo, Y. K., Philbrick, D. J., and Holub, B. J.,** Effects of dietary n-3 fatty acids on mass changes and (^{3}H)glycerol incorporation in various glycerolipid classes of rat kidney in vivo, *Biochim. Biophys. Acta*, 1006, 9, 1989.

332. **Rossoni, G., Berti, F., Buschi, A., et al.,** The ginkgolide BN 52021 antagonizes the immune release of histamine and other lipid mediators from guinea-pig isolated kidney, in *Ginkgolides: Chemistry, Biology, Pharmacology and Clinical Perspectives, Vol. 2*, Braquet, P., Ed., J. R. Prous, Barcelona, 1990, 521.

333. **Gomez-Chiarri, M., Egido, J., Gomez, C., et al.,** Production of PAF and cytokines by glomerular cells of rats with nephrotic syndrome. Effect of the PAF receptor antagonist BN 52021, in *Ginkgolides: Chemistry, Biology, Pharmacology and Clinical Perspectives, Vol. 2*, Braquet, P., Ed., J. R. Prous, Barcelona, 1990, 581.

334. **Lamas, S., Olivera, A., Lopez-Novoa, J. M., et al.,** Effect of BN 52021 on cyclosporine-induced glomerular function impairment, in *Ginkgolides: Chemistry, Biology, Pharmacology and Clinical Perspectives, Vol. 2*, Braquet, P., Ed., J. R. Prous, Barcelona, 1990, 549.

335. **Rodriguez-Puyol, D., Lamas, S., Olivera, A., et al.,** Actions of cyclosporin A on cultured rat mesangial cells, *Kidney Int.*, in press.

336. **Pavao dos Santos, O. F. P., Boim, M. A., Bregman, R., et al.,** Effect of platelet-activating factor antagonist on cyclosporine nephrotoxicity. Glomerular hemodynamics evaluation, *Transplantation*, 47, 592, 1989.

337. **Pavao dos Santos, O. F. P., Boim, M. A., Barros, E. J. G., et al.,** Effect of platelet-activating factor antagonist on cyclosporine nephrotoxicity: glomerular hemodynamics evaluation, in *Ginkgolides: Chemistry, Biology, Pharmacology and Clinical Perspectives, Vol. 2,* Braquet, P., Ed., J. R. Prous, Barcelona, 1990, 559.

338. **Egido, J., Mendiluce, A., Mampaso, F., et al.,** Protection against cyclosporin-induced nephropathy by PAF antagonists in rats, in *Ginkgolides: Chemistry, Biology, Pharmacology and Clinical Perspectives, Vol. 2,* Braquet, P., Ed., J. R. Prous, Barcelona, 1990, 569.

339. **Pavao dos Santos, O. F. P., Boim, M. A., Barros, E. J. G., et al.,** The CIS-diamminedi-chloroplatinum induced glomerular hemodynamic alterations are blunted by BN 52063, in *Ginkgolides: Chemistry, Biology, Pharmacology and Clinical Perspectives, Vol. 2,* Braquet, P., Ed., J. R. Prous, Barcelona, 1990, 541.

340. **Pirotzky, E., Guilmar, C., Sidoti, C., et al.,** Reduction of experimental CIS-diammine-dichloroplatinum-induced nephrotoxicity in the rat by the platelet-activation factor antagonist, BN 52021, in *Ginkgolides: Chemistry, Biology, Pharmacology and Clinical Perspectives, Vol. 2,* Braquet, P., Ed., J. R. Prous, Barcelona, 1990, 531.

341. **Page, C. and Abbott, A.,** PAF: new antagonists, new roles in disease and a major role in reproductive biology, *Trends Pharmacol. Sci.,* 10, 255, 1989.

342. **Abigosum, A. O., Braquet, P., and Tsafririr, A.,** The involvement of platelet activating factor in ovulation, *Science,* 243, 381, 1989.

343. **Daphna-Iken, D., Chun, S. Y., Abisogun, A. O., et al.,** Platelet-activating factor, ginkgolides and follicle rupture during ovulation, in *Ginkgolides: Chemistry, Biology, Pharmacology and Clinical Perspectives, Vol. 2,* Braquet, P., Ed., J. R. Prous., Barcelona, 1990, 835.

344. **Espey, L. L., Tanaka, N., Woodward, D. S., et al.,** Decrease in ovarian platelet-activating factor during ovulation in the gonadotropin-primed immature rat, *Biol. Reprod.,* 41, 104, 1989.

345. **Harper, M. J.,** Platelet-activating factor: a paracrine factor in preimplantation stages of reproduction?, *Biol. Reprod.,* 40, 907, 1989.

346. **Sueoka, K., Dharmarajan, A. M., Miyazaki, T., et al.,** Platelet activating factor-induced early pregnancy factor activity from the perfused rabbit ovary and oviduct, *Am. J. Obstet. Gynecol.,* 159, 1580, 1988.

347. **Minhas, B. S., Kumar, R., Ricker, D. D., et al.,** Effects of platelet activating factor on mouse oocyte fertilization *in vitro, Am. J. Obstet. Gynecol.,* 161, 1714, 1989.

348. **Collier, M., O'Neill, C., Ammit, A. J., et al.,** Biochemical and pharmacological characterization of human embryo-derived platelet activating factor, *Hum. Reprod.,* 3, 993, 1988.

349. **O'Neill, C., Collier, M., Ryan, J. P., et al.,** Embryo-derived platelet-activating factor, *J. Reprod. Fertil. Suppl.,* 37, 19, 1989.

350. **O'Neill, C., Ryan, J. P., Collier, M., et al.,** Supplementation of in vitro fertilization culture medium with platelet activating factor, *Lancet,* 2, 769, 1989.

351. **Spinks, N. R., O'Neil, C., Ryan, J. P., et al.,** Antagonists of platelet-activating factor (PAF) and their effects on early pregnancy, in *Ginkgolides: Chemistry, Biology, Pharmacology and Clinical Perspectives, Vol. 2,* Braquet, P., Ed., J. R. Prous, Barcelona, 1990, 805.

352. **Kodama, H., Muto, H., and Maki, M.,** Isolation and identification of embryo-derived platelet-activating factor in mice, *Nippon Sanka Fujinka Gakkai Zasshi,* 41, 899, 1989.

353. **Ryan, J. P., Spinks, N. R., O'Neill, C., et al.,** Platelet-activating factor (PAF) production by mouse embryos *in vitro* and its effect on embryonic metabolism, *J. Cell. Biochem.,* 40, 387, 1989.

354. **Geissler, F. T., Kuzan, F. B., Faustman, E. M., et al.,** Lipid mediator production by post-implantation rat embryos *in vitro, Prostaglandins,* 38, 145, 1989.

355. **Hansel, W., Stock, A., and Battista, P. J.,** Low molecular weight lipid-soluble luteotrophic factor(s) produced by conceptuses in cows, *J. Reprod. Fertil. Suppl.,* 37, 11, 1989.

356. **Hansel, W. and Hickey, G. L.,** Early pregnancy signals in domestic animals, *Ann. N.Y. Acad. Sci.,* 541, 472, 1988.

357. **Acker, G., Braquet, P., and Mencia-Huerta, J. M.,** Role of platelet-activating factor (PAF) in the initiation of the decidual reaction in the rat, *J. Reprod. Fertil.,* 85, 623, 1989.

358. **Acker, G., Braquet, P., and Mencia-Huerta, J. M.,** Role of platelet-activating factor (PAF) in ovoimplantation and decidual reaction in the rat: effect of the ginkgolide B (BN 52021), in *Ginkgolides: Chemistry, Biology, Pharmacology and Clinical Perspectives,* Braquet, P., Ed., J. R. Prous, Barcelona, 1990, 821.

359. **Kudolo, G. B. and Harper, M. J. K.,** Characterization of platelet-activating factor binding sites on the uterine membranes from pregnant rabbits, *Biol. Reprod.,* 41, 587, 1989.

360. **Kudolo, G. B. and Harper, M. J. K.,** Molecular heterogeneity of platelet-activating factor (PAF) receptors in rabbit endometrial membranes: autoradiographic and biochemical evidence, *Biol. Reprod.,* submitted.

361. **Ricker, D. D., Minhas, B. S., Kumar, R., et al.,** The effects of platelet-activating factor on the motility of human spermatozoa, *Fertil. Steril.,* 52, 655, 1989.

362. **Harper, M. J. K., Woodard, D. S., and Norris, C. J.,** Spermicidal effect of antagonists of platelet-activating factor, *Fertil. Steril.,* 51, 890, 1989.

363. **Adamus, W. S., Heuer, H., and Meade, C. J.,** PAF-induced platelet aggregation ex vivo as a method for monitoring pharmacological activity in healthy volunteers, *Meth. Find. Exp. Clin. Pharmacol.,* 11, 415, 1989.

364. **Adamus, W. S., Heuer, H., Meade, C. J., et al.,** Safety, tolerability and pharmacologic activity of multiple doses of the new platelet-activating factor antagonist WEB 2086 in human subjects, *Clin. Pharmacol. Ther.,* 45, 270, 1989.

365. **Bonvoisin, B. and Guinot, Ph.,** Clinical studies of BN 52063 a specific PAF antagonist, in *Ginkgolides: Chemistry, Biology, Pharmacology and Clinical Perspectives, Vol. 2,* Braquet, P., Ed., J. R. Prous, Barcelona, 1990, 845.

366. **Guinot, Ph., Hosford, D., Brambilla, C., et al.,** Effects of the specific PAF antagonist, BN 52063, in asthma: a multicenter study, *J. Lipid Med.,* in press.

367. **Roberts, N. M. and Barnes, P. J.,** Evaluation of BN 52063 in man, in *Ginkgolides: Chemistry, Biology, Pharmacology and Clinical Perspectives, Vol. 2,* Braquet, P., Ed., J. R. Prous, Barcelona, 1990, 855.

368. **Charpentier, B., Guinot, Ph., Hosford, D., et al.,** Tolerance and immunological effects of repeated administration of BN 52063 in healthy volunteers, in *Ginkgolides: Chemistry, Biology, Pharmacology and Clinical Perspectives, Vol. 2,* Braquet, P., Ed., J. R. Prous, Barcelona, 1990, 905.

369. **Duchier, J., Cournot, A., Hosford, D., et al.,** Clinical studies on the tolerance and effects of BN 52021 on PAF-induced platelet aggregation and skin reactivity in healthy volunteers, in *Ginkgolides: Chemistry, Biology, Pharmacology and Clinical Perspectives, Vol. 2,* Braquet, P., Ed., J. R. Prous, Barcelona, 1990, 897.

370. **Chiu, C. P. and Hsieh, K. H.,** Pulmonary response to platelet-activating factor (PAF) and PAF antagonist in allergic asthmatic children, in *Ginkgolides: Chemistry, Biology, Pharmacology and Clinical Perspectives, Vol. 2,* Braquet, P., Ed., J. R. Prous, Barcelona, 1990, 871.

371. **Hopp, R. J., Bewtra, A. K., Agrawal, D. K., et al.,** Effect of platelet-activating factor inhalation on nonspecific bronchial reactivity in man, *Chest,* 96, 1070, 1989.

372. **Skvortsev, A. A., Gabbasov, Z. A., Popov, E. G., et al.,** New approaches to the study of thrombocyte aggregation in patients with dilated cardiomyopathy, *Ter. Arkh.,* 61, 95, 1989.

373. **Burke, L. A. and Lee, T. H.,** Effect of BN 52063 on clinical and histological effects of PAF in atopic skin, in *Ginkgolides: Chemistry, Biology, Pharmacology and Clinical Perspectives, Vol. 2,* Braquet, P., Ed., J. R. Prous, Barcelona, 1990, 879.

374. **Bevan, J., Heptinstall, S., Vathenen, A. S., et al.,** Diurnal variation in platelet aggregation and the effect of a PAF antagonist, *Clin. Pharmacol. Ther.,* in press.

375. **Guinot, P., Caffrey, E., Lambe, R., et al.,** Tanakan inhibits platelet-activating factor-induced platelet aggregation in healthy male volunteers, *Haemostasis,* 19, 219, 1989.

376. **Lemaire, C., Peraudeau, P., and Guinot, P.,** Interaction of BN 52063 and flunitrazepam by the technique of quantified electroencephalography, in *Ginkgolides: Chemistry, Biology, Pharmacology and Clinical Perspectives, Vol. 2,* Braquet, P., Ed., J. R. Prous, Barcelona, 1990, 887.

377. **Beutler, B., Milsark, I. W., and Cerami, A. C.,** Passive immunisation against cachectin/tumor necrosis factor protects mice from lethal effects of endotoxin, *Science,* 229, 869, 1985.

378. **Tracey, K. J., Beutler, B., Lowry, S. F., et al.,** Shock and tissue injury induced by recombinant human cachectin, *Science* 234, 470, 1986.

379. **Braquet, P., Hosford, D., Paubert-Braquet, M., et al.,** Role of cytokines and platelet-activating factor in microvascular immune injury, *Int. Arch. Allergy Appl. Immunol.,* 88, 88, 1989.

380. **Braquet, P., Paubert-Braquet, M., Bourgain, R., et al.,** PAF/cytokine autogenerated feedback networks in microvascular immune injury: consequences in shock, ischemia and graft rejection, *J. Lipid Med.,* 1, 75, 1989.

381. **Malech, H. L. and Gallin, J. I.,** Neutrophils in human diseases, *N. Engl. J. Med.,* 11, 687, 1987.

382. **Wardlaw, A. J. and Kay, A. B.,** PAF-aether is a potent chemotactic factor for human eosinophils, *J. Allergy Clin. Immunol.,* 77, 236, 1986.

383. **Bonavida, B., Mencia-Huerta, J. M., and Braquet, P.,** Effect of platelet-activating factor (PAF) on monocyte activation and production of tumour necrosis factor (TNF), *Int. Arch. Allergy Appl. Immunol.,* 88, 157, 1989.

384. **Pignol, B., Henane, S., Mencia-Huerta, J. M., et al.,** Effect of PAF-acether (platelet-activating factor) and its specific antagonist, BN 52021, on interleukin 1 (IL 1) synthesis and release by rat monocytes, *Prostaglandins,* 33, 931, 1987.

385. **Barrett, M. L., Lewis, G. P., Ward, S., et al.,** activating factor induces interleukin-1 production from human adherent macrophages, *Br. J. Pharmacol.,* 90, 113, 1987.

386. **Ward, S. G., Lewis, G. P., Westwick, J., et al.,** Platelet-activating factor stimulates interleukin 1 production from human adherent monocyte-macrophages, in *New Trends in Lipid Mediator Research,* Vol. 1, Braquet, P., Ed., S. Karger, Basel, 1988, 6.

387. **Salem, P., Dulioust, A., Derickz, S., et al.,** PAF-acether (Platelet-activating factor) increases interleukin 1 (IL 1) secretion by human monocytes, *Fed. Proc.,* 46, 922, 1987.

388. **Barthelson, R., Valone, F. H., Debs, R., et al.,** Synergy in interleukin 1 (IL 1) release by human monocytes stimulated with platelet-activating factor (PAF) plus gamma interferon (IFN gamma) or tumor necrosis factor (TNF), *FASEB J.,* 2, 1228, 1988.

389. **Valone, F. H. and Epstein, L. B.,** Biphasic platelet-activating factor (PAF) synthesis by human monocytes stimulated with interleukin 1β (IL 1β) and tumor necrosis factor (TNF), *FASEB J.,* 2, 878, 1988.

390. **Pignol, B., Henane, S., Sorlin, B., et al.,** Effect of long-term in vivo treatment with platelet-activating factor on interleukin 1 and interleukin 2 production by rat splenocytes, in *New Trends in Lipid Mediator Research,* Vol. 1, Braquet, P., Ed., S. Karger, Basel, 1988, 38.

391. **Braquet, P. and Rola-Pleszczynski, M.,** Platelet-activating factor and cellular immune responses, *Immunology Today,* 8, 345, 1987.

392. **Hosford, D., Mencia-Huerta, J. M., and Braquet, P.,** The role of platelet-activating factor and structurally related alkyl phospholipids in immune and cytotoxic processes, in *Eicosanoids, Lipid Peroxidation and Cancer,* Nigham, S. and Slater, T. F., Eds., Springer-Verlag, Heidelberg, 1988, 53.

393. **Rola-Pleszczynski, M., Pignol, B., Pouliot, C., et al.,** Inhibition of human lymphocyte proliferation and interleukin 2 production by platelet-activating factor (PAF-acether): reversal by a specific antagonist, BN 52021, *Biochem. Biophys. Res. Commun.,* 142, 754, 1987.

394. **Berkow, R. L., Wang, D., Larrich, J. W., et al.,** Enhancement of neutrophil superoxide production by preincubation with recombinant human tumor necrosis factor, *J. Immunol.,* 139, 378, 1987.

395. **Strosberg, A. M., Johnson, L. G., Wood, L., et al.,** Cardiovascular effects of interleukin-1β in anesthetized rhesus monkeys, *FASEB J.,* 3, 317, 1989.

396. **Weinberg, J. R., Wright, D. J. M., and Guz, A.,** Interleukin-1β and tumor necrosis factor cause hypotension in the conscious rabbit, *Clin. Sci.,* 75, 251, 1988.

397. **Whatley, R. E., Zimmerman, G. A., McIntyre, T. M., et al.,** Endothelium from diverse vascular sources synthesizes platelet-activating factor, *Arteriosclerosis,* 8, 321, 1988.

398. **Bussolino, F., Camussi, G., Baglioni, C., et al.,** Synthesis and release of platelet-activating factor by human vascular endothelial cells treated with tumor necrosis factor or interleukin 1α, *J. Biol. Chem.,* 263, 11856, 1988.

399. **DiPersio, J. F., Billing, P., Williams, R., et al.,** Human granulocyte-macrophage colony-stimulating factor and other cytokines primes human neutrophils for enhanced arachidonic acid release and leukotriene B_4 synthesis, *J. Immunol.,* 140, 4315, 1988.

400. **Dahinden, C. A., Zirgg, I., Malif, F. E., et al.,** Leukotriene production in human neutrophils primed by recombinant human granulocyte/macrophage colony-stimulating factor and stimulated with the complement component C5A and FMLP as second signals, *J. Exp. Med.,* 167, 1281, 1988.

401. **McColl, S. H., Krump, E., Naccache, P. H., et al.,** Granulocyte-macrophage colony-stimulating factor enhances the synthesis of leukotriene B_4 by human neutrophils in response to PAF-acether, *J. Lipid Med.,* 2, S119, 1990.

402. **Silberstein, D. J., Owen, W. F., Gasson, J. C., et al.,** Enhancement of human eosinophil cytotoxicity and leukotriene synthesis by biosynthetic (recombinant) granulocyte-macrophage colony stimulating factor, *J. Immunol.,* 137, 3290, 1986.

403. **Cannistra, S. A., Vellenga, E., Groshek, P., et al.,** Human granulocyte-monocyte colony-stimulating factor and interleukin 3 stimulate monocyte cytotoxicity through a tumor necrosis factor-dependent mechanism, *Blood,* 71, 672, 1988.

404. **Thom, R.,** *Structural Stability and Morphogenesis* (transl. D. H. Fowler), Benjamin-Addison Wesley, New York, 1975.

405. **Zeeman, E. C.,** A catastrophe machine, in *Towards a Theoretical Biology,* Vol. 4, Waddington, C. H., Ed., Edinburgh University Press, Edinburgh, 1972, 276.

406. **Heuer, H., and Letts, G.,** Priming of effects of PAF in vivo by tumor necrosis factor and endotoxin, *J. Lipid Med.,* in press.

407. **Sirois, M. G., Plante, G. E., Oppenheim, J. J., et al.,** Tumor necrosis factor primes the effects of platelet activating factor on rat vascular permeability, *J. Lipid Med.,* 2, S109, 1990.

408. **Howat, D., Desa, F., Chander, C., et al.,** The synergism between PAF and interleukin-1 on cartilage breakdown, *J. Lipid Med.,* 2, S143, 1989.

409. **Shimokawa, H., Aarhus, L. L., and Vanhoutte, P. M.,** Porcine coronary arteries with regenerated endothelium have a reduced endothelium-dependent responsiveness to aggregating platelets and serotonin, *Circ. Res.,* 61, 256, 1987.

410. **Deby-Dupont, G., Etienne, A., Braquet, P., et al.,** Effect of ginkgolide (BN 52021) on the enzymatic activity of bovine and human trypsins, *Arch. Int. Physiol. Biochim.,* 94, 7P, 1986.
411. **Etienne, A., Hecquet, F., Guilmard, C., et al.,** Inhibition of rat endotoxin-induced lethality by BN 52021 and BN 52063, compounds with PAF-acether antagonistic effect and protease-inhibitory activity, *Int. J. Tissue Reac.,* 9, 19, 1987.
412. **Hosford, D. and Braquet, P.,** Antagonists of platelet-activating factor: chemistry, pharmacology and clinical applications, in *Prog. Med. Chem., Vol.* 27, Ellis, G. P. and West, G. B. Eds., 325, 80, 1990.

Chapter 2

PAF ANTAGONISTS FROM MICROBIAL ORIGIN: STRUCTURE-ACTIVITY RELATIONSHIP OF DIKETOPIPERAZINE DERIVATIVES

Keiji Hemmi, Norihiko Shimazaki, Ichiro Shima, Masanori Okamoto, Keizo Yoshida, and Masashi Hashimoto

INTRODUCTION

Platelet-activating factor (PAF), an endogenous phospholipid generated and secreted by a number of different cell types, i.e., neutrophil, mast cell, platelet, and basophil, was first discovered and characterized as a potent platelet-aggregating agent. Since synthetic PAF became available, a wide range of activities in various biological systems have been evaluated. PAF has been reported to be a mediator of anaphylaxis, inflammation, endotoxin shock, hypotension, and other conditions. It was also suggested that the binding of PAF to its specific receptor sites is a first step in its biological function. These demonstrations have generated considerable impact in the search for PAF inhibitors or antagonists which are likely to have therapeutic effects in these diseases.[1]

Several PAF antagonists have been reported recently, and can be classified into three categories. The first group is PAF-related phospholipids having a heteroaromatic quaternary ammonium function such as CV 3988,[2] and SRI 63-441.[3] The second group is synthetic compounds such as 52770 RP,[4] L-652,731,[5] and WEB 2086.[6] The third group is natural products. The Institut Henri Beaufour has concentrated on development of a terpenoid, BN 52021, isolated from a Chinese tree, *Gingko biloba*.[7] Merck has been developing a lignan, kadsurenone, isolated also from a Chinese plant, *Pipa kutokadsurae*.[8]

We are also interested in the pathophysiological function of PAF and have started to search for PAF antagonists from microbial origin. Here we will discuss the structure-activity relationship of the novel natural products and related compounds which contain diketopiperazine as a common structural unit.

FR49175 AND ITS DERIVATIVES

In our screening programs for potent PAF antagonists, a wide range of fermented broths have been tested for inhibitory effects against PAF-induced rabbit platelet aggregation.

The activity was found in the culture filtrate of *Penicillium terlikowskii* No. 5348, and *Penicillium citrinum* No. 2973, and active compounds were identified as bisdethiodi(methylthio)gliotoxin (**1**), designated FR49175, and 3,6-bismethylthio-3-hydroxymethyl-6-phenylmethylpiperazine-2,5-dione (**2**), designated FR106969, respectively (Figure 1).[9-11] Although compound (**1**) had been previously isolated from cultures of the wood fungus *Gliocladium delquescens* as an antifungal and antiviral agent, its PAF-inhibitory activity was not reported. These two compounds were both moderately active with an IC_{50} of 4.4 $\times$ 10^{-6} M and 1.7 $\times$ 10^{-5} M, respectively. Compound (**1**) slightly inhibited collagen-induced aggregation with an IC_{50} of 8.4 $\times$ 10^{-5} M, but had no effect on the aggregation induced by arachidonic acid and adenosine diphosphate at a concentration of 400 μM.

In order to clarify the structure-activity relationship, we tried the chemical modification of FR49175 (**1**) and examined the inhibitory effect on PAF (0.1 μM) induced rabbit platelet aggregation (Figure 2).

Acetylation of (**1**) with acetic anhydride gave the diacetyl derivative (**3**). Treatment of

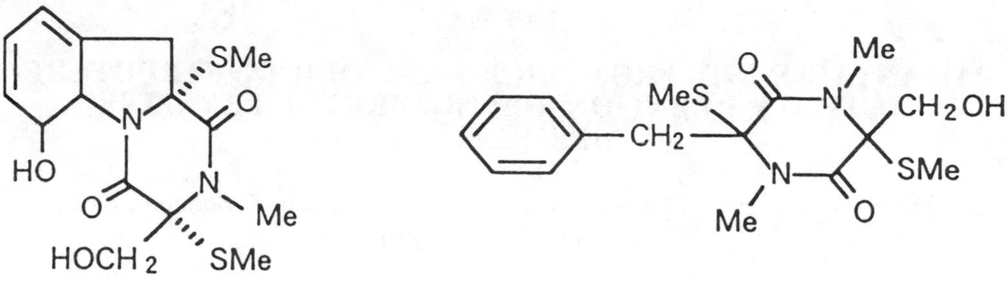

1 (FR49175) **2 (FR106969)**

FIGURE 1. Structure of FR49175 and FR106969.

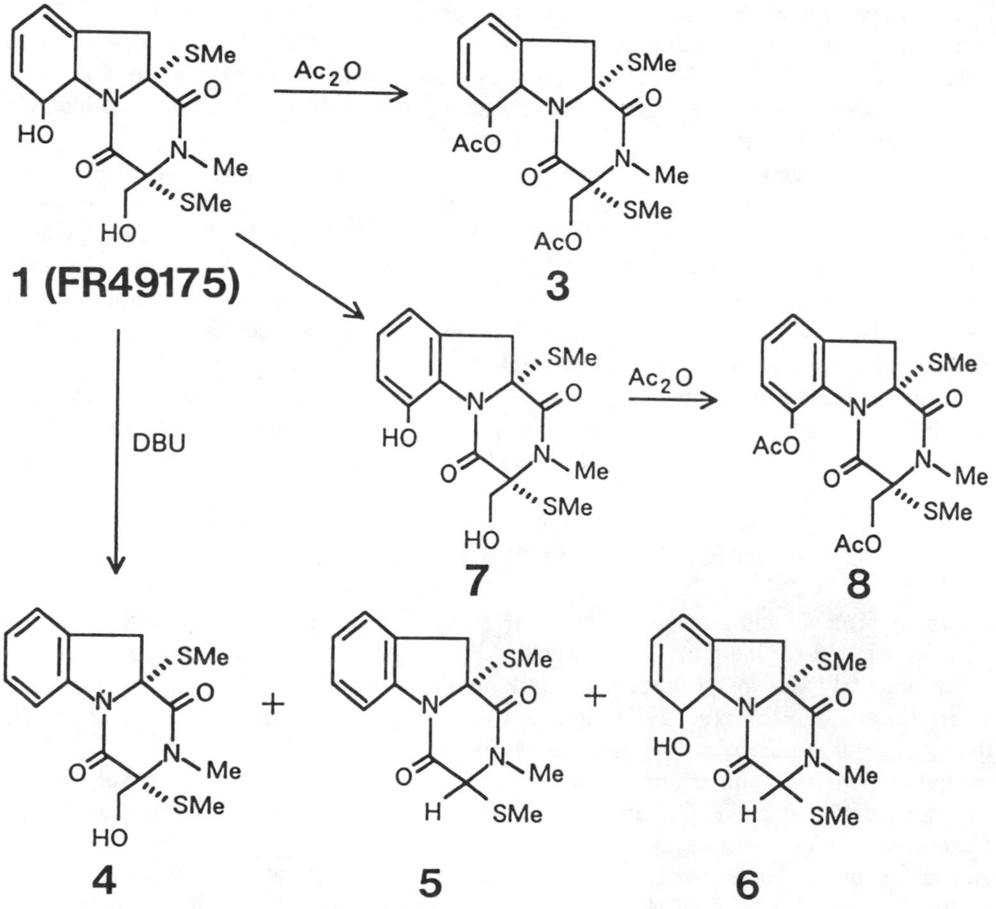

FIGURE 2. Chemical modification of FR49175.

(1) with base (DBU) gave a mixture of compounds **(4)**, **(5)**, and **(6)**. Compound **(7)** was prepared from **(1)** by Kirby's method.[12] Successive acetylation of **(7)** gave compound **(8)**.

The IC_{50} values of these derivatives are shown in Table 1. Acetylation of the hydroxy group of **(1)** and **(7)** reduced the inhibitory activity. The dihydrobenzene ring system seems

TABLE 1
Inhibitory Activity of FR49175 and Relative Compounds

Compounds	IC$_{50}$ (M)
FR49175	8.4×10^{-6}
FR106969	1.7×10^{-5}
3	3.0×10^{-5}
4	4.4×10^{-6}
5	3.9×10^{-5}
6	4.9×10^{-5}
7	1.7×10^{-5}
8	6.9×10^{-5}

not to be essential for the activity since the phenolic dihydroxy compound (**7**) still showed a potent activity. The hydroxymethyl group seems to play an important role for the inhibitory activity since the dehydroxymethylated compounds (**5**) and (**6**) were less active than the corresponding compounds (**4**) and (**1**), respectively.

FR900452 AND DIKETOPIPERAZINE DERIVATIVES

The new compound, designated FR900452, was isolated from the culture broth of *Streptomyces phaeofaciens* No. 7739.[13,14] The compound showed a high potency with an IC$_{50}$ of 3.7×10^{-7} M. The structure of this natural product was presumed on the basis of chemical and spectroscopic evidence and finally confirmed by X-ray crystal analysis of the dihydro derivative (Figure 3).[15] The absolute structure was established on the basis of the isolation of S-methyl-L-cysteine by acid hydrolysis.

The structure of the natural product FR900452 is unique in that it has the oxocyclopentylidene group incorporated as a vinylogous amide in the diketopiperazine skeleton. We speculated that the vinylogous diketopiperazine moiety might contribute to the ability of the molecule to bind to PAF receptor sites. In order to examine this point, we prepared structurally simpler analogs incorporating the diketopiperazine skeleton. This approach appeared reasonable because the two natural products described above have the diketopiperazine skeleton.[16] On the synthesis of diketopiperazine derivatives, we focused on the following points: (1) stereochemistry of diketopiperazine, (2) modification of oxindole part, (3) modification of S-methyl cysteine part, and (4) effect of β-methyl group (Figure 4).

First, the structurally simpler compounds, which lacked the β-methyl group in the

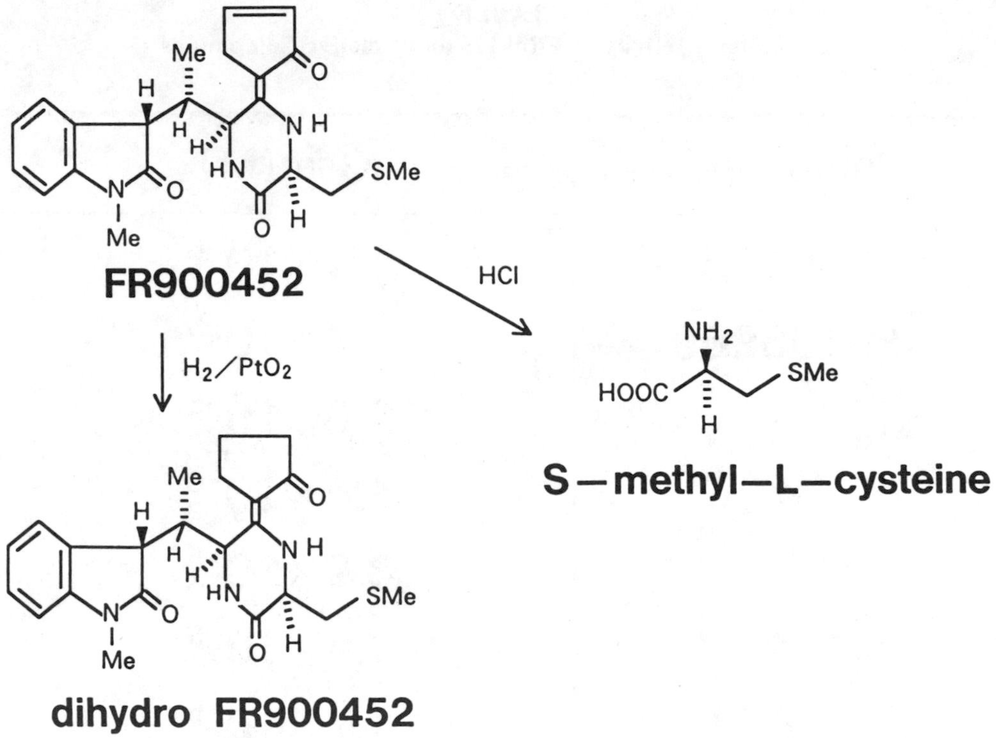

FIGURE 3.   Structure of FR900452 and dihydro FR900452.

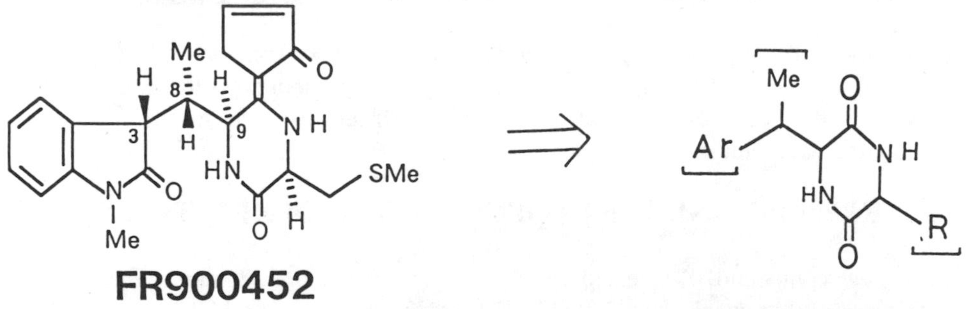

FIGURE 4.   Chemical modification of FR900452.

tryptophan moiety, were synthesized in order to examine which stereochemistry of dike-topiperazine is required for the inhibitory activity.

All of the four stereoisomers (**9a—d**) of the diketopiperazine with L-L, D-L, L-D, and D-D configuration were prepared starting from N-Boc-1-methyl-L- and D-tryptophan and S-methyl-L- and D-cysteine ethyl ester.

The inhibitory activities of these compounds are shown in Table 2. Of the four stereoisomers, compound (**9d**) with D-D configuration was found to be the most active and the other diastereoisomers were less potent or virtually inactive. It is thus concluded that the D-D form is preferable in this diketopiperazine series. The corresponding methionine derivative (**10**) with D-D configuration, which was similarly prepared from D-methionine, was more potent than the S-methyl cysteine derivative (**9d**). Further modification of this cysteine part of the molecule will be described later.

Subsequently, we examined the possibility of replacement of oxindole to the other

TABLE 2
Inhibitory Activity of Diketopiperazines 9a—d and 10

Compound	Configuration of		IC_{50} (M)
	C-3	C-6	
9a	L	L	2.5×10^{-4}
9b	D	L	3.6×10^{-5}
9c	L	D	1.4×10^{-4}
9d	D	D	7.9×10^{-6}
10	D	D-methionine	2.3×10^{-6}

TABLE 3
Inhibitory Activity of Diketopiperazines 11-13

Compound	Ar	IC_{50} (M)
11		4.3×10^{-5}
12		1.5×10^{-6}
13		4.3×10^{-5}
10		2.3×10^{-6}

simpler aromatic nuclei. Some diketopiperazines were synthesized from D-methionine and aromatic D-amino acid such as D-phenylalanine, D-naphthylalanine, and D-tryptophan. The inhibitory activities are shown in Table 3.

The naphthyl derivative (**12**) was more potent than the phenyl derivative (**11**) and the

TABLE 4
Inhibitory Activity of Diketopiperazines 14-17

Compound	R	IC_{50} (M)
14	$-CH_2CH_2CH_2CH_3$	1.9×10^{-6}
15	$-CH_2-\langle\!\!\!\!\bigcirc\!\!\!\!\rangle$	2.5×10^{-6}
16	$-CH_2OH$	1.5×10^{-4}
17	$-CH_2-\langle\!\!\!\!\bigcirc\!\!\!\!N\rangle$	5.4×10^{-6}
9d	$-CH_2SCH_3$	7.9×10^{-6}
10	$-CH_2CH_2SCH_3$	2.3×10^{-6}

1-methylindole derivative (10) was more potent than the indole derivative (13). The activity of the naphthyl derivative (12) was almost the same as that of the 1-methylindole derivative (10). This result showed that the oxindole nuclei could be replaced by hydrophobic aromatic nuclei. It could be speculated that the aromatic portion could occupy the hydrophobic region of the PAF receptor.

In order to modify the S-methylcysteine part of the natural product, we prepared alkyl, hydroxyalkyl, and aryl derivatives with D-D configuration of the diketopiperazine nucleus. The inhibitory activities are shown in Table 4.

The activities of the *n*-butyl (14) and benzyl (15) derivatives were as potent as that of the methionine derivative (10). The pyridylmethyl derivative (17) showed moderate activity. Although the hydroxymethyl group seems to play an important role for the activity of FR49175, the hydroxymethyl derivative (16) reduced the activity.

Finally, we tried to clarify the effect of the β-methyl group in the tryptophan residue, whether the methyl group is necessary for the activity and, if so, which configuration is preferable.

The (7R)-methyl derivative (18a) was prepared starting from *dl*-erythro-β-methyltryptophan(αR,βR).[17] The corresponding (7S)-methyl derivative (18b) was similarly prepared starting from *dl*-threo-β-methyltryptophan(αR,βS). Table 5 shows the activities of the four stereoisomers. Compound (18a) with the (7R)-methyl and D-D diketopiperazine configurations was the most active of the four diastereoisomers. Its potency was more than that of the corresponding desmethyl derivative (10) by about threefold. The (7S)-methyl counterpart (18b) showed a somewhat decreased potency which was about fivefold less potent than that of compound (18a). The *trans* diketopiperazine derivatives (18c) and (18d) were again considerably less active.

TABLE 5
Inhibitory Activity of Diketopiperazines 18a—d

Compound	Configuration of			IC_{50} (M)
	C-7	C-3	C-6	
18a	R	R(D)	R(D)	7.0×10^{-7}
18b	S	R(D)	R(D)	3.6×10^{-6}
18c	S	S(L)	R(D)	$>2.3 \times 10^{-4}$
18d	R	S(L)	R(D)	$>2.3 \times 10^{-4}$

At this stage, we can summarize from the results of the above chemical modifications that the compound (18a) with (3R, 6R, 7R)-configurations is the most active and that hydrophobic aromatic nuclei is preferable for the binding of the diketopiperazine nucleus to the PAF receptor.

For further chemical modifications, the pyridylmethyl derivative (17) was selected as a lead compound because acid salt of (17) was more soluble in aqueous solution as compared with the other alkyl or aryl derivatives. We planned the synthesis of compounds (19a—f) (Table 6). For this purpose a stereospecific synthesis of (αR,βR)-1,β-dimethyltryptophan was required. We succeeded in the regio- and stereospecific synthesis of the β-methyltryptophan from indole and aziridine carboxylate derived from D-threonine. Using this optically active amino acid, we prepared various derivatives which have substituents on the indole nuclei.

The inhibitory activities of the compounds (19a—f) are shown in Table 6. The activity of compound (19a) was about ninefold more potent than that of compound (17). The N-ethyl derivative (19b) showed an increased potency compared with the N-methyl derivative (19a). The effect of substituents on the indole moiety seems to contribute to the activity. Compound (19f) which was substituted with electron withdrawing group was about threefold more potent than compound (17c) which was substituted with electron donating group. We could conclude that the compounds having hydrophobic and electron withdrawing substituent on the indole moiety showed potent inhibitory activities.

SUMMARY

In this review, we discussed the structure-activity relationship of the diketopiperazine compounds which derived from the natural products of microbial origin FR49175, FR106969, and FR900452. It is concluded that the stereochemistry of the diketopiperazine moiety is

TABLE 6
Inhibitory Activity of Diketopiperazines 19a—f

Compound	X	R	IC_{50} (M)
19a	H	Me	4.4×10^{-7}
19b	H	Et	1.6×10^{-7}
19c	OMe	Me	5.1×10^{-7}
19d	Me	Me	2.1×10^{-7}
19e	F	Me	4.7×10^{-7}
19f	Cl	Me	1.5×10^{-7}

an important factor for PAF inhibitory activity and that the hydrophobic aromatic portion plays an important role for the binding of diketopiperazines to the PAF receptor in this series.

Among the derivatives, we selected compound (19a), designated FR76600, for more detailed biological evaluation after taking into consideration their activities and physiological properties. FR76600 inhibits PAF-induced hypotension with an ED_{50} of 4.2 mg/kg,i.v., in rats and bronchoconstriction with an ED_{50} of 2.8 mg/kg,p.o., in guinea pigs.[18]

REFERENCES

1. For reviews on PAF and PAF antagonists, see, e.g., (a) Braquet, P., Touqui, L., Shen, T. Y., and Vargaftig, B. B., Perspectives in platelet-activating factor research, *Pharmacol. Rev.*, 39, 97, 1987. (b) Chang, M. N., PAF and PAF antagonists, *Drugs Future*, 11, 869, 1986. (c) Godfroid, J. J. and Braquet, P., PAF-acether specific binding sites. I. Quantitative SAR study of PAF-acetherisosters, *Trends Pharmacol. Sci.*, 7, 368, 1986. (d) Braquet, P., and Godfroid, J. J., PAF-acether specific binding sites. II. Design of specific antagonists, *Trends Pharmacol. Sci.*, 8, 398, 1986.
2. **Terashita, Z., Tsushima, S., Yoshioka, Y., Nomura, H., Inada, Y., and Nishikawa, K.,** CV 3988, a specific antagonist of platelet activating factor (PAF), *Life Sci.*, 32, 1975, 1983.
3. **Handley, D. A., Van Valen, R. G., Melden, M. K., Deacon, R. W., Farley, C., Saunders, R. N., and Tomesch, J. C.,** Inhibition by SRI 63-441 of endotoxin- and PAF-induced responses in the rat and dog (abstract), in *2nd Int. Conf. on Platelet-Activating Factor and Structurally Related Alkyl Ether Lipids*, Gatlinburg, TN, October 1986, 111.

4. Cavero, L., Lave, D., Marquis, O., and Robaut, C., [^{3}H]-52770RP: a novel ligand for PAF-receptor sites in rabbit platelet preparation, *Br. J. Pharmacol.*, 90, 116, 1987.
5. Biftu, T., Gamble, N. F., Daebber, T., Hwang, S. B., Shen, T. Y., Snyder, J., Springer, J. P., and Stevenson, R., Conformation and activity of tetrahydrofuran lignans and analogues as specific platelet activating factor antagonists, *J. Med. Chem.*, 29, 1917, 1986.
6. Casals-Stenzel, J., Muacevic, G., and Weber, K. H., WEB 2086, a new and specific antagonist of platelet-activating factor (PAF), *Arch. Pharmacol. (Suppl.)*, 334, R44, 1986.
7. Braquet, P., Spinnewyn, B., Braquet, M., Bourgain, R. H., Taylor, J. E., Etienne, A., and Drieu, K., BN 52021 and related compounds: a new series of highly specific PAF-acether receptor antagonists isolated from *Ginkgo biloba, Blood Vessels*, 16, 559, 1985.
8. Shen, T. Y., Hwang, S. B., Chang, M. N., Doebber, T. W., Lam, M. H., Wu, M. S., Wang, X., Han, G. Q., and Li, R. Z., Characterization of platelet-activating factor antagonist isolated from haifenteng *(Piper futokadsura):* specific inhibitor of in vitro and in vivo platelet-activating factor-induced effects, *Proc. Natl. Acad. Sci. U.S.A.*, 82, 672, 1985.
9. Okamoto, M. Yoshida, K., Uchida, I., Nishikawa, M., Kohsaka, M., and Aoki, H., Studies of platelet-activating factor (PAF) antagonist from microbial products. I. Bisdethiobis(methylthio)gliotoxin and its derivatives, *Chem. Pharm. Bull.*, 34, 340, 1986.
10. Okamoto, M., Yoshida, K., Uchida, I., Kohsaka, M., and Aoki, H., Studies of platelet-activating factor (PAF) antagonists from microbial product. II. Pharmacological studies of FR49175 in animal models, *Chem. Pharm. Bull.*, 34, 345, 1986.
11. Shimazaki, N., Shima, I., Hemmi, K., Tsurumi, Y., and Hashimoto, M., Diketopiperazine derivatives, a new series of platelet-activating factor inhibitor, *Chem. Pharm. Bull.*, 35, 3527, 1987.
12. Kirby, G. W., Robins, D. J., Sefton, M. A., and Talekar, R. R., Biosynthesis of bisdethiobis(methylthio)gliotoxin, a new metabolite of *Gliocladium deliquesens, J. Chem. Soc., Perkin 1*, 1980, 119.
13. Okamoto, M., Yoshida, K., Nishikawa, K., Ando, T., Iwami, M., Kohsaka, M., and Aoki, H., FR900452 a specific antagonist of platelet-activating factor (PAF) produced by *Streptomyces phaeofaciens*. I. Taxonomy, fermentation, isolation, and physicochemical and biological characteristics, *J. Antibiotics*, Tokyo, 39, 198, 1986.
14. Okamoto, M., Yoshida, K., Nishikawa, M., Hayashi, K., Uchida, I., Kohsaka, M., and Aoki, H., Studies of platelet-activating factor (PAF) antagonists from microbial products. III. Pharmacological studies of FR900452 in animal models, *Chem. Pharm. Bull.*, 34, 3005, 1986.
15. Takase, S., Shigematsu, N., Shima, I., Uchida, I., Hashimoto, M., Toda, T., Koda, S., and Morimoto, Y., Structure of FR900452, a novel platelet-activating factor inhibitor from a *Streptomyces, J. Org. Chem.*, 52, 3485, 1987.
16. Shimazaki, N., Shima, I., Hemmi, K., Hashimato, M., Diketopiperazines as a new class of platelet-activating factor inhibitor, *J. Med. Chem.*, 30, 1706, 1987.
17. Gould, S. J., Chang, C. C., Darling, D. S., Roberts, J. D., and Squillacote, M., Streptonigrin biosynthesis. IV. Detail of the tryptophan metabolism, *J. Am. Chem. Soc.*, 102, 1707, 1980.
18. Shima, I., Shimazaki, N., Imai, K., Hashimoto, M., and Hemmi, K., in preparation.

Chapter 3

KADSURENONE TYPE NEOLIGNANS, POTENTIAL PAF ANTAGONISTS: CHEMISTRY AND DISTRIBUTION

Otto R. Gottlieb, Massayoshi Yoshida, and Paulete Romoff

INTRODUCTION

Many naturally occurring oxidative dimers of various $C_6.C_3$-phenols encompassing a benzofuranoid moiety have recently been discovered (Scheme 1). Although details concerning their biosynthetic origin remain to be clarified, it seems probable that their monomeric units are based on cinnamic acids, cinnamyl alcohols, propenylphenols, and allylphenols as alternative monomeric starting materials. This fact transpires by inspection of the structure such as hordatin (1.1)[1] from *Hordeum vulgare* (barley, family Poaceae), salvianolic acid (1.2)[2] from *Salvia miltiorrhiza* (Lamiaceae), fragransol-C (1.3)[3] from *Myristica fragrans* (Myristicaceae), olmecol (1.4)[4] from *Krameria cystisoides* (Krameriaceae), licarin-A (1.5)[5] from many species of Lauraceae, Magnoliaceae, Myristicaceae, Aristolochiaceae and Krameriaceae, eupomatenoid-6 (1.6)[6] from species of Eupomatiaceae and Krameriaceae. Since ratanhiaphenol-I (1.7)[7] from Krameriaceae and egonol (1.8)[8] from Styracaceae are probably generated by decarboxylation of C-8, compounds of this type also belong to the class of dimeric benzofuran lignoids.

The present review is restricted to still another group of such compounds, namely, oxidative dimers of propenylphenols *plus* allylphenols, which are, among the several groups of coupling products, certainly the most interesting ones. First, and in the context of the present book most conspicuously, their practical importance is enhanced by the discovery of one of their representatives, kadsurenone (1.9), as a specific and potent inhibitor of PAF-induced rabbit platelet aggregation.[10] The bioactivity of this and other benzofuranoid neolignans is supported by a striking chemical reactivity including several highly specific skeletal rearrangements.[1,11] Furthermore, such neolignans comprise a surprisingly varied series of structural types.[12] Finally, they are of considerable chemosystematic value, since their known natural occurrence is limited to a few angiosperm families of the magnolialean block.[13]

BIOGENETIC CLASSIFICATION

Natural distribution, structural comparison, reactivity and even synthesis of propenylphenol plus allylphenol derived neolignans are studied more conveniently through a biogenetic system of classification (Table 1). The formulation of such a system requires the original numbering of the two fundamental monomeric units (Scheme 2) to be maintained in the dimeric forms. This procedure is helpful in visualizing the putative oxidative coupling modes which lead to the specific compound types (Scheme 3). Clearly, many other types of couplings do occur among which chiefly 8.8-couplings of two propenylphenol derived radicals (2.1),[13] but the resulting compound types do not fall within the scope of this review. In all covered cases the structures of the end products are consistent with the intermediate existence of radicals. Nevertheless, such mechanisms, although convenient for the understanding of this area of natural product biogenesis, are so far purely hypothetical.

Initially, oxidation, i.e., abstraction of a hydrogen atom, from both types of phenols leads to phenoxide radicals (2.2, 2.5, 2.9). As revealed by the structure of the end products the only relevant mesomeric form of such radicals if derived from propenylphenols is 2.3. In the case of the allylphenol derived radicals phenoxide is operative directly and leads to the unusual 3-aryl-2-methyl derivatives of the chrysophyllone and chrysophyllin types. A

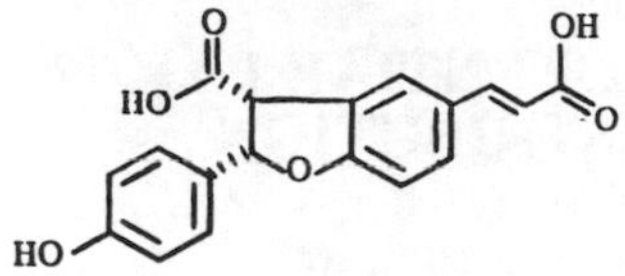

SCHEME 1.   Examples of benzofuranoid $C_6.C_3$-dimers.

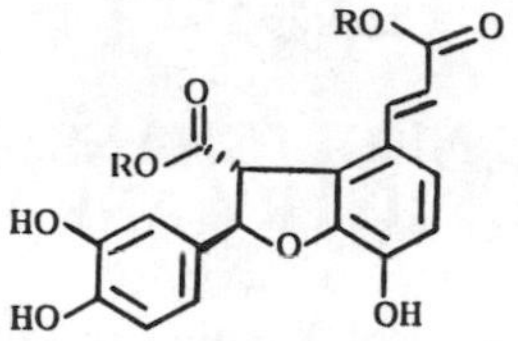

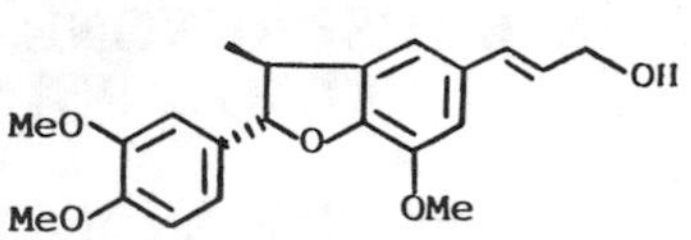

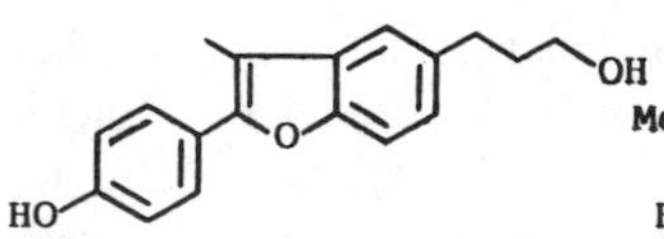

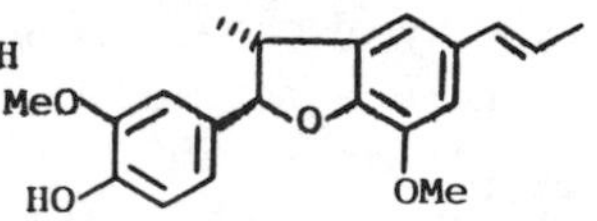

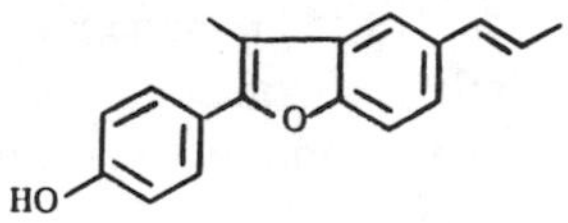

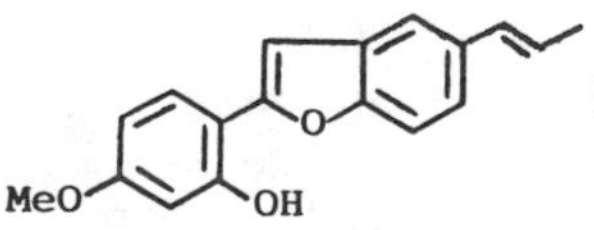

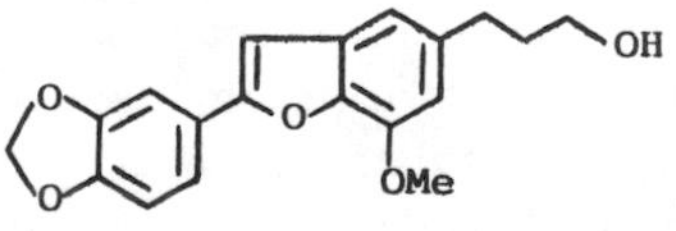

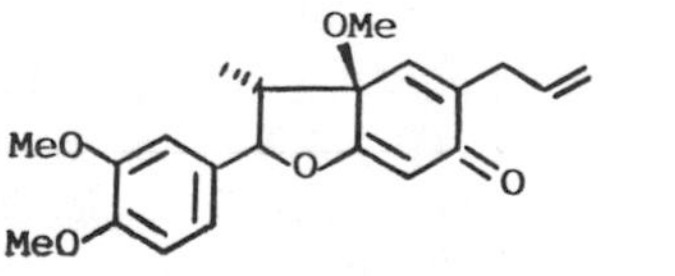

higher oxygenation pattern than featured in **2.9** seems to favor the intervention of the phenoxide radical in coupling with **2.3**. The pathways to the usual 2-aryl-3-methylbenzo-furanoid neolignans all involve one of the three possible mesomeric forms of *p*-phenoxy-allylphenol radicals of lesser, at most tri, oxygenation. These include one *para*-radical (e.g., **2.8**) and two *ortho*-radicals (e.g., **2.7** and **2.6**). The formation of the furan rings requires additional bridging through oxygen, leading in the 8.1′ dimers to the burchellin type (**3.1**) and the porosin type (**3.6**), in the 8.3′ dimers to the mirandin type (**3.8**) and the fargesone type (**3.11**), and in the 8.5′ dimers to the carinatin type (**3.12**) and the ferrearin type (**3.13**); or through carbon, leading in the 8.O.2′ dimers to the chrysophyllone type (**3.15**) and the chrysophyllin type (**3.18**). As indicated by their oxygenation patterns, some of the benzo-furanoids must have suffered allyl rearrangement. This is the case of the 8.1′,7.O.6′-coupled burchellin II-IV types (**3.2—3.4**), the 8.5′,7.O.4′-coupled ferrearin type (**3.13**) and the 8.O.2′,7.1′-coupled chrysophyllone II and III types (**3.17, 3.18**). In absence of additional bridging no furan moieties do of course result and 8.1′ dimers give the megaphone type (**4.1**) and, after 1′→3′ and 1′→O.4′ allyl rearrangements respectively the carinatonol (**4.2**) and the aurein (**4.3**) types, 8.3′ dimers give the lancifolin (**4.4a**) type and 8.5′ dimers give the carinatol (**4.5**) type.

The comprehensive display of propenylphenol *plus* allylphenol derived benzofuranoid

TABLE 1
Biogenetic Classification of the Propenylphenol *Plus* Allylphenol Derived Benzofuranoid Neolignan Types

Radical (2.3 plus radicals)	Coupling models	Allyl	Neolignans (types)
2.8, R=OH	8.1', 7.O.6'		burchellin I (3.1)
		1' → 3'	burchellin II (3.2)
		1' → O.4'	burchellin III (3.3)
		1' → 5'	burchellin IV (3.4)
		elimination	burchellin V (3.5)
2.8, R=H			porosin (3.6)
			dihydroporosin hydrate (3.7)
2.6, R=OH	8.3', 7.O.4'		mirandin (=kadsurenone) (3.8)
			mirandin hydrate (3.9)
2.6, R=H			dihydromirandin hydrate (3.10)
2.6, R=OH	8.3', 7.O.2'		fargesone (3.11)
2.7, R=H	8.5', 7.O.4'		carinatin (3.12)
		3' → 1'	ferrearin (3.13)
			dihydroferrearin (3.14)
2.9	7.1', 8.O.2'		chrysophyllone I (3.15)
		1' → 3'	chrysophyllone II (3.16)
		1' → O.4'	chrysophyllone III (3.17)
			chrysophylline (3.18)

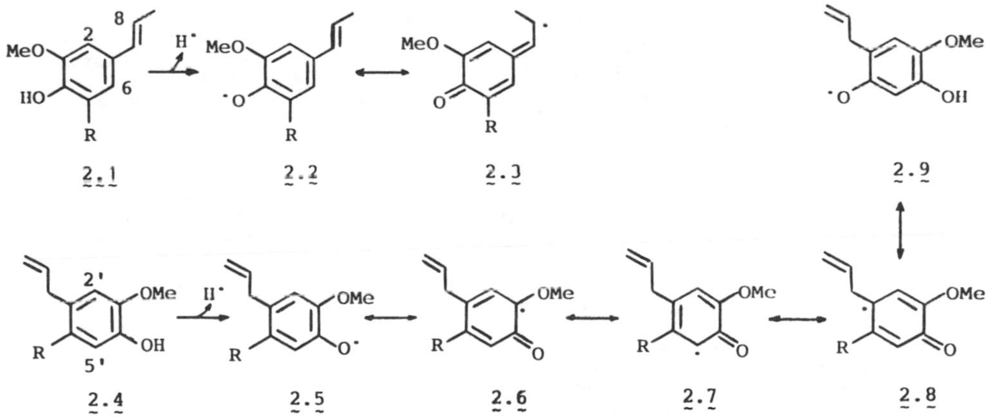

SCHEME 2. Oxidation of propenylphenols and allylphenols to mesomeric radicals.

neolignan types (Scheme 4), when used in combination with Table 2, allows access to the structures, trivial names, plant sources, and literature of all presently known derivatives.

CHEMICAL REACTIVITY

Burchellin I type neolignans (e.g., **5.1,6.1**) co-occur in plants with a series of isomers (Schemes 5 and 6) the formation of which can be imagined to imply transposition of the allyl group from position 1' alternatively to position 3' in burchellin II type (**5.2, 6.2**), O.4' in burchellin III type (**5.3,6.3**) and 5' in burchellin IV type (**5.4,6.4**). Such products should be formed by successive rearrangements involving Cope (**5.1→5.2, 6.1→6.2**), retro Claisen (**5.2→5.3, 6.2→6.3**) and Claisen (**5.3→5.4, 6.3→6.4**) mechanisms. Indeed the same series of products can be obtained by pyrolysis of burchellin I type compounds in the laboratory. The reaction sequence also explains the existence of trisnor neolignans ($C_6.C_3.C_6$ compounds)

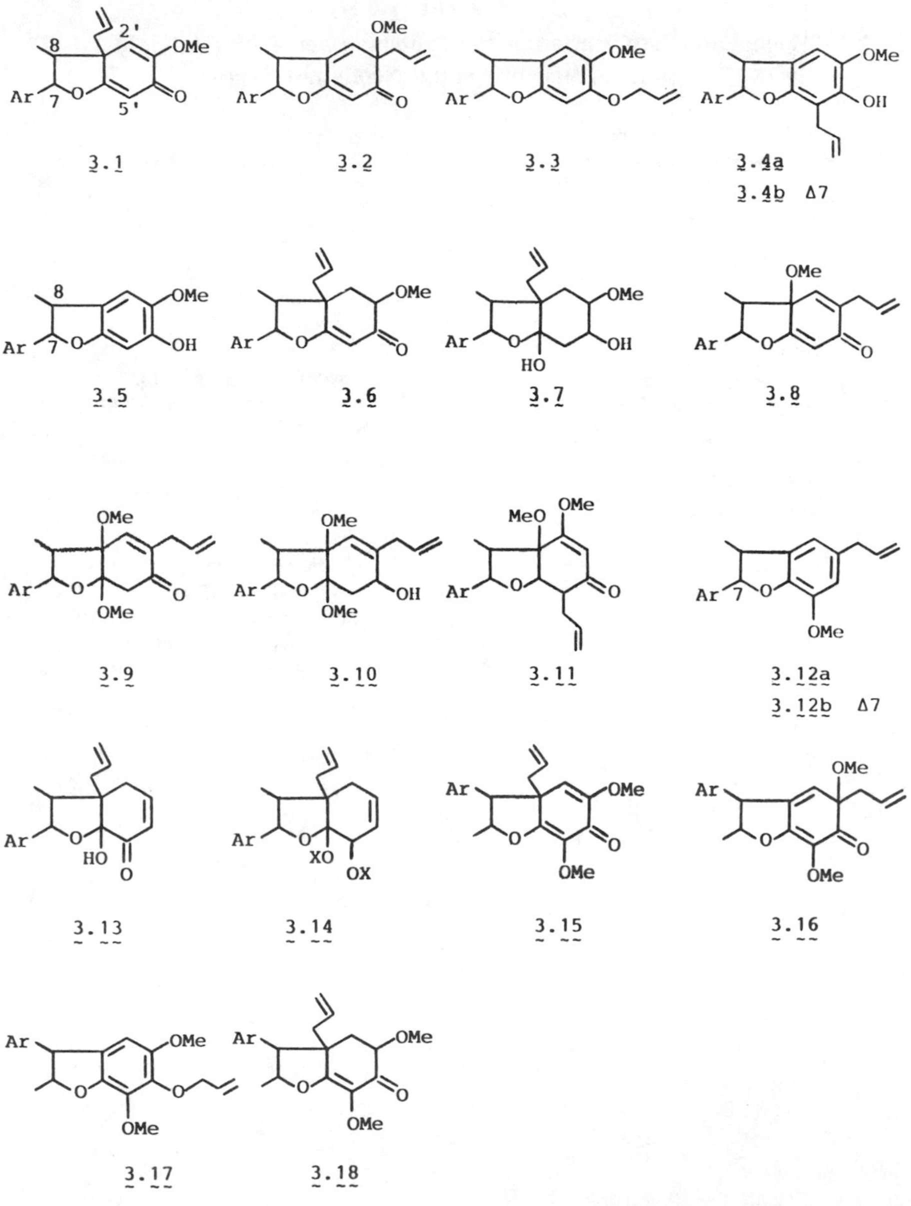

SCHEME 3.   Propenylphenol *plus* allylphenyl derived benzofuranoid neolignan types.

(5.5,6.5) which, *a priori,* without consideration of their preparation from neolignans, could be classified as flavonoids. Indeed, obtusafuran[14] and melanoxin,[15] two dihydrobenzofurans which even share oxygenation patterns with the neolignans, are undoubtedly flavonoids since they co-occur with neoflavonoids in the genus *Dalbergia* (Fabaceae).

Burchellin type neolignans also co-occur in plants with bicyclo[3.2.1]octanoid neolignans **(5.6,6.6)** and spiro[5.5]undecanoid neolignans **(6.7)**. In this case interconversion can be imagined to proceed by acid catalysis. It could be anticipated that in the laboratory, i.e., in absence of enzymes, treatment with acid should always promote the transformation of the latter type into the former **(5.6→5.1)**, since this possesses the most extensive conjugated system. Nevertheless electron conjugation cannot be the sole driving force for rearrangement. Reactions in the opposite direction have also been observed **(6.1→6.6)**. It is thus probable that the strains caused by specific chiralities should also intervene in the selection of the

TABLE 2
Structures and Occurrences of the Propenylphenol *Plus* Allylphenol Derived Benzofuranoid Neolignans

Types (Scheme 3)	Structural details	Trivial names	Occurrences	Ref.
3.1.1	R:1′,S:7,8; Ar:Pi	burchellin	LauAniaff	12
			LauAnifer	12
			LauAnisp	17
			LauAniter	12
			MagMagden	18
			MagMaglil	18
			LauMezita	19
			LauOcopor	20
			Laulicchr	21
2	R:1′,S:7,8; Ar:Ve		LauAniaff	12
			LauAnibur	18
			LauNecsp	22
3	R:1′,S:7,8; Ar:Tp		LauNecsp	18
4	R:1′,S:7,8; Ar:Ve; OMe:5′		LauAniaff	12
5	R:1′,S:7,8; Ar:Pi; OMe:5′		LauOcover	23
			LauOcoaci	24
6	S:7.8,1′; Ar:Pi		LauAnisp	17
			LauAniter	12
7	S:7,8,1′; Ar:Tp		LauAnisim	12
			LauNecmir	12
8	R:7,S:8,1′; Ar:Tp		LauAnisim	12
9	R:7,S:8,1′; Ar:Pi		LauAnisp	17
			LauAniter	12
			LauOcocat	18
			AnnDugsur	12
			LauMezita	19
			LauOcopor	20
			LauLicarm	25
10	R:7,S:8,1′; Ar:Mp		LauAnism	12
			LauLicarm	25
11	R:7,S:8,1′; Ar:Pi; OMe:5′		LauOcocat	18
			LauOcoaci	24
3.2.1	S:7,8,3′; Ar:Pi		LauAnibur	18
			LauAnisp	17
			LauAniter	12
			LauLicchr	21
			LauMezita	19
2	S:7,8,3′; Ar:Ve		LauAniaff	12
			LauAnibur	18
			AnnDugsur	12
3	R:3′,S:7,8; Ar:Mp		LauAnisim	12
			LauLicarm	25
4	R:3′,S:7,8; Ar:Mp; OMe:5′		LauAnisim	12
5	R:3′,S:7,8; Ar:Tp		LauAnisim	12
			LauNecmir	12
			LauNecsp	18
6	R:8,S:7,3′; Ar:Tp		LauAnicit	26
7	R:3′,S:7,8; Ar:Tp; OMe:5′		LauAnisim	12
8	R:3′,S:7,8; Ar:Pi; OMe:5′		LauOcover	18
			LauOcosp	23
9	R:3′,S:7,8; Ar:Pi		LauAnisp	17
			LauAniter	12
			LauOcover	18
			LauLicarm	25

TABLE 2 (continued)
Structures and Occurrences of the Propenylphenol *Plus* Allylphenol Derived Benzofuranoid Neolignans

Types (Scheme 3)	Structural details	Trivial names	Occurrences	Ref.
10	R:7,3′,S:8; Ar:Pi		LauAniaff	12,18
			LauAniter	12
			LauMezita	19
11	R:7,3′,S:8; Ar:Mp		LauAnisim	12
3.3.1	S:7,8; Ar:Pi		LauAnibur	18
			LauAniter	12
			LauLicchr	21
			LauMezita	19
2	S:7,8; Ar:Mp		LauAnisim	12
			LauLicarm	25
3	S:7,8; Ar:Tp		LauNecmir	12
4	S:7,8; Ar:Tp; OMe:5′		LauAnisim	12
5	S:7,8; Ar:Pi; OMe:5′		LauOcover	23
6	R:7,S:8; Ar:Mp		LauAnisim	12
3.4a.1	S:7,8; Ar:Pi		LauAniter	12
			LauMezita	19
2	S:7,8; Ar:Mp		LauAnisim	12
3	R:7,S:8; Ar:Pi		LauAniter	12
4	R:7,S:8; Ar:Mp		LauAnisim	12
3.4b.1	Ar:Pi		LauAniter	12
			LauMezita	19
2	Ar:Mp		LauAnisim	12
3	Ar:Tp		LauNecmir	12
3.5.1	S:7,8; Ar:Pi		products	27
2	S:7,8; Ar:Mp			27
3	S:7,8; Ar:Tp		of	27
4	R:7; S:8; Ar:Tp			27
5	R:7; S:8; Ar:Tp		pyrolysis	27
3.6.1	R:7,1′,3′,S:8; Ar:Ve	porosin A	LauLicarm	12
			LauOcopor	12,20
			LauUrbver	18
2	R:7,1′,3′,S:8; Ar:Pi	porosin B	LauOcopor	20
			LauUrbver	18
3	R:7′,1′,S:8,3′; Ar:Pi		LauOcopor	28
4	R:8,S:7,1′,3′; Ar:Mp; OMe:5′		LauAnifer	18
			LauAnisp	29
5	R:8,S:7,1′,3′; Ar:Pi; OMe:5′		LauAnifer	18
6	R:7,8,1′,3′; Ar:Pi; OMe:5′	canellin B	LauLiccan	12
7	R:7,8,1′,3′; Ar:Pi	canellin F	LauOcopor	28
8	R:1′,3′,S:7,8; Ar:Tp	armenin C	LauAnisp	30
9	R:7,8,1′,3′; Ar:Tp	canellin D	LauAnisp	30
10	R:7,8,1′,3′; Ar:Mp; OMe:5′	canellin E	LauAnisp	30
11	Ar:Pi	armenin A	LauLicarm	31
			LauOcoaci	24
12	Ar:Pi; Ome:5′	armenin B	LauLicarm	31
3.7.1	R:7,1′,3′,4′,S:8; Ar:Ve		LauOcopor	28
2	R:7,1′,3′,S:8,4′; Ar:Ve		LauOcopor	28
3.8.1	R:8,S:7,3′, Ar:Tp	mirandin A	LauNecmir	12
			LauNecsp	18
2	R:8,3′,S:7; Ar:Tp	mirandin B	LauNecmir	12
3	R:8,3′,S:7; Ar:Pi	denudatin A	MagMagden	18
			MagMaglil	18
			LauLicchr	21
4	R:8,3′,S:7; Ar:Ve	denudatin B	MagMagden	18
			MagMaglil	18

TABLE 2 (continued)
Structures and Occurrences of the Propenylphenol *Plus* Allylphenol Derived Benzofuranoid Neolignans

Types (Scheme 3)	Structural details	Trivial names	Occurrences	Ref.
5	R:7,3′,S:8; Ar:Ve	kadsurenone	PipPipfut	32
3.9.1	R:8,4′,S:7,3′; Ar:Ve	piperenone	MagMaglil	18
			PipPipfut	12
2	R:8,4′,S:7,3′; Ar:Gu	liliflone	MagMaglil	18
3	R:7,3′,S:8,4′; Ar:Pi	kadsurin A	PipPipfut	32
3.10.1	R:7,3′,S:8,4′; Ar:Pi	kadsurin B	PipPipfut	32
3.11.1	R:8,3′,S:7,1′; Ar:Pi	fargesone A	MagMagfar	33
2	R:8,1′,3′,S:7; Ar:Pi	fargesone B	MagMagfar	33
3.12a.1	S:7,8; Ar:Ve	dihydrocarinatin	MyrVircar*	18
2	S:7,8; Ar:Gu		MyrVircar	18
3.12b.1	Ar:Ve	carinatin	MyrVircar	18
2	Ar:Gu	carinatidin	MyrVircar	18
3.13.1	R:7,S:8,1′; Ar:Mp	ferrearin A	LauAnifer	
2	R:7,S:8,1′; Ar:Pi	ferrearin B	LauAnifer	
			LauOcoaci	24,34
3	S:7,8,1′; Ar:Pi	ferrearin C	LauOcoaci	34
3.14.1	S:7,8,1′; Ar:Pi; X:Me; Y:ll		LauOcopor	28
2	S:7,8,1′; Ar:Pi; X:Me; Y:Me; OMe:5′	ferrearin D	LauOcoaci	24
3.15.1	R:7,S:8,1′; Ar:Mp	chrysophyllone IA	LauLicchr	35
2	R:7,S:8,1′; Ar:Tp	chrysophyllone IB	LauLicchr	35
3	Ar:Mp		LauLicchr	16
3.16.1	R:7,3′,S:8; Ar:Tp	chrysophyllone IIA	LauLicchr	35
2	R:7,3′,S:8; Ar:Mp	chrysophyllone IIB	LauLicchr	35
3	R:8,3′,S:7; Ar:Mp		LauLicchr	16
3.17.1	R:7,S:8; Ar:Mp	chrysophyllone IIIA	LauLicchr	35
2	R:8,S:7; Ar:Tp	chrysophyllone IIIB	LauLicchr	35
3	R:8,S:7; Ar:Mp		LauLicchr	16
3.18.1	R:7,1′,5′,S:8; Ar:Mp	chrysophyllin A	LauLicchr	36
2	R:7,1′,5′,S:8; Ar:Tp	chrysophyllin B	LauLicchr	36

* Wrongly cited as a natural product from this source in Reference 18.

Note: (see pg. 19a for text)
Note: Glossary to Table 2

1. Aryl groups:
   Gu ... Guaiacyl (4-hydroxy-3-methoxyphenyl)
   Mp ... 4,5-Methylenedioxy-3-methoxyphenyl
   Pi ... Piperonyl (3,4-methylenedioxyphenyl)
   Tp ... 3,4,5-Trimethoxyphenyl
   Ve ... Veratryl (3,4-dimethoxyphenyl)

2. Plant family —
genus — species:

AnnDugsur ... Annonaceae	*Duguetia*	*surinamensis*
LauAniaff ... Lauraceae	*Aniba*	*affinis*
LauAnibur		*burchellii*
LauAnicit		*citrifolia*
LauAnifer		*ferrea*
LauAnimeg		*megaphylla*
LauAnisim		*simulans*
LauAnisp		sp
LauAnisp		sp 41
LauAniter		*terminalis*
LauLicarm	*Licaria*	*armeniaca*

TABLE 2 (continued)
Structures and Occurrences of the Propenylphenol *Plus* Allylphenol Derived
Benzofuranoid Neolignans

2. Plant family —
genus — species (cont.):

LauLiccan		*canella*
LauLicchr		*chrysophylla*
LauMezita	*Mezilaurus*	*itauba*
LauNecmir	*Nectandra*	*miranda*
LauNecsp		*sp*
LauOcoaci	*Ocotea*	*aciphylla*
LauOcocat		*catharinensis*
LauOcopor		*porosa*
LauOcosp		*sp*
LauOcover		*veraguensis*
LauUrbver	*Urbanodendron*	*verrucosum*
MagMagden ... Magnoliaceae	*Magnolia*	*denudata*
MagMagfar		*fargesii*
MagMaglil		*liliflora*
MyrVircar ... Myristicaceae	*Virola*	*carinata*
PipPipfut ... Piperaceae	*Piper*	*futokadsura*

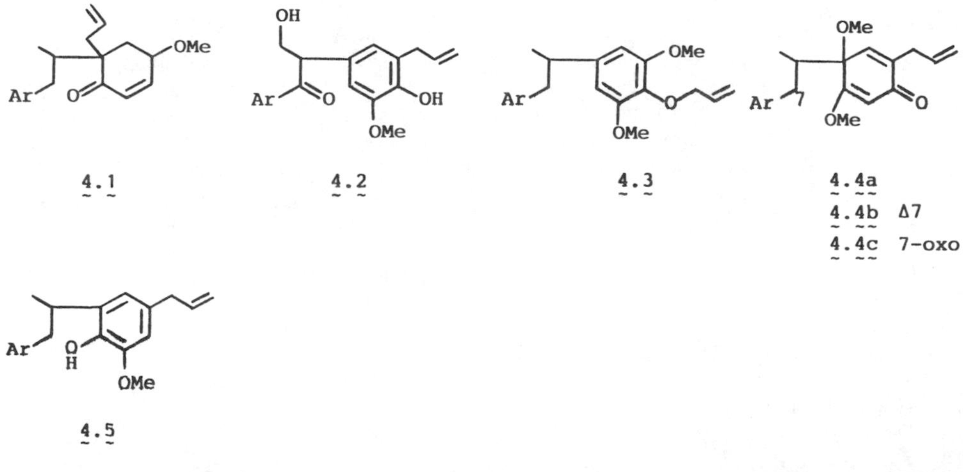

SCHEME 4.   Propenylphenol *plus* allylphenol derived neolignan types of close biogenetic relationship with the analogously derived benzofuranoid neolignans of Scheme 3.

nature of the transformation. The acid catalyzed conversions of the naturally abundant and substitutionally and configurationally varied burchellin type neolignans into bicyclo[3.2.1]octanoids and spiro[5.5]undecanoids is of preparative interest. All three 8.1′ neolignan types are accessible by an elegant synthetic approach (Scheme 7) with a ramification into the synthesis of substituted tropolones.

In the porosin series (**3.6**) the pyrolytic transposition of the allyl does of course not occur (Scheme 8). Acid treatment, however, leads again, as in the burchellin series, to spiro[5.5]undecanoids (**8.1→8.2**). Such dihydrofutoenone types have not yet been isolated from a natural source.

The burchellin II type neolignans (**3.2**), formed by a Cope rearrangement of burchellin I type compounds, possess the same carbon-skeleton as the mirandin type (**3.8**), one of the two possible direct 8.3′ coupling products. Mirandins again co-occur with bicy-

SCHEMES 5 and 6. Rearrangements in the burchellin series.

clo[3.2.1]neolignans *in vivo* and also undergo the hydrobenzofuranoid-bicy-clo[3.2.1]octanoid rearrangement by acid treatment *in vitro* (Scheme 9).

A neat distinction between rearranged neolignans primarily derived by 8.1' coupling (**3.1**) and neolignans derived by direct 8.3' coupling (**3.8,3.12**) results by the comparison of the oxygenation pattern of their allylphenol derived moieties with the oxygenation pattern of the eugenol type (**2.4**) precursor. The same argument is again employed in the classification of the singular neolignans of the ferrearin type (**3.13**). As suggested by their oxygenation pattern, the compounds should not be formed by direct 8.1' coupling, but by 8.3' coupling followed by a 3'→1' allyl rearrangement (**10.2→10.3**) (Scheme 10). Interestingly, treatment of the ferrearins with a trace of acid in methanol produces, besides two ketals (**10.4b, 10.5**), a compound (**10.6**) which reveals the allyl to have returned to its original position.

As burchellin I type neolignans, chrysophyllone I type compounds also co-occur in nature with isomers and the same considerations justifying pyrolytic *in vivo* and *in vitro* allyl rearrangements are applicable (Scheme 11).

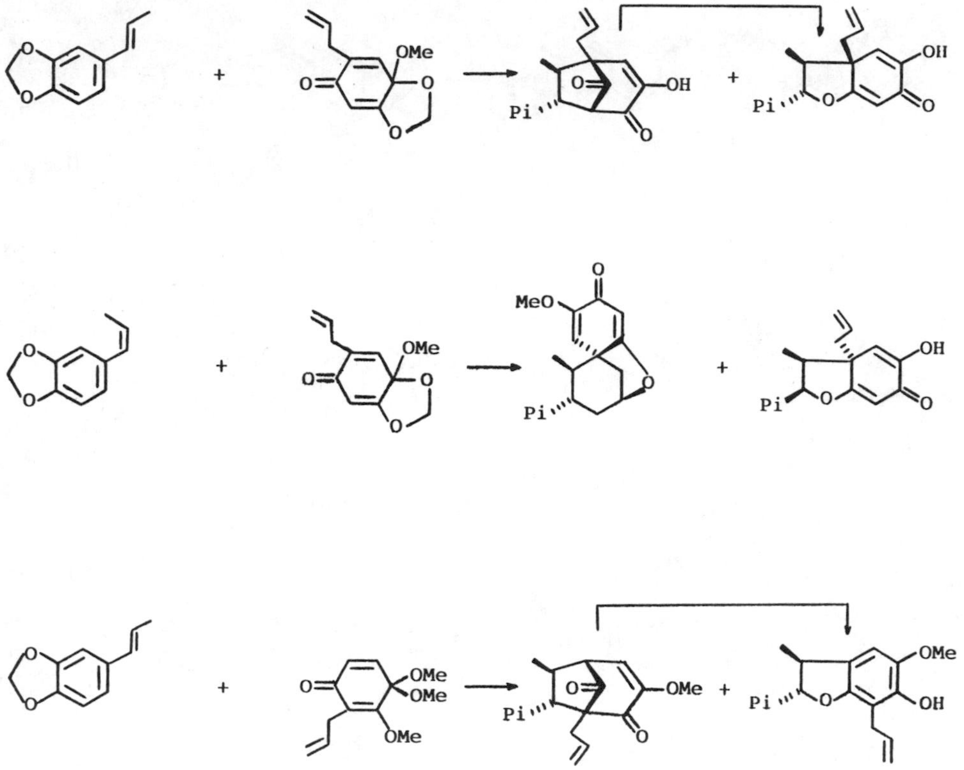

SCHEME 7.   Syntheses of propenylphenol *plus* allylphenol derived neolignan types.

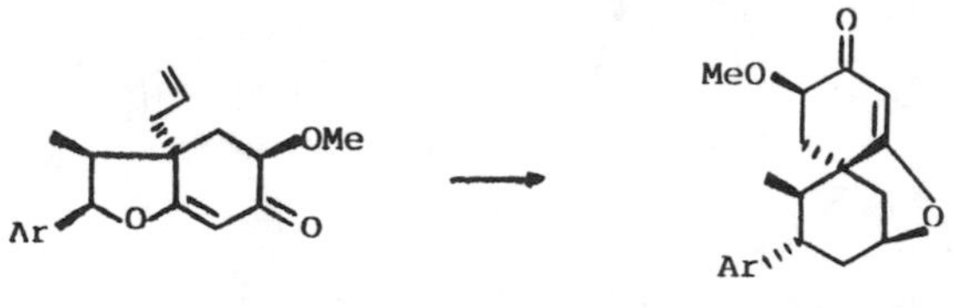

8.1   8.2

SCHEME 8.   Rearrangement in the porosin series.

CONCLUSION

The present review was limited to propenylphenol *plus* allylphenol derived neolignans. As shown in Table 2, all known compounds of this type occur mainly in the family Lauraceae, a few having been isolated also from the Magnoliaceae, Myristicaceae, and Piperaceae. The identification in a species of Annonaceae needs confirmation. Precisely the same distribution, limited to a few families of the magnolialean block has been noted for some biosynthetically related coupling products exempt of a heterocycle with one (Scheme 4) or two (Schemes 5, 6) carbon – carbon bonds bridging the two different monomeric phenol types. Still other propenylphenol *plus* allylphenol derived neolignans, now involving one (e.g., the virolongins[16]) or two (e.g., the eusiderins[16]) also have so far been located in Lauraceae, Magnoliaceae, and Myristicaceae, as well as in Aristolochiaceae and Krameriaceae.

Allylphenol *plus* allylphenol derived neolignans are also known and occur as 5.5′-dimers again in the former three families and the Eupomatiaceae, or as oxidative methoxylation

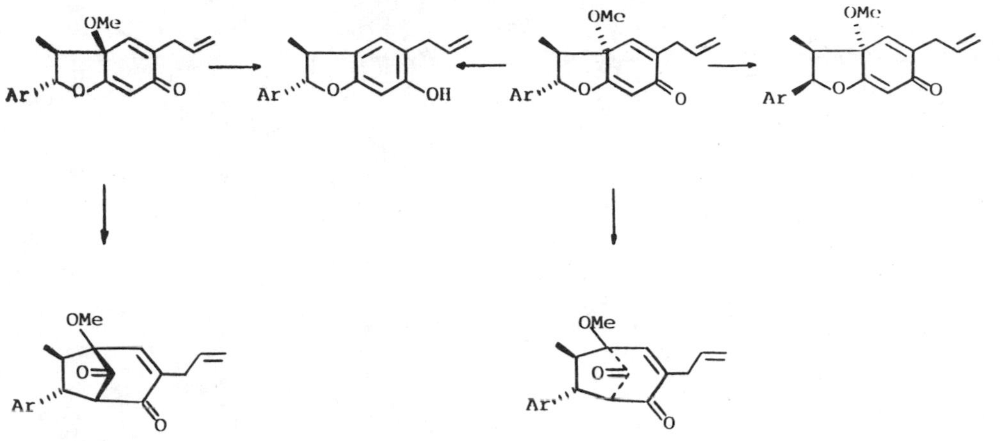

SCHEME 9.   Rearrangements in the mirandin series.

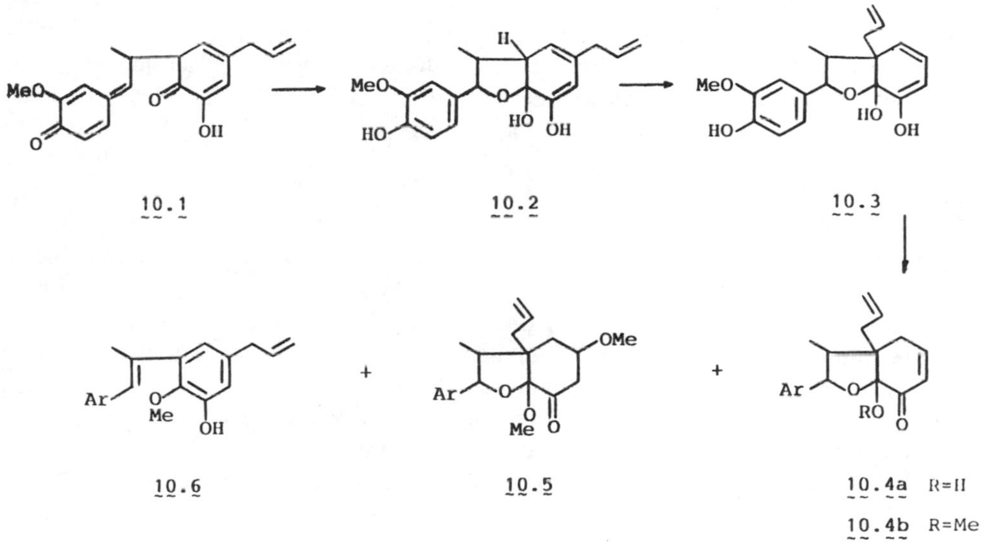

SCHEME 10.   Biogenesis and laboratory methylation of the ferrearin type.

products in the Aristolochiaceae. Both these latter families also belong to the magnolialean block.

Propenylphenol *plus* propenylphenol derived neolignans can also be divided into benzofuranoid (8.5′,7.O.4′-coupled) and other types, the latter involving primarily 8.8′-coupling (without or with additional bridges linking positions 7.O.7′; 7.O.9′; 7.7′; 6.7′; 2.7′; 2.7′ and 3.O.6′; 2.7′ *plus* rearrangements; 2.2′; 2.2′; and 7.O.7′; 2.1′). And again, both the benzofuranoids and the other C_6C_3-dimers occur chiefly in Lauraceae, Magnoliaceae, Myristicaceae, and Eupomatiaceae. The primarily 8.8′-coupled compounds occur additionally in Araceae, Austrobaileyaceae, Himantandraceae, Piperaceae, Schizandraceae, and Trimeniaceae which also all belong to the magnolialean block of the angiosperms. Among the few exceptions to this preferential distribution is the registry of benzofuranoids in Combretaceae, Krameriaceae, Styracaceae, and Polemoniaceae and of 8.8′-coupled compounds in Combretaceae, Krameriaceae, Verbenaceae, and Zygophyllaceae. Not only are these oc-

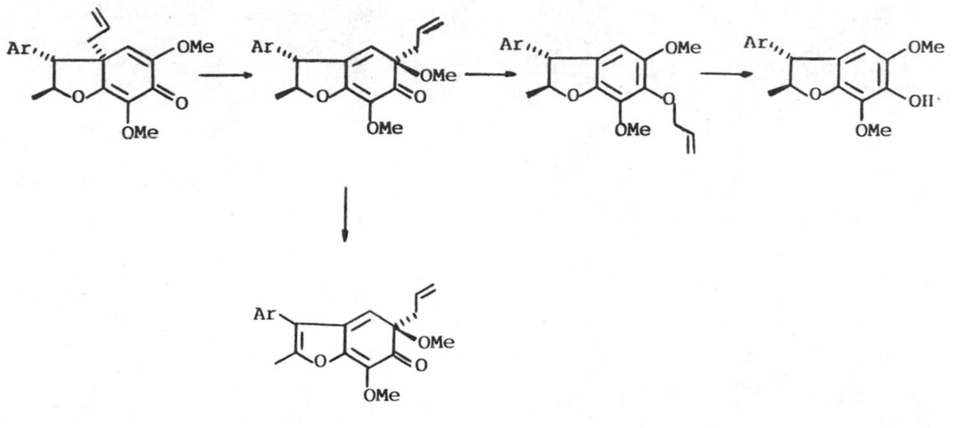

SCHEME 11. Rearrangements in the chrysophyllone series.

currences relatively few in number, but they refer frequently to structurally modified (e.g., side-chain degraded) representatives.

A completely different distribution pattern persists for the cinnamic acid and/or cinnamyl alcohol derived oxidative dimers (lignans). They have been noted in Pteridophyta (Pteridaceae) and Gymnospermae (Araucariaceae, Cupressaceae, Ephedraceae, Pinaceae, Podocarpaceae, Taxaceae, and Taxodiaceae) and are very widespread in Angiospermae. Here they do not occur only in most of the magnolialean families mentioned above, but also in some others, viz., Cannellaceae, Hernandiaceae, Monimiaceae, Saururaceae, Berberidaceae, and Menispermaceae. No doubt, however, in this case the generality of distribution in angiosperms is no exception since lignans have been found also in many of the families of the rosiflorean block, viz., Acanthacaeae, Apiaceae, Apocynaceae, Araliaceae, Asteraceae, Betulaceae, Bignoniaceae, Burseraceae, Combretaceae, Cucurbitaceae, Ebenaceae, Ericaceae, Eucommiaceae, Euphorbiaceae, Globulariaceae, Hydrangeaceae, Lamiaceae, Loganiaceae, Oleaceae, Pedaliaceae, Polygalaceae, Rosaceae, Rutaceae, Scrophulariaceae, Thymeleaceae, Ulmaceae, Urticaceae, Verbenaceae, and Viscaceae. Indeed the extraordinarily restricted distribution of the neolignans, as opposed to the general occurrence of the lignans[13] is the most convincing evidence for the separation of neolignans and lignans into separate biosynthetic classes.

REFERENCES

1. **Gottlieb, O. R. and Yoshida, M.,** Lignóides, com atenção especial à química das neolignanas, *Química Nova* (SBQ, São Paulo), 7, 250, 1984.
2. **Ai, C.-B. and Li, L.-N.,** Stereostructure of salvianolic acid B and isolation of salvianolic acid C from *Salvia miltiorrhiza, J. Nat. Prod.,* 51, 145, 1988.
3. **Massao, H., Yang, X.-W., Shu, Y.-Z., Kakiuchi, N., Tezuka, Y., Kikuchi, T. and Namba, T.,** New constituents of the aril of *Myristica fragrans, Chem. Pharm. Bull.,* 36, 648, 1988.
4. **Achenbach, H., Grob, J., Dominguez, X. A., Cano, G., Star, J. V., Brussolo, L. D., Muñoz, G., Salgado, F., and Lopes, L.,** Lignans, neolignans and norneolignans from *Krameria cystisoides, Phytochemistry,* 26, 1159, 1987.
5. **Aiba, C. J., Corrêa, R. G. C., and Gottlieb, O. R.,** Natural occurrence of Erdtman's dehydrodiisoeugenol, *Phytochemistry,* 12, 1163, 1973.
6. **Bowden, B. F., Ritchie, E., and Taylor, W. C.,** Isolation and structure determination of further eupomatenoid lignans from the bark of *Eupomatia laurina, Austr. J. Chem.,* 25, 2659, 1972.
7. **Stahl, E. and Ittel, I.,** Neue lipophile Benzofuranderivate aus Ratanhiawurzel, *Planta Med.,* 42, 144, 1981.

8. **Takanishi, M. and Takisawa, Y.,** New benzofurans related to egonol from immature seeds of *Styrax obassia, Phytochemistry,* 27, 1224, 1988.

9. **Gottlieb, O. R.,** Chemistry of neolignans with potential biological activity, in *New Natural Products and Plant Drugs with Pharmacological, Biological or Therapeutical Activity,* Wagner, H. and Wolff, P., Eds., Springer-Verlag, Berlin, 1977.

10. **Shen, T.-Y., Hwang, S.-B., Chang, M.-N., Doebber, T. W., Lam, M. H., Wu, M.-S., Wang, X., Han, G.-Q., and Li, R.-Z.,** Characterization of a platelet-activating factor receptor antagonist isolated from haifenteng *(Piper futokadsura):* specific inhibition of *in vitro* and *in vivo* platelet-activating factor-induced effects. *Proc. Natl. Acad. Sci U.S.A.,* 82, 672, 1985.

11. **Alvarenga, M. A. de, Brocksom, U., Gottlieb, O. R., Yoshida, M., Braz-Filho, R., and Figliuolo, R.,** Hydrobenzofuranoid-bicyclo[3.2.1]octanoid neolignan rearrangement, *J. Chem. Soc. Chem. Commun.,* 831, 1978.

12. **Gottlieb, O. R.,** Neolignans, *Prog. Chem. Org. Nat. Prod.,* 35, 1, 1978.

13. **Gottlieb, O. R. and Yoshida, M.,** Lignans and neolignans, in *Natural Products of Woody Plants—Chemicals Extraneous to the Lignocellulosic Cell Wall,* Rowe, J. W., Ed., Springer-Verlag, Berlin, 1989, Chap. 7.3.

14. **Gregson, M., Ollis, W. D., Redman, B. T., Sutherland, I. O., Dietrichs, H. H., and Gottlieb, O. R.,** Obtusastyrene and obtustyrene, cinnamylphenols from *Dalbergia retusa, Phytochemistry,* 17, 1395, 1978.

15. **Donnelly, B. J., Donnelly, D. M. X., O'Sullivan, A. M., and Prendergast, J. P.,** The isolation and structure of melanoxin. A new dihydrobenzofuran from *Dalbergia melanoxylon* Guill. and Perr. (Leguminosae), *Tetrahedron,* 25, 4409, 1969.

16. **Silva, M. S. da, Barbosa-Filho, J. M., Yoshida, M., and Gottlieb, O. R.,** Benzodioxane and β-aryloxy-arylpropane neolignans from *Licaria chrysophylla, Phytochemistry,* 28, 3477, 1989.

17. **Martinez V., J. C., Maia, J. G. S., Yoshida, M., and Gottlieb, O. R.,** Neolignans from an *Aniba* species, *Phytochemistry,* 19, 474, 1980.

18. **Whiting, D. A.,** Lignans and neolignans, *Nat. Prod. Rep.,* 2, 191, 1985.

19. **Yanez, X., de Diaz, A. M. P., and Diaz D. P. P.,** Neolignans from *Mezilaurus itauba, Phytochemistry,* 25, 1953, 1986.

20. **de Carvalho, M. G., Yoshida, M., Gottlieb, O. R., and Gottlieb, H. E.,** Bicyclooctanoid, carinatone and megaphone type neolignans from *Ocotea porosa, Phytochemistry,* 27, 2319, 1988.

21. **Boralle, N.,** Neolignanas e cinamoilamidas de *Licaria chrysophylla,* Dissertação de Mestrado, Instituto de Química da Universidade de São Paulo, São Paulo, 1986.

22. **Braz-Filho, R., Figliuolo, R., and Gottlieb, O. R.,** Neolignans from a *Nectandra* species, *Phytochemistry,* 19, 659, 1980.

23. **Khan, M. R., Gray, A. I., and Waterman, P. G.,** Neolignans from stem bark of *Ocotea veraguensis, Phytochemistry,* 26, 1155, 1987.

24. **Felicio, J. D'A., Motidome, M., Yoshida, M., and Gottlieb, O. R.,** Further neolignans from *Ocotea aciphylla, Phytochemistry,* 25, 1707, 1986.

25. **Barbosa-Filho, J. M., Yoshida, M., and Gottlieb, O. R.,** Neolignans from the fruits of *Licaria armeniaca, Phytochemistry,* 26, 319, 1987.

26. **Trevisan, L. M. V., Yoshida, M. and Gottlieb, O. R.,** Neolignans from *Aniba citrifolia, Phytochemistry,* 23, 701, 1984.

27. **Aiba, C. J., Fernandes, J. B., Gottlieb, O. R., and Maia, J. G. S.,** Neolignans from an *Aniba* species, *Phytochemistry,* 14, 1597, 1975.

28. **Dias, D. A., Yoshida, M., and Gottlieb, O. R.,** Further neolignans from *Ocotea porosa, Phytochemistry,* 25, 2613, 1986.

29. **Dias, S. M. C., Fernandes, J. B., Maia, J. G. S., Gottlieb, O. R., and Gottlieb, H. E.,** Eusiderins and other neolignans from an *Aniba* species, *Phytochemistry,* 25, 213, 1986.

30. **Trevisan, L. M. V., Yoshida, M., and Gottlieb, O. R.,** Hexahydrobenzofuranoid neolignans from an *Aniba* species, *Phytochemistry,* 23, 661, 1984.

31. **Aiba, C. J., Gottlieb, O. R., Maia, J. G. S., Pagliosa, F. M., and Yoshida, M.,** Benzofuranoid neolignans from *Licaria armeniaca, Phytochemistry,* 17, 2038, 1978.

32. **Chang, M.-N., Han, G.-Q., Arison, B. H., Springler, J. P., Hwang, S.-B., and Shen, T.-Y.,** Neolignans from *Piper futokadsura, Phytochemistry,* 24, 2079, 1985.

33. **Chen, C.-C., Huang, Y.-L., Chen, Y.-P., Hsu, H.-Y., and Kuo, Y.-H.,** Three new neolignans, farge-sones A, B and C, from the flower buds of *Magnolia fargesii, Chem. Pharm. Bull.,* 36, 1791, 1988.

34. **Romoff, P., Yoshida, M., and Gottlieb, O. R.,** Neolignans from *Ocotea aciphylla, Phytochemistry,* 23, 2101, 1984.

35. **Lopes, M. N., da Silva, M. S., Barbosa-Filho, J. M., Ferreira, Z. S., Yoshida, M., and Gottlieb, O. R.,** Unusual benzofuranoid neolignans from *Licaria chrysophylla, Phytochemistry,* 25, 2609, 1986.

36. **Ferreira, Z. S., Roque, N. F., Gottlieb, O. R., and Gottlieb, H. E.,** An unusual porosin type neolignan from *Licaria chrysophylla, Phytochemistry,* 21, 2756, 1982.

Part II
Synthetic PAF Antagonists

Chapter 4

STRUCTURE ACTIVITY RELATIONSHIPS IN CV-3988 AND CV-6209 PAF ANTAGONISTS SERIES

Muneo Takatani and Susumu Tsushima

INTRODUCTION

Since the identification of platelet activating factor (PAF) as glycero-3-phosphocholine,[1-3] a number of constitutional analogs of PAF have been reported.[4] They have been synthesized for three main purposes: (1) to prove the structural requirements for activity; (2) to enhance the desirable biological activities (e.g., hypotension), while diminishing or eliminating undesirable effects (e.g., platelet aggregation, anaphylaxis); and (3) to discover PAF antagonists.

Over the last several years we have also been involved in structure-activity studies of this important phospholipid. In these studies, we found CV-3988[5] (the first PAF antagonist) and CV-6209[6-7] (one of the most potent PAF antagonists known to date). In this chapter we have described the process used to find these PAF antagonists, their structure-activity relationships, and their biological activities.

BIOASSAY OF ANTI-PAF ACTION

PAF has a wide variety of potent biological actions: stimulation of platelets and leukocytes, bronchoconstriction, hypotension, negative inotropic cardiac effects, and effects which increase vascular permeability.[8-9]

To evaluate PAF antagonistic activities of compounds, we first examined their inhibitory effect on PAF-induced rabbit platelet aggregation *in vitro* as a first screening using the method of Born.[10] In the case of CV-6209, we then examined their inhibitory effects on PAF-induced hypotension in rats and PAF-induced death in mice as a second method of screening.

CV-3988

DISCOVERY OF CV-3988

Alkyl ether phospholipids of both natural and synthetic origin have attracted much attention in recent years due to their interesting biological activities. The most striking development in this field was, of course, the discovery of platelet activating factor (PAF). Another interesting development in this field was the discovery of the tumor inhibiting effects of the octadecyl ether analog of lysolecithin, ET-18-OMe (Figure 1) by Munder et al.[11] This compound has been shown to destroy tumor cells selectively and to have prophylactic and therapeutic effects on several experimental tumors. Tumor destruction by this compound is considered to be due to the disturbance of phospholipid metabolism in the tumor cells and activation of macrophages in the host.

In search of a better therapeutic agent, we focused our attention on a new series of synthetic phospholipids differing structurally from ET-18-OMe. Alkyl and alkylcarbamoyl phospholipids with a variety of aliphatic chains and polar head groups were synthesized for this purpose. These derivatives were found to possess antimicrobial activities (antifungal and antiprotozoal).[12-13] Subsequently, some alkyl phospholipids were found to induce differentiation of tumor cells *in vitro*[14] and to activate guinea pig peritoneal macrophages.[15]

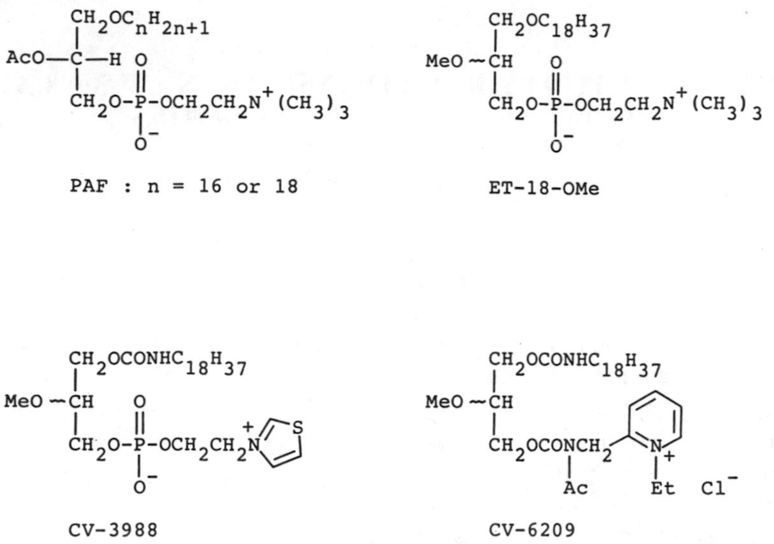

$CH_2OC_nH_{2n+1}$
AcO—C—H O
CH_2O-P-$OCH_2CH_2N^+(CH_3)_3$
O⁻

PAF : n = 16 or 18

$CH_2OC_{18}H_{37}$
MeO~CH O
CH_2O-P-$OCH_2CH_2N^+(CH_3)_3$
O⁻

ET-18-OMe

$CH_2OCONHC_{18}H_{37}$
MeO~CH O
CH_2O-P-$OCH_2CH_2N^+$⟨S⟩
O⁻

CV-3988

$CH_2OCONHC_{18}H_{37}$
MeO~CH
$CH_2OCONCH_2$-⟨N^+⟩ Cl⁻
Ac   Et

CV-6209

FIGURE 1.   Chemical structure of PAF-related compounds.

In the course of these studies, the determination of the structure of PAF was reported. We were very interested in the similarity of the structures of our compounds to that of PAF, so they were tested for their PAF-agonistic and antagonistic activities. CV-3988, the first PAF specific antagonist, was found among them.

STRUCTURE-ACTIVITY RELATIONSHIPS[16]

Phospholipid analogs and their PAF antagonist activities are shown in Table 1. Only compounds possessing an aromatic heterocycle such as thiazolium and pyridinium as the quaternary polar head base showed antagonist activity, while the phosphorylcholine derivatives had no inhibitory activity. Among those compounds, CV-3988 was the most potent.

The contribution of the glycerol backbone to the antagonist activity was also investigated. Modification of the glycerol moiety of CV-3988 led to complete loss of activity (Figure 2). From this result, it follows that in the phospholipid analogs the glycerol skeleton is also important for antagonist activity.

SYNTHESIS OF CV-3988[16]

The synthetic pathway for CV-3988 is shown in Figure 3A—C. For large scale production, we investigated alternative routes to prepare the alcohol 4 and CV-3988 more efficiently.

In our previous report,[5] benzylidene acetal 3 was hydrolyzed to 2-methylglycerol 5 and then treated with isocyanate. But in this reaction, the disubstituted analog 8 was also produced, and separation by chromatography was necessary. In an alternative route, compound 3 was treated with NBS in the presence of water to give benzoylglycerol 6, which was then treated with isocyanate followed by hydrolysis with a base to afford the desired alcohol 4. The overall yield from 3 was improved to 76%.

The other step that has been improved is the final one. Generally, phosphorylcholine analogs are synthesized by the reaction of bromoethyl phosphate and trimethylamine. In this case, the yield is generally satisfactory. But the reaction of bromoethyl phosphate with aromatic heterocycles, especially thiazole, is slow and the yield is poor. In the improved method, the phosphate 10 was condensed with the hydroxyethylthiazolium salt 11 using mesitylenesulfonyl chloride as a coupling reagent. The tosylate 11 is better in this reaction

TABLE 1

Lysolecithin Analogs and their Inhibitory Activity on PAF-Induced Rabbit Platelet Aggregation

$$CH_2\text{-}O\text{-}R_1$$
$$CH\text{-}O\text{-}R_2$$
$$CH_2O\text{-}\overset{O}{\underset{O}{P}}\text{-}OCH_2CH_2N^+(R_3)_3$$

R_1	R_2	$N^+(R_3)_3$	inhibition of PAF-induced platelet aggregation (%)	
			$3 \times 10^{-6} M$	$3 \times 10^{-5} M$
$CONHC_{18}H_{37}$	Me (CV-3988)	[1,3-thiazolium]	45	100
$CONHC_{18}H_{37}$	Me	[pyridinium]		95
$CONHC_{18}H_{37}$	Et	[1,3-thiazolium]		85
$C_{18}H_{37}$	Me	[pyridinium]		83
$CONHC_{18}H_{37}$	CH_2Ph	[1,3-thiazolium]		79
$CONHC_{18}H_{37}$	Me	[imidazolium-NMe]		56
$CONHC_{18}H_{37}$	Me	[isoquinolinium]		37
$CONHC_{18}H_{37}$	Me	N^+Me_3		0
$C_{18}H_{37}$	Me	N^+Me_3		0 (weak agonist)
$CONHC_{18}H_{37}$	Me	[N-Me pyrrolidinium]		0

than the halide, for it is more soluble in an organic solvent. The isolated yield was improved to 68%.

BIOLOGICAL ACTIVITY OF CV-3988
PAF Antagonist Activity of CV-3988 *In Vitro* and *In Vivo*[5]

CV-3988 inhibits PAF-induced platelet aggregation, but has no effect on the aggregation induced by arachidonic acid, ADP, collagen, or calcium ionophore (Figure 4).

As shown in Figure 5, PAF(1 μg/kg i.v.)-induced hypotension in rats was also inhibited dose dependently by the administration of CV-3988(0.05—1 mg/kg i.v.). The hypotensive action induced by acetylcholine, arachidonic acid, bradykinin, isoprotenerol, and histamine was not suppressed by CV-3988.

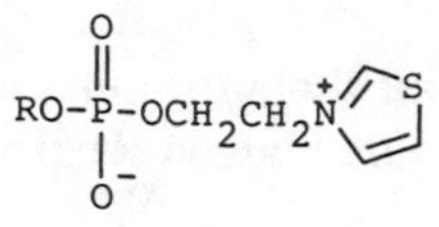

$$RO-\overset{\overset{\displaystyle O}{\|}}{\underset{\underset{\displaystyle O^-}{|}}{P}}-OCH_2CH_2\overset{+}{N}\diagdown S$$

R	R
$CH_2OCONHC_{18}H_{37}$ CH_2 CH_2-	$CH_2OCONHC_{18}H_{37}$ CH_2-
	$CH_2OCH_2CH_2OC_{18}H_{37}$ CH_2-
$CH_2OC_9H_{19}$ $CHOC_9H_{19}$ CH_2-	$C_{18}H_{37}-$

FIGURE 2.   Analogs of CV-3988. No inhibitory activity at 3×10^{-5} *M*.

Effects of CV-3988 on Endotoxin-Induced Hypotension and Death in Rats[17]

In experimental animal models, CV-3988 has been utilized to demonstrate important evidence for the involvement of PAF in several diseases. The possible role of PAF in endotoxin shock has been reported by researchers in our Biology Laboratories.

As shown in Figure 6, endotoxin (*E. coli* No.0111 B4, Difco, 15 mg/kg,i.v.) gradually reduced blood pressure which reached a nadir 5 to 10 min after the injection. Thereafter the pressure recovered slowly but recovery was not complete even after 60 min. This endotoxin-induced hypotension was reversed rapidly by CV-3988 in a dose-related manner. Similar results have been reported using the other PAF antagonists, kadsurenone,[18] SRI-63-072,[19] BN-52021,[20] and WEB 2086.[21]

Figure 7 shows the time course of the survival rate during the 30 h following the simultaneous injection of endotoxin (5 mg/kg i.v.) and CV-3988 (1 to 10 mg/kg i.v.). CV-3988 at a dose of 10 mg/kg improved the survival rate for 20 h or more after endotoxin injection. The survival rates at 20 h were 29% for the control (endotoxin alone) and 67% for the group treated with CV-3988.

These results suggest that PAF might be an endogenous mediator and play a pivotal role in the pathogenesis of endotoxin shock.

Effect of CV-3988 on Endotoxin-Induced Disseminated Intravascular Coagulation in Rats[22]

Disseminated intravascular coagulation (DIC) is a pathophysiological syndrome induced by endotoxemia and neoplasia. The formation of fibrin thrombi, the consumption of specific plasma proteins, reduction of platelets and activation of the fibrinolytic system occur in cases of DIC.

The i.v. infusion of endotoxin (0.25 mg/kg/h for 4 h) induced DIC in rats; thrombocytopenia, prolongation of prothrombin time and partial thromboplastin time, hypofibrinogenemia and elevated levels of fibrinogen/fibrin degradation products were observed. As shown in Figure 8, CV-3988(2 mg/kg bolus 5 min before endotoxin and 1 or 2 mg/kg/h infusion for 4 h with endotoxin) improved all the parameters that had been altered by endotoxin.

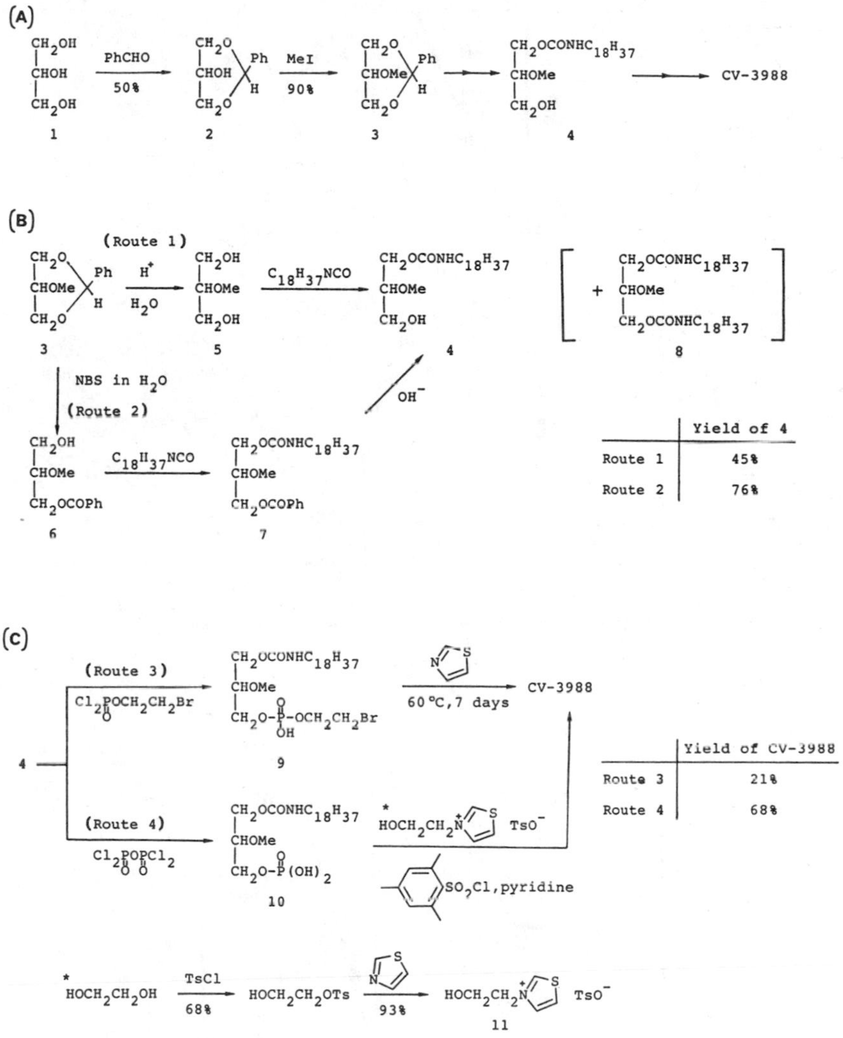

(A)

CH_2OH / $CHOH$ / CH_2OH — $\xrightarrow[50\%]{PhCHO}$ — CH_2O/$CHOH$/CH_2O $\diagdown$Ph$\diagup$H — $\xrightarrow[90\%]{MeI}$ — CH_2O/$CHOMe$/CH_2O $\diagdown$Ph$\diagup$H — $\longrightarrow$ — $CH_2OCONHC_{18}H_{37}$/$CHOMe$/CH_2OH — $\longrightarrow$ CV-3988

1   2   3   4

(B)

(Route 1)

CH_2O/$CHOMe$/CH_2O $\diagdown$Ph$\diagup$H — $\xrightarrow[H_2O]{H^+}$ — CH_2OH/$CHOMe$/CH_2OH — $\xrightarrow{C_{18}H_{37}NCO}$ — $CH_2OCONHC_{18}H_{37}$/$CHOMe$/CH_2OH — $\left[+ \quad CH_2OCONHC_{18}H_{37}/CHOMe/CH_2OCONHC_{18}H_{37} \right]$

3   5   4   8

NBS in H_2O

(Route 2)

CH_2OH/$CHOMe$/CH_2OCOPh — $\xrightarrow{C_{18}H_{37}NCO}$ — $CH_2OCONHC_{18}H_{37}$/$CHOMe$/CH_2OCOPh $\xrightarrow{OH^-}$ (to 4)

6   7

	Yield of 4
Route 1	45%
Route 2	76%

(C)

(Route 3)

$Cl_2POCH_2CH_2Br$ (with O) — from 4 — $CH_2OCONHC_{18}H_{37}$/$CHOMe$/$CH_2O-\overset{O}{\underset{OH}{P}}-OCH_2CH_2Br$ — $\xrightarrow[60°C, 7 days]{N\diagdown S}$ — CV-3988

9

(Route 4)

Cl_2POPCl_2 (with O O) — $CH_2OCONHC_{18}H_{37}$/$CHOMe$/$CH_2O-\overset{O}{P}(OH)_2$

10

$HOCH_2CH_2\overset{+}{N}\diagdown S$ TsO⁻ , SO_2Cl, pyridine

	Yield of CV-3988
Route 3	21%
Route 4	68%

$HOCH_2CH_2OH$ — $\xrightarrow[68\%]{TsCl}$ — $HOCH_2CH_2OTs$ — $\xrightarrow[93\%]{N\diagdown S}$ — $HOCH_2CH_2\overset{+}{N}\diagdown S$ TsO⁻

11

FIGURE 3. (A) Synthetic route for CV-3988. (B) Improvement of the step 3→4. (C) Improvement of the step 4→CV-3988.

Protective Effect of CV-3988 on IgE-Mediated Anaphylactic Shock in Mice[23]

Mice, immunized with bovine serum albumin (BSA) and killed *Bordetella pertussis*, died within 60 min after a challenge with BSA. CV-3988 (1 to 10 mg/kg) improved the survival rate of mice partially, but significantly, in a dose-dependent manner (Figure 9).

CV-6209

In a continuation of our effort to prepare more potent PAF antagonists, we began examining the compounds in which the charged phosphate moiety of PAF was replaced with another functional group.[24-26] Several groups reported PAF antagonists in which the phosphate moiety of CV-3988 was replaced with an ether or ester linkage (Ro 18-7953, Ro 18-8736, Ro 19-1400, Ro 19-3704, SRI 63-119, ONO-6240).[27-29] Among these antagonists, ONO-6240 is about ten times more potent than CV-3988 *in vitro*. However, the inhibitory effect of ONO-6240 on PAF-induced hypotension in rats is only 1.5 to 2.5 times more potent than that of CV-3988.[6]

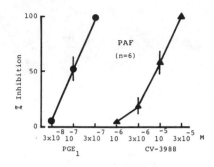

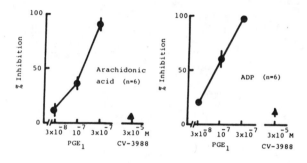

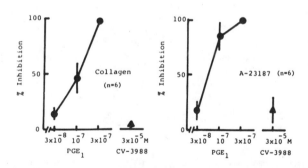

FIGURE 4. Effects of CV-3988 and PGE_1 on rabbit platelet aggregation induced by various drugs. The experiments were done with PRP obtained from six rabbits. The concentration of the drugs and percent aggregation are as follows: PAF, 0.03 μM, 62 ± 2%; arachidonic acid, 80—100 μM, 70 ± 1%; ADP, 10 μM, 52 ± 4%; collagen, 10—30 $\mu g/ml$, 72 ± 3%; A-23187, 3 μM, 68 ± 2%.

In order to obtain more potent PAF antagonists both *in vitro* and *in vivo,* we undertook the synthesis of the new analogs of PAF in which the phosphate moiety were replaced with a carbamoyl linkage (Figure 10).

SYNTHESIS OF *N*-ACETYLCARBAMOYL DERIVATIVE OF PAF

In the acetylation of the hydroxy group of the intermediate **13**, the carbamoyl group at the 3-position was acetylated simultaneously to give the diacetyl compound **14**, which was then converted to the quaternary derivative **15** by the reaction with methyl iodide. Compound **15** was found to have potent inhibitory activity on PAF-induced rabbit platelet aggregation *in vitro,* that is, about nine times more potent than that of CV-3988. The corresponding

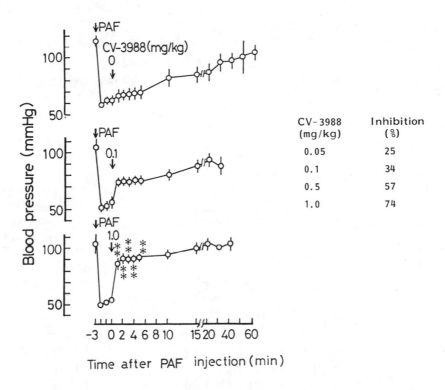

FIGURE 5. Reversal of PAF-induced hypotension by CV-3988 in anesthetized rats. PAF(1 µg/kg) was given at −3 min and CV-3988(dose in mg/kg,iv) at zero min. ** $p < 0.01$. vs. the values of the control (Student's t-test).

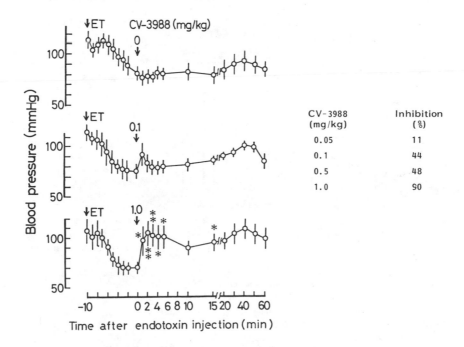

FIGURE 6. Reversal of endotoxin (ET)-induced hypotension by CV-3988 in anesthetized rats. ET(15 mg/kg) was given at −10 min and CV-3988(dose in mg/kg,iv) at zero min. * $p < 0.05$, ** $p < 0.01$ vs. the values of the control (Student's t-test).

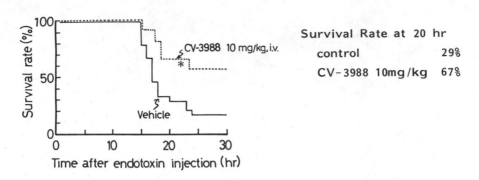

FIGURE 7. Protective effects of CV-3988 on endotoxin-induced death in conscious rats. Endotoxin(15 mg/kg) and CV-3988 were given simultaneously. * $p < 0.05$ vs. the values of the control (X^2-test).

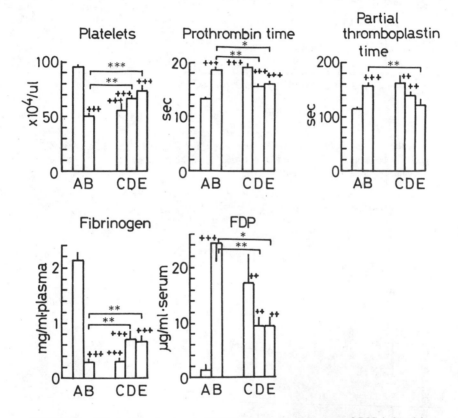

FIGURE 8. Effects of pretreatment of CV-3988 on the parameters of DIC induced by endotoxin(ET) in anesthetized rats. ET and CV-3988 were given in bolus or infusion in the rats.

A (n = 9): 0.9 % saline (0.6 ml/h) was infused for 4 h (normal group).

B (n = 26): ET(0.25 mg/kg/h) was infused for 4 h (control group).

C (n = 9): CV-3988(2 mg/kg, bolus) was given before ET.

D (n = 11): CV-3988(2 mg/kg, bolus) was given before ET and infused (1 mg/kg/h) for 4 h with ET.

E (n = 8): CV-3988(2 mg/kg, bolus) was given before ET and infused (2 mg/kg/h) for 4 h with ET.

[++] $p < 0.01$, [+++] $p < 0.001$ as compared with the normal group A (Student's t-test).

* $p < 0.05$, ** $p < 0.01$, *** $p < 0.001$ as compared with the control group B (Student's t-test). FDP: fibrinogen and fibrin degradation products.

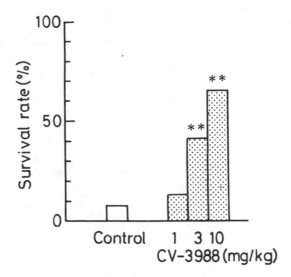

FIGURE 9. Protective effects of CV-3988 on IgE-mediated anaphylactic shock in mice. ** $p<0.01$ vs. the value of the control (X^2-test).

carbamoyl derivative **19** was synthesized in a different manner. This compound also showed PAF antagonist activity *in vitro,* but was less potent than **15**.

On the basis of this finding, a study was carried out to elucidate the structure-activity profile of the PAF analogs in which the phosphate moiety had been replaced with an acylcarbamoyl group as PAF specific antagonists.

The mechanism of the acetylation of the carbamoyl group at the 3-position was not further investigated; however, it was revealed that the reaction rate was strongly affected by the nature of the amino group, basicity of the tertiary amine and the distance between the carbamoyl group and the amino group (Table 2). Thus the acetylation of compounds **27 c,e** bearing a weakly basic amino group as the polar head moiety required considerably longer reaction time and higher reaction temperature than did compounds **21a** and **27a** which possess a more basic amino group. The reaction rate of the dimethylaminoethyl derivative **21a** was much faster than that of the dimethylaminopropyl derivative **21b**. In the case of acetylation of **21a,b** and **27a—g**, the carbamoyl group at the 1-position was not acetylated under the reaction conditions. From these results, the mechanism of this acetylation reaction might be explained as shown in Figure 11.

The tertiary amino group of A is acetylated with acetic anhydride to afford the quaternary ammonium salt (B), then the acetyl group is transferred to the carbamoyl group by an intramolecular rearrangement to give the acetylcarbamoyl derivative (C). A similar rearrangement reaction of quaternary ammonium salt has been reported.[30]

SYNTHESIS AND STRUCTURE-ACTIVITY RELATIONSHIPS OF N-ACYLCARBAMOYL DERIVATIVES OF CV-3988

The different types of PAF analogs modified in the phosphate moiety were synthesized by the method shown in Figure 12. Since variation of the substituents at the 1- and 2-positions did not cause marked change in inhibitory activity, as seen in the comparison of **26a** with **15**, modification of the substituent at the 3-position was explored using the same substituent pattern at the 1- and 2-positions as in CV-3988 in subsequent studies.

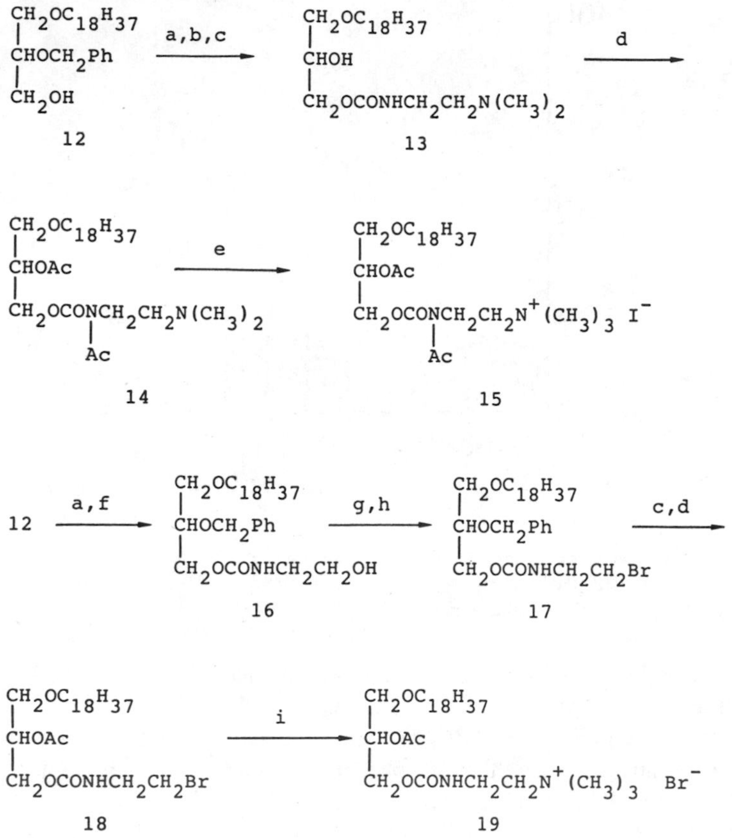

$$\begin{array}{c}
\text{CH}_2\text{OC}_{18}\text{H}_{37} \\
\text{CHOCH}_2\text{Ph} \\
\text{CH}_2\text{OH}
\end{array}
\quad \xrightarrow{\text{a,b,c}} \quad
\begin{array}{c}
\text{CH}_2\text{OC}_{18}\text{H}_{37} \\
\text{CHOH} \\
\text{CH}_2\text{OCONHCH}_2\text{CH}_2\text{N(CH}_3)_2
\end{array}
\quad \xrightarrow{\text{d}}$$

12   13

$$\begin{array}{c}
\text{CH}_2\text{OC}_{18}\text{H}_{37} \\
\text{CHOAc} \\
\text{CH}_2\text{OCONCH}_2\text{CH}_2\text{N(CH}_3)_2 \\
\quad\quad\;\;\, |\\
\quad\quad\;\;\, \text{Ac}
\end{array}
\quad \xrightarrow{\text{e}} \quad
\begin{array}{c}
\text{CH}_2\text{OC}_{18}\text{H}_{37} \\
\text{CHOAc} \\
\text{CH}_2\text{OCONCH}_2\text{CH}_2\overset{+}{\text{N}}(\text{CH}_3)_3 \; \text{I}^- \\
\quad\quad\;\;\, |\\
\quad\quad\;\;\, \text{Ac}
\end{array}$$

14   15

$$12 \quad \xrightarrow{\text{a,f}} \quad
\begin{array}{c}
\text{CH}_2\text{OC}_{18}\text{H}_{37} \\
\text{CHOCH}_2\text{Ph} \\
\text{CH}_2\text{OCONHCH}_2\text{CH}_2\text{OH}
\end{array}
\quad \xrightarrow{\text{g,h}} \quad
\begin{array}{c}
\text{CH}_2\text{OC}_{18}\text{H}_{37} \\
\text{CHOCH}_2\text{Ph} \\
\text{CH}_2\text{OCONHCH}_2\text{CH}_2\text{Br}
\end{array}
\quad \xrightarrow{\text{c,d}}$$

16   17

$$\begin{array}{c}
\text{CH}_2\text{OC}_{18}\text{H}_{37} \\
\text{CHOAc} \\
\text{CH}_2\text{OCONHCH}_2\text{CH}_2\text{Br}
\end{array}
\quad \xrightarrow{\text{i}} \quad
\begin{array}{c}
\text{CH}_2\text{OC}_{18}\text{H}_{37} \\
\text{CHOAc} \\
\text{CH}_2\text{OCONHCH}_2\text{CH}_2\overset{+}{\text{N}}(\text{CH}_3)_3 \quad \text{Br}^-
\end{array}$$

18   19

a): $ClCO_2Ph$, pyridine;   b): $H_2NCH_2CH_2N(CH_3)_2$; c): H_2, Pd/C;

d): Ac_2O, Et_3N; e): CH_3I; f): $H_2NCH_2CH_2OH$; g): p-TsCl/Et_3N;

h): LiBr; i): Me_3N/toluene

FIGURE 10.   Synthesis of *N*-acetyl derivatives of PAF.

The Effects of the Distance Between the *N*-Acetylcarbamoyl Group and the Polar Head Moiety

Compound **26b**, which has three methylene bridges between the *N*-acetylcarbamoyl group and the polar head moiety, was synthesized from **20** by the reaction with 3-dimethyl-aminopropylamine followed by acetylation with acetic anhydride in pyridine at 100°C and treatment with methyl iodide. As shown in Table 3, increasing the distance between the *N*-acetylcarbamoyl group and the polar head moiety (compound **26b**) resulted in a decrease in PAF induced platelet aggregation *in vitro*, compared to **26a**.

The Effects of the N-Substituent on the Carbamoyl Moiety at the 3-Position

To confirm the contribution of the acetyl group on the carbamoyl moiety to PAF an-tagonist activity, compound **21a** was converted to the quaternary derivative **23** with methyl iodide. Next, the effects of the N-substituent on the carbamoyl moiety were examined by replacing the acetyl group with methyl, propionyl, butyryl, methoxycarbonyl, and some carbamoyl groups (Figure 12).

As shown in Table 3, the carbamoyl derivatives of PAF (**19** and **23**) showed comparable PAF antagonist activity *in vitro* to CV-3988. It was evident that introduction of an acetyl

TABLE 2

N-Acetylation of the Carbamoyl Group at the 3-Position with Acetic Anhydride in Pyridine

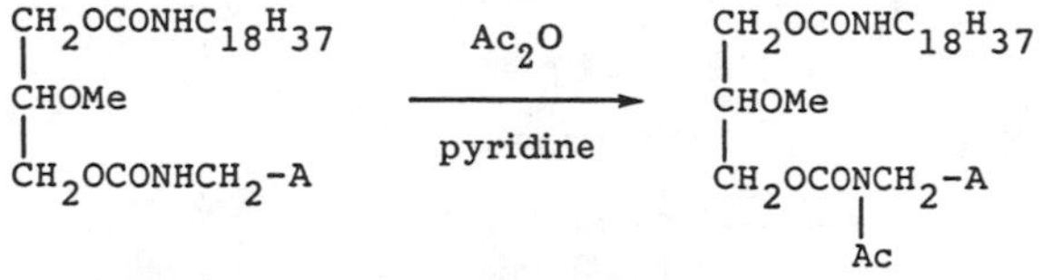

$$
\begin{array}{c}
CH_2OCONHC_{18}H_{37} \\
| \\
CHOMe \\
| \\
CH_2OCONHCH_2-A
\end{array}
\xrightarrow[\text{pyridine}]{Ac_2O}
\begin{array}{c}
CH_2OCONHC_{18}H_{37} \\
| \\
CHOMe \\
| \\
CH_2OCONCH_2-A \\
| \\
Ac
\end{array}
$$

compd	A	Reaction Conditions	Yield[a], %
21a	CH_2NMe_2	RT^b , 6h	95
21b	$CH_2CH_2NMe_2$	RT^b	NR^c
		100 °C , 24 h	29
27a	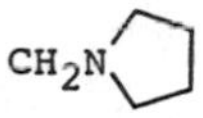 CH_2N⟨ ⟩	RT^b , 6 h	89
27c	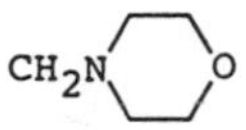 CH_2N⟨ O⟩	RT^b	NR^c
		100 °C , 24 h	43
27e	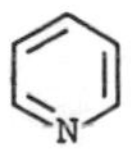 (pyridine)	110 °C , 72 h	80

[a] Yields were not optimized.
[b] RT = room temperature.
[c] NR = no reaction.

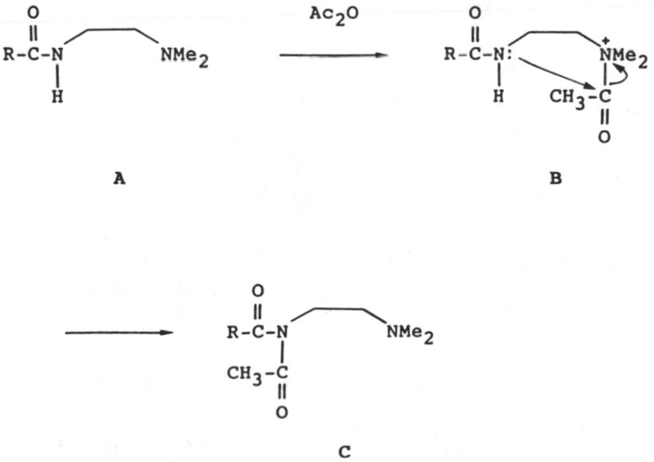

FIGURE 11. Proposed mechanism of trans-acetylation.

group into the carbamoyl moiety at the 3-position resulted in a large increase in potency in blocking PAF induced platelet aggregation *in vitro* (**15** and **26a**, compared with **19** and **23**, respectively). Replacement of the acetyl group on the carbamoyl moiety with methyl, pro-pionyl, butyryl, methoxycarbonyl, or some carbamoyl groups resulted in a decrease in PAF

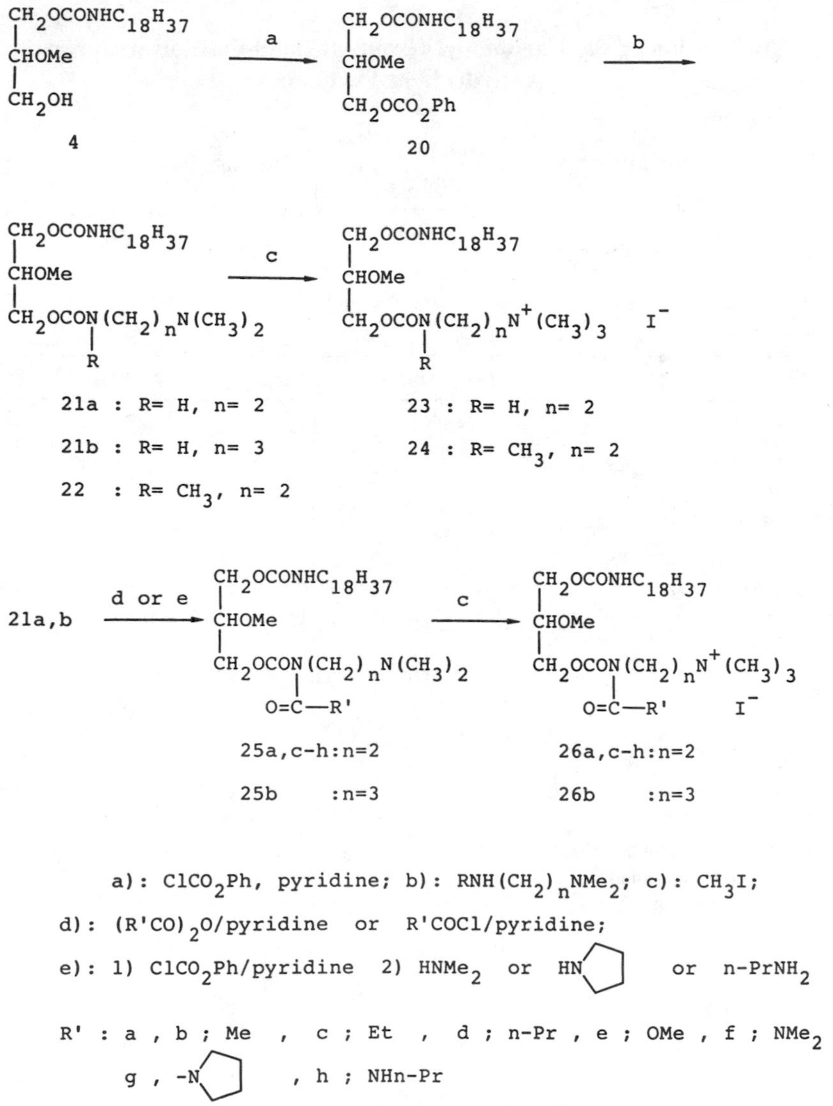

$$\underset{4}{\overset{\displaystyle CH_2OCONHC_{18}H_{37}}{\underset{\displaystyle CH_2OH}{\overset{\displaystyle |}{\underset{\displaystyle |}{CHOMe}}}}} \quad \xrightarrow{\text{a}} \quad \underset{20}{\overset{\displaystyle CH_2OCONHC_{18}H_{37}}{\underset{\displaystyle CH_2OCO_2Ph}{\overset{\displaystyle |}{\underset{\displaystyle |}{CHOMe}}}}} \quad \xrightarrow{\text{b}}$$

$$\overset{\displaystyle CH_2OCONHC_{18}H_{37}}{\underset{\displaystyle CH_2OCON(CH_2)_nN(CH_3)_2}{\overset{\displaystyle |}{\underset{\displaystyle | \atop R}{CHOMe}}}} \quad \xrightarrow{\text{c}} \quad \overset{\displaystyle CH_2OCONHC_{18}H_{37}}{\underset{\displaystyle CH_2OCON(CH_2)_nN^+(CH_3)_3 \quad I^-}{\overset{\displaystyle |}{\underset{\displaystyle | \atop R}{CHOMe}}}}$$

21a : R= H, n= 2   23 : R= H, n= 2

21b : R= H, n= 3   24 : R= CH$_3$, n= 2

22 : R= CH$_3$, n= 2

$$21a,b \quad \xrightarrow{\text{d or e}} \quad \overset{\displaystyle CH_2OCONHC_{18}H_{37}}{\underset{\displaystyle \underset{O=C-R'}{CH_2OCON(CH_2)_nN(CH_3)_2}}{\overset{\displaystyle |}{\underset{\displaystyle |}{CHOMe}}}} \quad \xrightarrow{\text{c}} \quad \overset{\displaystyle CH_2OCONHC_{18}H_{37}}{\underset{\displaystyle \underset{O=C-R' \quad I^-}{CH_2OCON(CH_2)_nN^+(CH_3)_3}}{\overset{\displaystyle |}{\underset{\displaystyle |}{CHOMe}}}}$$

25a,c-h:n=2   26a,c-h:n=2

25b   :n=3   26b   :n=3

a): ClCO$_2$Ph, pyridine; b): RNH(CH$_2$)$_n$NMe$_2$; c): CH$_3$I;

d): (R'CO)$_2$O/pyridine or R'COCl/pyridine;

e): 1) ClCO$_2$Ph/pyridine 2) HNMe$_2$ or HN⬠ or n-PrNH$_2$

R' : a , b ; Me , c ; Et , d ; n-Pr , e ; OMe , f ; NMe$_2$

g , -N⬠   , h ; NHn-Pr

FIGURE 12.   Synthesis of *N*-acylcarbamoyl derivatives of CV-3988.

antagonist potency. The introduction of methyl or larger acyl substituents such as butyryl, pyrrolidinocarbonyl, or *n*-propylcarbamoyl group led to even greater decreases in potency (**24**, **26d**, **26g**, and **26h**).

The Effects of the Polar Head Base

To evaluate the effects of the polar head base on PAF antagonist activity, compounds possessing a cyclic ammonium moiety as the polar head group were synthesized (Figure 13).

As shown in Tables 4 and 5, compounds **29d,e** in which the nitrogen atom of the polar head was incorporated into the ring system showed more potent PAF antagonist activity than the trimethylammonium derivative **26a**. Especially, the pyridinium methyl derivative **29e** was ten times more potent than **26a** (Table 4). Since the thiazolium group was the best polar head base for PAF antagonist activity in the case of CV-3988, thiazolium derivatives

TABLE 3
Inhibitory Activity on PAF-Induced Rabbit Platelet Aggregation

$$CH_2-O-R_1$$
$$CH-O-R_2$$
$$CH_2OCON(CH_2)_mN^+(CH_3)_3 \quad X^-$$
$$R_3$$

compd	R_1	R_2	R_3	X	m	platelet IC_{50} (μM)
CV-3988						7.8 (n=6)
15	$C_{18}H_{37}$	Ac	Ac	I	2	0.88 (n=2)
19	$C_{18}H_{37}$	Ac	H	Br	2	8.4 (n=2)
23	$CONHC_{18}H_{37}$	Me	H	I	2	14 (n=2)
24	$CONHC_{18}H_{37}$	Me	Me	I	2	8.2 (n=2)
26a	$CONHC_{18}H_{37}$	Me	Ac	I	2	1.5 (n=2)
26b	$CONHC_{18}H_{37}$	Me	Ac	I	3	8.5 (n=2)
26c	$CONHC_{18}H_{37}$	Me	COEt	I	2	5.6 (n=2)
26d	$CONHC_{18}H_{37}$	Me	COnPr	I	2	7.8 (n=2)
26e	$CONHC_{18}H_{37}$	Me	CO_2Me	I	2	2.3 (n=2)
26f	$CONHC_{18}H_{37}$	Me	$CONMe_2$	I	2	5.8 (n=2)
26g	$CONHC_{18}H_{37}$	Me	CON⬠	I	2	8.6 (n=2)
26h	$CONHC_{18}H_{37}$	Me	CONHnPr	I	2	> 30 (n=2)

Note: The n values are the number of experiments.

29f and **29g** were synthesized. These compounds had approximately the same potency as the corresponding pyridinium derivative **29e** (Table 5).

The Effects of the Substituent on the Nitrogen Atom of the Pyridinium Moiety

To investigate the effects of the substituent on the nitrogen atom of the pyridinium moiety, compounds **30, 31**, and **32** were prepared by the reaction of **28e** with ethyl iodide, n-propyl iodide and n-butyl iodide, respectively, followed by treatment with ion exchange resin. The thiazolium derivatives **33** and **34** which were substituted with an ethyl group at the nitrogen atom of the polar head moiety were also synthesized by the reaction of **28f,g** with ethyl iodide, followed by treatment with ion exchange resin (in the case of **28g**).

As shown in Table 5, modification of the substituent on the nitrogen atom of the pyridinium moiety resulted in an increase in reducing PAF induced platelet aggregation (**30, 31**, and **32**), and the ethyl group appeared to be optimal. Similarly, the thiazolium derivatives substituted with an ethyl group at the nitrogen atom also had strong PAF antagonist activity (**33** and **34**).

Compounds with strong PAF antagonist activity *in vitro* were further evaluated by measuring their inhibitory effect on PAF induced hypotension in rats. As shown in Table 5, compounds **30, 33**, and **34** completely inhibited PAF induced hypotension at a dose of 0.1 mg/kg after 5 min. It was noteworthy that these N-ethyl derivatives were about ten times

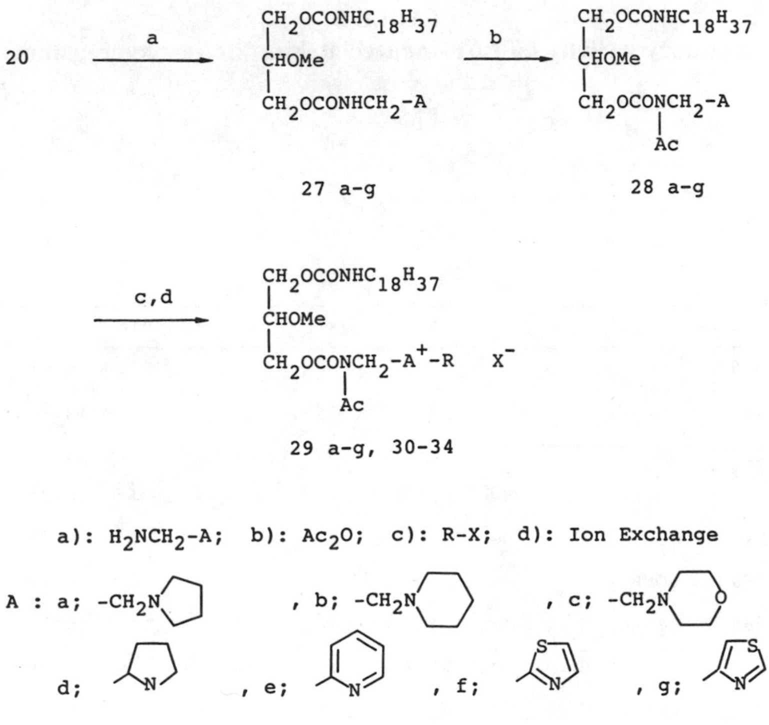

$$20 \xrightarrow{a} \begin{array}{l} CH_2OCONHC_{18}H_{37} \\ | \\ CHOMe \\ | \\ CH_2OCONHCH_2\text{-}A \end{array} \xrightarrow{b} \begin{array}{l} CH_2OCONHC_{18}H_{37} \\ | \\ CHOMe \\ | \\ CH_2OCONCH_2\text{-}A \\ \qquad\qquad | \\ \qquad\qquad Ac \end{array}$$

27 a-g   28 a-g

$$\xrightarrow{c,d} \begin{array}{l} CH_2OCONHC_{18}H_{37} \\ | \\ CHOMe \\ | \\ CH_2OCONCH_2\text{-}A^+\text{-}R \quad X^- \\ \qquad\qquad | \\ \qquad\qquad Ac \end{array}$$

29 a-g, 30-34

a): H_2NCH_2-A;   b): Ac_2O;   c): R-X;   d): Ion Exchange

A : a; -CH₂N⟨pyrrolidine⟩   , b; -CH₂N⟨piperidine⟩   , c; -CH₂N⟨morpholine⟩

d; ⟨pyrrolidine-N⟩   , e; ⟨pyridine-N⟩   , f; ⟨thiazole⟩   , g; ⟨thiazole⟩

FIGURE 13.   Modification of the polar head base.

TABLE 4
Inhibitory Activity of PAF-Induced Rabbit
Platelet Aggregation

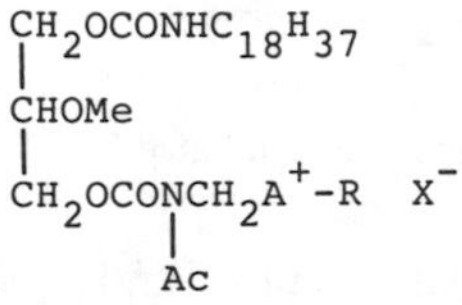

$$\begin{array}{l} CH_2OCONHC_{18}H_{37} \\ | \\ CHOMe \\ | \\ CH_2OCONCH_2A^+\text{-}R \quad X^- \\ \qquad\qquad | \\ \qquad\qquad Ac \end{array}$$

compd	A^+-R	X	platelet IC_{50} (μM)
29a	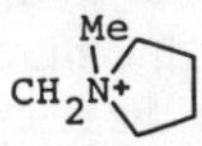 CH_2N^+⟨pyrrolidine, Me⟩	I	1.1 (n=2)
29b	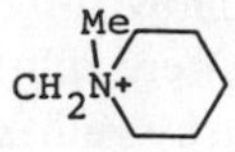 CH_2N^+⟨piperidine, Me⟩	I	5.4 (n=2)
29c	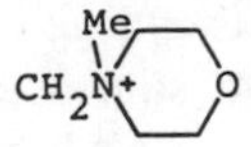 CH_2N^+⟨morpholine, Me⟩	I	9.2 (n=2)
29d	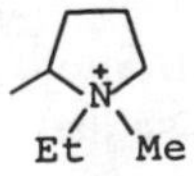 ⟨pyrrolidine ring N^+, Et, Me⟩	I	0.67 (n=2)
29e	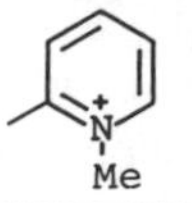 ⟨pyridine N^+, Me⟩	Cl	0.20 (n=2)

Note: The n values are the number of experiments.

TABLE 5
Inhibitory Activity on PAF-Induced Rabbit Platelet Aggregation and PAF-Induced Hypotension in Rats

$$CH_2OCONHC_{18}H_{37}$$
$$CHOMe$$
$$CH_2OCONCH_2\text{-(pyridinium)}N^+\text{-}R \quad X^-$$
$$Ac$$

29e,30-32

$$CH_2OCONHC_{18}H_{37}$$
$$CHOMe$$
$$CH_2OCONCH_2\text{-(thiazolium)}N^+\text{-}R \quad X^-$$
$$Ac$$

29f,33

$$CH_2OCONHC_{18}H_{37}$$
$$CHOMe$$
$$CH_2OCONCH_2\text{-(thiazolium)}N^+\text{-}R \quad X^-$$
$$Ac$$

29g,34

Compd	R	X	Platelet IC$_{50}$ (μM)	Inhibition of PAF hypotention (%)[a]			
				dose (mg/kg)	5 min	60 min	120 min
29e ⇌	Me	Cl	0.20 (n = 2)	1.0 (n = 2)	82	39	33
30 ⇌	Et	Cl	0.075 (n = 8)	0.1 (n = 5)	100	55	34
(R)-(−)-30	Et	Cl	0.084 (n = 2)	0.1 (n = 3)	100	36	20
(S)-(+)-30	Et	Cl	0.091 (n = 2)	0.1 (n = 2)	100	54	17
31	nPr	Cl	0.094 (n = 2)	0.1 (n = 2)	45	0	
32	nBu	Cl	0.11 (n = 2)	1.0 (n = 2)	100	0	
29f	Me	I	0.41 (n = 2)	1.0 (n = 1)	100	100	30
				0.1 (n = 2)	43	6	0
33	Et	I	0.096 (n = 2)	0.1 (n = 2)	100	3	0
29g	Me	I	0.10 (n = 2)	1.0 (n = 2)	92	29	4
34	Et	Cl	0.092 (n = 2)	0.1 (n = 2)	100	40	14

Note: The n values are the number of experiments.

[a] PAF(0.3 μg/kg,i.v.) was first injected twice at an interval of 20 min. Twenty minutes after the second injection, test compounds (one dose per rat for one compound) were given i.v. and PAF was injected 5, 60, and 120 min after the compound. The hypotension induced by the second injection of PAF was defined as 100 and the percent inhibition of the PAF-induced hypotension by test compounds was estimated. The standard deviation of the mean of these results were less than 5%.

more potent than the corresponding *N*-methyl derivatives. Consequently, compounds **30** and **34** were selected for further evaluation, and their protective effect against PAF-induced sudden death in mice was evaluated. Since a long-lasting effect is desirable for pharmaceutical usage, the duration of action was evaluated in this assay. As shown in Table 6, the duration of action of the pyridinium derivative **30** was longer than that of the thiazolium derivative **34**. The protective effect of **30** at a dose of 1 mg/kg continued even after 24 h.

SYNTHESIS AND PAF ANTAGONIST ACTIVITIES OF (R)-(−)- AND (S)-(+)-CV-6209

PAF has the R configuration at the 2-position. Reversing of the chiral center to the S configuration leads to a great decrease in the activity of PAF.[31] In order to examine the enantiospecificity at the 2-position in PAF antagonist activities, (R)-(−)-6209 and (S)-(+)-6209 were synthesized from (S)-(−)-**4** and (R)-(+)-**4** which were prepared as outlined in Figure 14.

As shown in Table 5, no significant differences were observed in the PAF antagonist activity *in vitro* or in the inhibitory effect on PAF induced hypotension *in vivo* between (RS)-6209 and its stereoisomers (R)-(−)-6209 and (S)-(+)-6209. Similar results have been reported by the Sandoz group (SRI 63-072 and SRI 63-119[28]) and by the Universite Paris/Roussel-Uclaf group.[32] Recently, Leo Pharmaceutical Products' group reported two achiral PAF antagonists, GS-1065-180 and GS-1160-180.[33] Thus, these results suggest that

TABLE 6
Time Course of Protecting Effect of 30
and 34 on PAF-Induced Death in Mice

Compound	Dose (mg/kg)	Survival rate (%)[a]	
		8 h	24 h
30	1	100**[b]	69**
34	1	75**	25

[a] Test compounds were given i.v. 8 and 24 h before the injection of PAF (50 $\mu g/kg$,i.v.). Numbers of mice were 142(control) and 16(30 and 34). The survival rate was recorded 60 min after the injection of PAF and was 22% for control.

[b] **$p < 0.01$ vs. the value of the control (X^2-test).

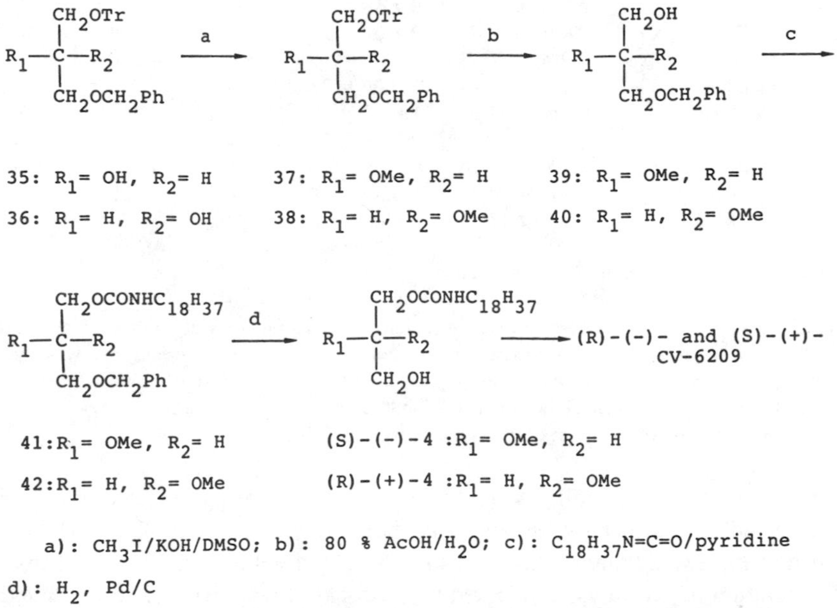

R_1—C—R_2 diagrams:

35: R_1= OH, R_2= H   37: R_1= OMe, R_2= H   39: R_1= OMe, R_2= H

36: R_1= H, R_2= OH   38: R_1= H, R_2= OMe   40: R_1= H, R_2= OMe

41: R_1= OMe, R_2= H   (S)-(-)-4 : R_1= OMe, R_2= H

42: R_1= H, R_2= OMe   (R)-(+)-4 : R_1= H, R_2= OMe

a): $CH_3I/KOH/DMSO$; b): 80 % $AcOH/H_2O$; c): $C_{18}H_{37}N=C=O$/pyridine

d): H_2, Pd/C

FIGURE 14.   Synthesis of (R)-(−)- and (S)-(+)-CV-6209.

the chirality of the carbon atom which mimics the 2-position of PAF may not be important to PAF antagonist activity.

From the results of biological evaluation, 2-[[N-acetyl-N-[[2-methoxy-3-[(octadecylcarbamoyl)oxy]propoxy]carbonyl]amino]methyl]-1-ethylpyridinium chloride **(30)**(CV-6209) was selected for further pharmacological characterization.[6]

PAF ANTAGONIST ACTIVITIES OF CV-6209 *IN VITRO* AND *IN VIVO*
Effects on Aggregation of Rabbit and Human Platelets

CV-6209 in final concentrations of 3×10^{-8} to 3×10^{-7} *M* (rabbit) or 3×10^{-8} to 3×10^{-6} *M* (human) inhibited the PAF-induced platelet aggregation, in a dose-dependent manner (Figure 15a and b): the IC_{50} value of CV-6209 was 7.5×10^{-8} *M* for rabbit platelets and 1.7×10^{-7} *M* for human platelets, (104 and 94 times, respectively, more potent than CV-3988). ONO-6240,[27] Ginkgolide B(BN-52021)[34] and etizolam[35] also inhibited the PAF-induced aggregation of rabbit platelets with IC_{50} values of 7.0×10^{-7}, 5.8×10^{-7}, and

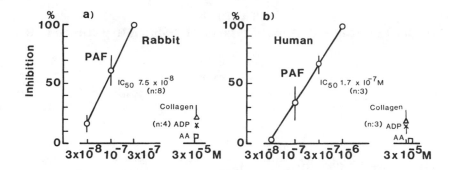

FIGURE 15. Effect of CV-6209 on aggregation of rabbit (a) and human (b) platelets induced by PAF and various agents. (a) Experiments were done with PRP obtained from eight(for PAF) or four(for other agents) rabbits. Concentrations of aggregation inducers and extent of aggregation were as follows: PAF, 2—5 nM, 67 ± 2%; AA, 1.67 mM 70 ± 2%; ADP, 3—5 μM, 50 ± 3%; collagen, 3—10 μg/ml, 75 ± 3%. (b) Experiments were done with PRP obtained from three volunteers for each agent. Concentrations of aggregation inducers and extent of aggregation were as follows: PAF, 0.3—1 μM, 77 ± 7%; AA, 0.6 mM, 90 ± 4%; ADP, 5—6 μM, 74 ± 7%; collagen, 1—3 μg/ml, 83 ± 2%.

1.9×10^{-7} M, respectively; CV-6209 was 9, 8, and three times more potent than ONO-6240, Ginkgolide B, and etizolam, respectively. CV-6209 at a high dose of 3×10^{-5} M showed little inhibitory effect on the aggregation of rabbit and human platelets, as induced by ADP, AA, and collagen (Figure 15a and b). CV-6209 (3×10^{-5} M) had no effect on shape change or weak aggregation of rabbit and human platelets as induced by 5-hydroxy-tryptamine(3×10^{-6} M). CV-6209 alone even at 10^{-4} M did not induce aggregation or shape change in the rabbit and human platelets. Thus, CV-6209 potently and specifically inhibited the aggregation of rabbit and human platelets induced by PAF.

Effects on [³H]Serotonin Release

CV-6209 inhibited the [³H]serotonin release from rabbit platelets stimulated by 3×10^{-8} M PAF in a dose-related manner. The inhibitions at concentrations of 3×10^{-8}, 10^{-7}, and 3×10^{-7} M of CV-6209 were 30 ± 9, 67 ± 24, and 93 ± 4%, respectively. These inhibitions by CV-6209 were similar to those shown in the platelet aggregation experiments above.

Effects on Hypotension Induced by PAF

As shown in Table 7, CV-6209 potently inhibited the hypotension induced by PAF (0.3 μg/kg, i.v.) compared with the other four drugs. Five minutes after the injection of drugs, the ID$_{50}$ values of CV-6209, CV-3988, ONO-6240, Ginkgolide B, and etizolam were 0.009, 0.73, 0.52, 3.1, and 2.6 mg/kg, respectively. Thus, CV-6209 was 81, 58, 344, and 289 times more potent than CV-3988, ONO-6240, Ginkgolide B, and etizolam, respectively. Even 60 min after the injection, CV-6209 inhibited the PAF-induced hypotension with an ID$_{50}$ value of 0.08 mg/kg. CV-6209 at doses of 1 and 10 mg/kg (i.v.) induced a slight and transient hypotension: 5 ± 0 and 49 ± 2 mmHg, respectively. The half-life of the hypotension induced by 10 mg/kg of CV-6209 was about 5 min.

Figure 16 shows the reversing effects of PAF antagonists on the hypotension induced by PAF (1 μg/kg,i.v.) in rats. CV-6209 potently reversed the hypotension with an ED$_{50}$ of 0.0046 mg/kg. CV-3988, ONO-6240, and Ginkgolide B also reversed the PAF-induced hypotension with ED$_{50}$ values of 0.34, 0.094, and 0.85 mg/kg, respectively; CV-6209 was 74, 20, and 185 times more potent than CV-3988, ONO-6240, and ginkgolide B, respectively. Etizolam at the high dose of 10 mg/kg reversed the hypotension by 41 ± 8%. CV-6209 was over 2100 times more potent than etizolam.

TABLE 7
Inhibitory Effects of PAF Antagonists on PAF-Induced Hypotension in Rats

Drugs	Dose (mg/kg/iv)	Inhibition of PAF-Induced Hypotension				n
		5 min[a] (%)	ID_{5050} (mg/kg)	60 min[a] (%)	ID (mg/kg)	
CV-6209	0.001	9 ± 5				5
	0.01	52 ± 8**		5 ± 3		5
	0.1	100**	0.009	55 ± 9**	0.08	5
	1	100**		100**		4
CV-3988	0.1	14 ± 5				5
	1	55 ± 5**	0.73	10 ± 5	4.1	5
	10	95 ± 2**		75 ± 4**		5
ONO-6240	0.1	4 ± 3				5
	1	68 ± 11**	0.52	11 ± 7	9.4	5
	10	94 ± 3**		51 + 15**		3
Ginkgolide B	1	13 ± 5				5
	10	88 ± 8**	3.1	23 ± 15		3
Etizolam	1	32 ± 4**				5
	10	75 ± 9**	2.6	35 ± 10**		5

Note: Values were mean ± SEM. Analysis of variance and subsequent t tests were used to examine the differences between vehicle and drug-treated groups at 5 and 60 min after the injection of drugs.

[a] PAF(1 μg/kg i.v.) was injected −5, 5, and 60 min after the i.v. injection of drugs. The n values are the number of rats.

** $p < 0.01$ vs. the values of the control (Student's t-test).

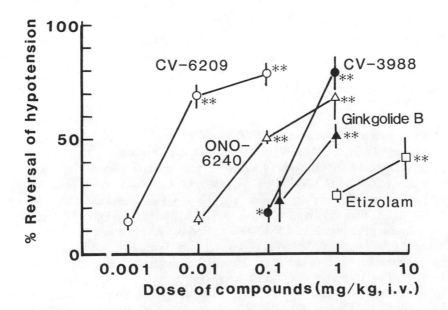

FIGURE 16.   Reversal of PAF-induced hypotension by various PAF antagonists in anesthetized rats. PAF antagonists were injected 3 min after injection of PAF (1 μg/kg,i.v.). Values are means ± SEM. Dunnett's or Scheffe's test was used for the statistical analysis of the recovery of blood pressure with PAF antagonists. Number of animals was five to seven except for the group treated with 1 mg/kg of ONO-6240 (n = 4). * $p < 0.05$, ** $p < 0.01$ vs. the values of the control.

a) Dose response curve

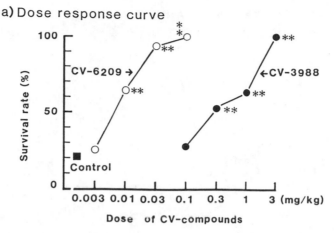

b) Time course

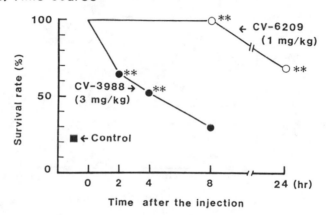

FIGURE 17. Protective effects of CV-6209 and CV-3988 on PAF-induced death in mice. (a) Drugs were given i.v. 5 min before the injection of PAF(50 μg/kg i.v.). Number of mice was 101 (control), 8-17 (CV-6209) and 18-30 (CV-3988). (b) CV-6209(1 mg/kg i.v.) and CV-3988(3 mg/kg i.v.) were given i.v. 2 to 24 h before the injection of PAF(50 μg/kg i.v.). Number of mice was 109 (control), 16 (CV-6209) and 24—27 (CV-3988). ** $p < 0.01$ vs. the values of the control (X^2-test).

Effects on PAF-Induced Death in Mice and Rats

As mentioned previously, CV-6209 protected the mice from PAF-induced death, with an ID_{50} value of 0.009 mg/kg (i.v.), and CV-3988 was also protective with an ID_{50} value of 0.80 mg/kg; CV-6209 was 89 times more potent than CV-3988 (Figure 17a). The protective effect of CV-6209 at a dose of 1 mg/kg continued for over 24 h (Figure 17b); the survival rates of the control, CV-6209-treated group (8 h after the injection) and CV-6209-treated group (24 h after the injection) were 22,100 ($p < 0.01$), and 69% ($p < 0.01$), respectively. PAF also has lethal effects in rats, which are more sensitive to PAF than are mice; PAF at a dose of 20 μg/kg is 100% lethal to rats. As shown in Figure 18a, CV-6209 protected rats from PAF-induced death with an ID_{50} value of 0.014 mg/kg (i.v.), and CV-3988 did so with an ID_{50} value of 0.65 mg/kg; CV-6209 was 46 times more potent than CV-3988. The protective effect of 3 mg/kg of CV-6209 continued for over 24 h (Figure 18b); survival rates of the control, CV-6209-treated group (8 h after the injection) and CV-6209-treated group (24 h after the injection) were 1, 100($p < 0.01$), and 25% ($p < 0.01$), respectively.

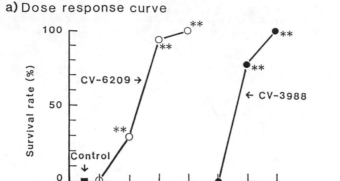

a) Dose response curve

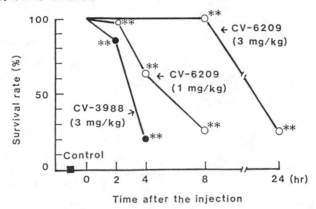

b) Time course

FIGURE 18. Protective effects of CV-6209 and CV-3988 on PAF-induced death in rats. (a) Drugs were given i.v. 5 min before the injection of PAF(20 μg/kg i.v.). Number of rats was 52 (control), 6-18 (CV-6209) and 6-18 (CV-3988). (b) Drugs(1 mg/kg i.v.) and CV-3988(3 mg/kg i.v.) were given i.v. 2 to 24 h before the injection of PAF(20 μg/kg i.v.). Number of rats was 74 (control), 8 (CV-6209), and 14 (CV-3988). ** p <0.01 vs. the values of the control (X^2-test).

CONCLUSION

From our studies on synthetic lysolecithin analogs, we found the first PAF-specific antagonist, CV-3988. This antagonist has been used by many researchers and has contributed to clarify the role of PAF.

CV-6209 was found during our studies on the structure-activity relationships of PAF analogs in which the phosphate moiety of PAF was replaced with the *N*-acetylcarbamoyl moiety. CV-6209 is one of the most potent PAF antagonists *in vitro* and *in vivo*.

Biological evaluation of CV-3988, CV-6209, and the other PAF antagonists (ONO-6240, ginkgolide B, and etizolam) gave us interesting results. That is, the relative potency of the PAF antagonistic action of PAF-related analogs (CV-3988, CV-6209, and ONO-6240) differed little between the assays of the inhibition of PAF-induced platelet aggregation and the reversal of PAF-induced hypotension. However, the relative PAF-antagonistic action of non-PAF analogs (ginkgolide B and etizolam) differed greatly under conditions of standardization with CV-6209. These results can be explained by the differences in the affinity of PAF antagonists for the PAF receptors of platelets and nonplatelets; the former mediates platelet aggregation and the latter mediates PAF-induced hypotension. PAF-related analogs (CV-3988, CV-6209, and ONO-6240) might have similar affinity for the receptor of both platelets and nonplatelets. Affinity of ginkgolide B and etizolam for the PAF (platelet) receptor might be higher than that to the PAF (nonplatelet) receptor. Lambrecht and Parnham[36] suggested the heterogeneity of PAF receptors in polymorphonuclear leukocytes and macrophages, determined using another PAF antagonist, kadsurenone. The relationship between their classification of PAF receptors and our classification remains to be clarified.

In conclusion, we hope that CV-3988 and CV-6209 may be useful drugs for investigating the pathophysiological role of PAF in diseases and beneficial drugs for treating diseases such as anaphylaxis, disseminated intravascular coagulation and endotoxin shock.

ACKNOWLEDGMENT

The authors are grateful to Drs. K. Nishikawa, Z. Terashita, and Y. Imura for permission to use data in the figures and tables, and for helpful suggestions concerning the text.

REFERENCES

1. **Benveniste, J., Tence, M., Varennce, P., Bidault, J., Boullet, C., and Polonsky, J.,** Semi-synthese et structure purposee du facteur activant les plaquettes (P.A.F.); PAF acether, un alkyl ether analogue de la lysophophatidylcholine, *C. R. Acad. Sci. D. (Paris)*, 289, 1037, 1979.
2. **Blank, M. L., Snyder, F., Byers, L. W., Brooks, B., and Muirhead, E. E.,** Antihypertensive activity of an alkyl ether analogue of phosphatidylcholine, *Biochim. Biophys. Res. Commun.*, 90, 1194, 1979.
3. **Demopoulos, C. A., Pinckard, R. N., and Hanahan, D. J.,** Platelet-activating factor. Evidence for 1-O-alkyl-2-acetyl-sn-glyceryl-3-phosphorylcholine as the active component (a new class of lipid chemical mediators), *J. Biol. Chem.*, 254, 9355, 1979.
4. **Lee, T.-C. and Snyder, F.,** Function, metabolism, and regulation of platelet activating factor and related ether lipids, in *Phospholipids and Cellular Regulation*, Vol. II, Kuo, J. F., Ed., CRC Press, Boca Raton, 1985, 1.
5. **Terashita, Z., Tsushima, S., Yoshioka, Y., Nomura, H., Inada, Y., and Nishikawa, K.,** CV-3988: a specific antagonist of platelet activating factor (PAF), *Life Sci.*, 32, 1975, 1983.
6. **Terashita, Z., Imura, Y., Takatani, M., Tsushima, S., and Nishikawa, K.,** CV-6209, a highly potent antagonist of platelet activating factor in vitro and in vivo, *J. Pharmacol. Exp. Ther.*, 242, 263, 1987.
7. **Takatani, M., Yoshioka, Y., Tasaka, A., Terashita, Z., Imura, Y., Nishikawa, K., and Tsushima, S.,** Platelet activating factor antagonists: synthesis and structure-activity studies of novel PAF analogues modified in the phosphorylcholine moiety, *J. Med. Chem.*, 32, 56, 1989.
8. **Benveniste, J. and Vargaftig, B. B.,** Platelet-activating factor: An ether lipid with biological activity, in *Ether Lipids: Biochemical and Biomedical Aspects*, Mangold, H. K. and Paltauf, F., Eds. Academic Press, New York, 1983, 355.
9. **Hanahan, D. J.,** Platelet activating factor: a biologically active phosphoglyceride, *Annu. Rev. Biochem.*, 55, 483, 1986.
10. **Born, G. V. R.,** Aggregation of blood platelets by adenosine diphosphate and its reversal, *Nature (London)*, 194, 927, 1962.
11. **Berdel, W. E., Andreesen, R., and Munder, P. G.,** Synthetic alkyl-phospholipid Analogs: a new class of antitumor agents, in *Phospholipids and Cellular Regulation*, Vol. II, Kuo, J. F., Ed., CRC Press, Boca Raton, FL, 1985, 1.
12. **Tsushima, S., Yoshioka, Y., Tanida, S., Nomura, H., Nojima, S., and Hozumi, M.,** Syntheses of alkyl lysophospholipids, *Chem. Pharm. Bull.*, 30, 3260, 1982.
13. **Tsushima, S., Yoshioka, Y., Tanida, S., Nomura, H., Nojima, S., and Hozumi, M.,** Syntheses and biological activities of N-alkyl- and N-alkenylcarbamoyl phospholipids, *Chem. Pharm. Bull.*, 32, 2700, 1984.
14. **Honma, Y., Kasukabe, T., Hozumi, M., Tsushima, S., and Nomura, H.,** Induction of differentiation of cultured human and mouse myeloid leukemia cells by alkyl-lysophospholipids, *Cancer Res.*, 41, 3211, 1981.

15. **Hayashi, H., Kudo, I., Inoue, K., Onozaki, K., Tsushima, S., Nomura, H., and Nojima, S.,** Activation of guinea pig peritoneal macrophages by platelet activating factor (PAF) and its agonists, *J. Biochem.,* 97, 1737, 1985.

16. **Nishikawa, K., Terashita, Z., Yoshioka, Y., and Tsushima, S.,** Discovery of a specific PAF antagonist, CV-3988, and an analysis of the pathophysiological roles of PAF, *J. Takeda Res. Lab.,* 46, 1, 1987.

17. **Terashita, Z., Imura, Y., Nishikawa, K., and Sumida, S.,** Is platelet activating factor (PAF) a mediator of endotoxin shock?, *Eur. J. Pharmacol.,* 109, 257, 1985.

18. **Doebber, T. W., Wu, M. S., Robbins, J. C., Choy, B. M., Chang, M. N., and Shen, T. Y.,** Platelet activating factor (PAF) involvement in endotoxin-induced hypotension in rats. Studies with PAF-receptor antagonist kadsurenone, *Biochem. Biophys. Res. Commun.,* 127, 799, 1985.

19. **Van Valen, R. G., Melden, M. K., Lee, M. K., Saunders, R. N., and Handley, D. A.,** Reversal by SRI 63-072 of endotoxin and immune aggregate-induced hypotension in the rats, in *New Horizons in Platelet Activating Factor Res.,* Palmetto Dunes Resort, Hilton Head Island, SC, October 15 to 18, 1985, abstr. 26.

20. **Etienne, A., Hecquet, F., Soulard, C., Spinnewyn, B., Clostre, F., and Braquet, P.,** In vivo inhibition of plasma protein leakage and salmonella enteritidis-induced mortality in the rat by a specific paf-acether antagonist: BN 52021, *Agents Action,* 17, 368, 1986.

21. **Casals-Stenzel, J., Muacevic, G., and Heuer, H.,** Modulation of the endotoxin shock and anaphylactic lung reaction by WEB 2086, a new potent antagonist of PAF, *2nd Int. Conf. on Platelet-Activating Factor and Structurally Related Alkyl Ether Lipids,* Gatlinburg, TN, October 26 to 29, 1986, abstr., 107.

22. **Imura, Y., Terashita, Z., and Nishikawa, K.,** Possible role of platelet activating factor(PAF) in disseminated intravascular coagulation (DIC), evidenced by use of a PAF antagonist, CV-3988, *Life Sci.,* 39, 111, 1986.

23. **Terashita, Z., Imura, Y., Shino, A., and Nishikawa, K.,** A lethal role of platelet activating factor in anaphylactic shock in mice, *J. Pharmacol. Exp. Ther.,* 243, 378, 1987.

24. **Moschidis, M. C., Demopoulos, C. A., and Kritikou, L. G.,** Phosphono-platelet activating factor I. Synthesis of 1-O-hexadecyl-2-O-acetylglyceryl-3-(2-trimethylammoniumethyl)phosphonate and its platelet activating potency, *Chem. Phys. Lipids,* 33, 87, 1983.

25. **Wissner, A., Kohler, C. A., and Goldstein, B. M.,** Analogues of platelet activating factor. III. Replacement of the phosphate moiety with a sulfonylbismethylene group, *J. Med. Chem.,* 28, 1365, 1985.

26. **Wissner, A., Schaub, R. E., Sum, P.-E., Kohler, C. A., and Goldstein, B. M.,** Analogues of platelet activating factor. IV. Some modifications of the phosphocholine moiety, *J. Med. Chem.,* 29, 328, 1986.

27. **Miyamoto, T., Ohno, H., Yano, T., Okada, T., Hamanaka, N., and Kawasaki, A.,** ONO-6240: a new potent antagonist of platelet-activating factor, in *Adv. Prostaglandin, Thromboxane, and Leukotriene Res.,* Hayaishi, O. and Yamamoto, S., Eds., 15, 719, 1985.

28. **Burri, K., Barner, R., Cassal, J. M., Hadvary, P., Hirth, G., and Muller, K.,** PAF: from agonists to antagonists by synthesis, *Prostaglandins,* 30, 691, 1985.

29. **Winslow, C. M., Anderson, R. C., D'Aries, F. J., Frisch, G. E., DeLillo, A. K., Lee, M. L., and Saunders, R. N.,** Toward understanding the mechanism of action of PAF receptor antagonists, in *Proc. of the 1st Sandoz Research Symposium, New Horizons in Platelet Activating Factor Research,* Winslow, C. M. and Lee, M. L., Eds., John Wiley, & Sons, London, 1987, 153.

30. **Willstatter, R.,** Ueber betaine, *Ber.,* 35, 584, 1902.

31. **Heymans, F., Michel, E., Borrel, M. C., Wichroeski, B., Godfroid, J.-J., Convert, O., Coeffier, E., Tence, M., and Benveniste, J.,** New total synthesis and high resolution 1H NMR spectrum of platelet-activating factor, its enantiomer and racemic mixtures, *Biochim. Biophys. Acta,* 666, 230, 1981.

32. **Wichrowski, B., Jouquey, S., Broquet, C., Heymans, F., Godfroid, J.-J., Fichelle, J., and Worcel, M.,** Structure-activity relationship in PAF-acether. IV. Synthesis and biological activities of carboxylate isosteres, *J. Med. Chem.,* 31, 410, 1988.

33. **Grue-Sorensen, G., Nielsen, I. M., and Nielsen, C. K.,** Derivatives of 2-methylenepropane-1,3-diol as new antagonists of platelet activating factor, *J. Med. Chem.,* 31, 1174, 1988.

34. **Braquet, P., Spinnewyn, B., Braquet, M., Bourgain, R. H., Taylor, J. E., Etienne, A., and Drieu, K.,** BN 52021 and related compounds: a new series of highly specific PAF-acether receptor antagonists isolated from Ginkgo biloba, *Blood Vessel,* 16, 559, 1985.

35. **Takehara, S., Mikashima, H., Terasawa, M., Muramoto, Y., Yasuda, H., Kurihara, A., Okumoto, T., Tahara, T., and Maruyama, Y.,** An antagonistic activity of etizolam (Depas) on platelet activating factor (PAF). I. Effects on platelet and leukocyte aggregation, in *Proc. of 59th General Meeting Japanese Pharmacological Soc., (Supplementum),* 40, 89, 1986.

36. **Lambrecht, G. and Parnham, M. J.,** Kadsurenone distinguishes between different platelet activating factor receptor subtypes on macrophages and polymorphonuclear leukocytes, *Br. J. Pharmacol.,* 87, 287, 1986.

Chapter 5

AMINOACYLATES AND AMINOCARBAMATES OF 2-SUBSTITUTED 4-HYDROXYMETHYL 1,3-DIOXOLANS: STRUCTURE ACTIVITY RELATIONSHIPS AND BIOLOGICAL ACTIVITY AS PAF-ANTAGONISTS

Colette Broquet, Annie Etienne, Caroline Touvay, Bernadette Pignol, Jean-Michel Mencia-Huerta, and Pierre Braquet

INTRODUCTION

Platelet-activating factor (1-O-alkyl-2-O-acetyl-*sn*-glyceryl-phosphorylcholine, PAF) is an endogenous ether phospholipid mediator with a wide range of biological activities.[1] This autacoid is generated in inflammatory and allergic responses,[2] and promotes platelet and neutrophil aggregation, induces bronchoconstriction and hypotension and increases vascular permeability.[3-5]

An intensive effort to find products blocking PAF effect has resulted in the discovery of a number of specific PAF antagonists, the first antagonist described being CV 3988 (Takeda).[6-8] These molecules have been classified as (i) charged PAF-like antagonists with an open chain or cyclic structure, (ii) natural products from plants and (iii) synthetic poly-cyclic compounds. We report here the synthesis and biological activity of new PAF-related antagonists with a constrained framework: aminoacylates and aminocarbamates of 2-substituted 4-hydroxymethyl dioxolans.

Several analogs were synthesized and investigated to establish which elements of their structure contribute to activity in inhibiting platelet aggregation induced by PAF. This work led to the optimization of the structural requirement for PAF antagonistic activity in this series. The most active compounds were submitted to further tests *in vitro* and *in vivo*.

Two compounds, BN 52111 and BN 52115, were found to display a very high potency in antagonizing the effects of PAF. These two antagonists were selected for further development based on their "in vivo" profile (Figure 1).

CHEMISTRY

The syntheses of 2-substituted 4-ammonio-acyl and ammonio-carbamoyl hydroxymethyl 1,3-dioxolan halogenides were accomplished according to the reactional Schemes 1 and 2. These are convenient methods for a multigram preparation. 2-substituted 4-hydroxymethyl 1,3 dioxolans **2** were obtained, as previously described, by reacting the corresponding carbonyl compound **1** with glycerol in the presence of *p*-toluene sulfonic acid.[9] Esterification of **2** by a ω-halogeno acid chloride yielded 2-substituted 4-(ω-halogeno acyl) oxymethyl 1,3-dioxolans **3** which were converted to I, II, or III by treatment with organic tertiary bases such as pyridine at 80°C (Figure 2).

Condensation of **2** with a ω halogeno alkyl isocyanate in the presence of pyridine at 80°C directly gave the corresponding ω-pyridinium alkyl carbamate (IV_a, IV_b). At 40°C, the ω-halogeno alkyl carbamate **4** was obtained and quaternarization of **4** by tertiary amines yielded the other carbamates (IV_c, IV_d) (Figure 3).

The different compounds were obtained as mixtures of diastereoisomers in equal proportions, as calculated by [^{1}H]NMR. A small amount of one diastereoisomer was separated by HPLC from BN 52115. No significant difference was found in its ability to inhibit platelet aggregation induced by PAF (IC_{50} 0.24 10^{-6} M and 0.3 10^{-6} M for the mixture).

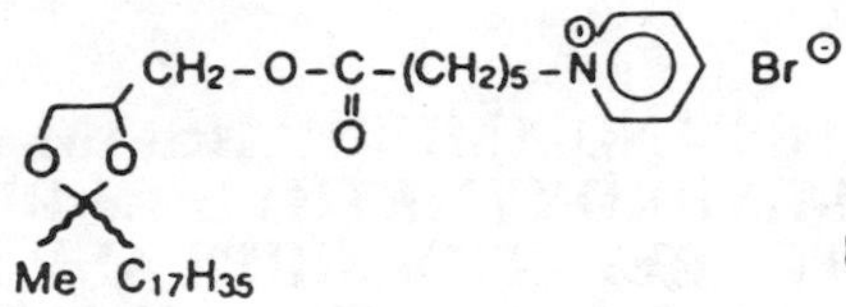

FIGURE 1.   Chemical structure of BN 52111 and BN 52115.

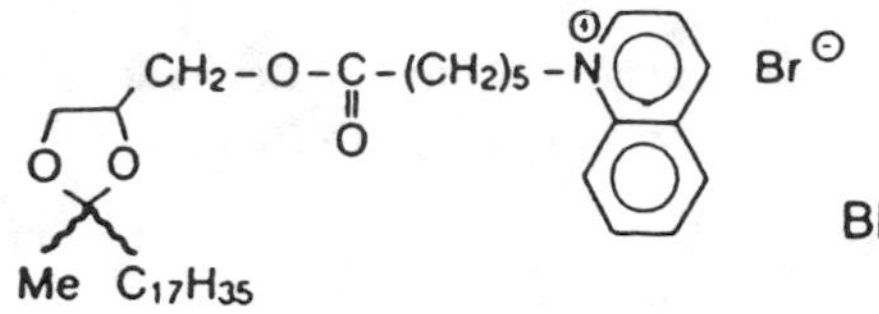

BIOLOGICAL RESULTS

IN VITRO STUDIES
Platelet Aggregation in Platelet Rich Plasma (PRP)

The compounds were tested *in vitro* for their ability to inhibit platelet aggregation induced by PAF. A structure activity relationship was established. Only the most active were tested on other aggregating agents.

Antagonism of PAF induced aggregation in PRP was performed according to Reference 10. The antagonist activity of the different compounds against PAF occurs between 3.1×10^{-5} and 3×10^{-7} M (Tables 1 and 2 summarize the IC_{50} values). None of them presents agonistic activity on platelet aggregation at 10^{-3} M.

The most active compounds were tested on other aggregating agents such as ADP, AA or A 23187; they did not show any important antagonistic effect (Table 3).

Structure-Activity Relationship

It is of interest to note the effect of chain hydrophobicity for R_1 and R_2. With respect to R_1, BN 52111 ($R_1 = C_{17}H_{35}$) is about 3.5 times more potent than BN 52120 ($R_1 = C_9H_{19}$). BN 52102 ($R_1 = C_{17}H_{35}$) is 10 times more potent than BN 52110 ($R_1 = C_6H_2(OCH_3)_3$).

The difference is less pronounced for R_2: BN 52101 ($R_2 = H$), BN 52102 ($R_2 = CH_3$) and BN 52109 ($R_2 = C_3H_7$). The best results were obtained for $R_2 = CH_3$ and $R_1 = C_{17}H_{35}$.

The substituent in the 4 position seems to play a more important role.

(a)   With ester function

When the distance between the ester group and the polar head moiety increases, no significant difference in IC_{50} is observed for n = 3 and 4 carbon atoms. (I_b and I_d); the best results are obtained with n = 5 (I_e); with n = 10 (I_g) the antagonistic activity dramatically decreases.

A polar head seems to be necessary and the nature of the charge transfer groups plays an important role. If the replacement of pyridinium by quinolinium moiety does not significantly affect the IC_{50} activity, isoquinolinium or thiazolium gives products about 100-fold less potent (Table 1).

(b)   With carbamate function

The change from ester moiety to an acylcarbamoyl moiety with the same length of acyl chain (n = 5, I_e to IV_a) does not lead to significant decrease of IC_{50} (two times less).

However, the PAF antagonistic activity is strongly influenced by the chain length, IV_a is about 30 more active than IV_b (n = 2). Moreover, trimethyl ammonium group is about thirty less active than a pyridinium polar head (Table 2).

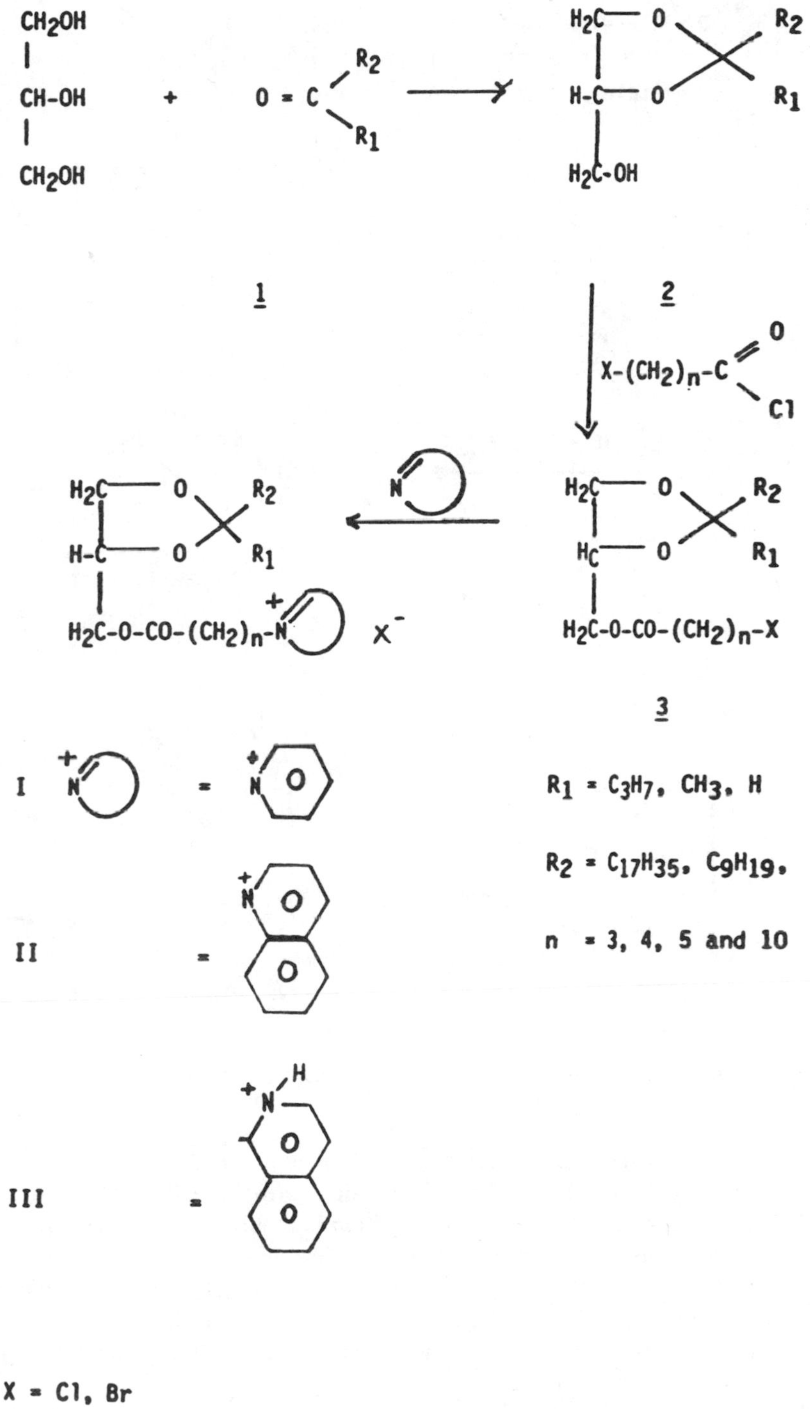

FIGURE 2. General synthetic scheme of aminoacylates of dioxolans (compounds I, II, and III).

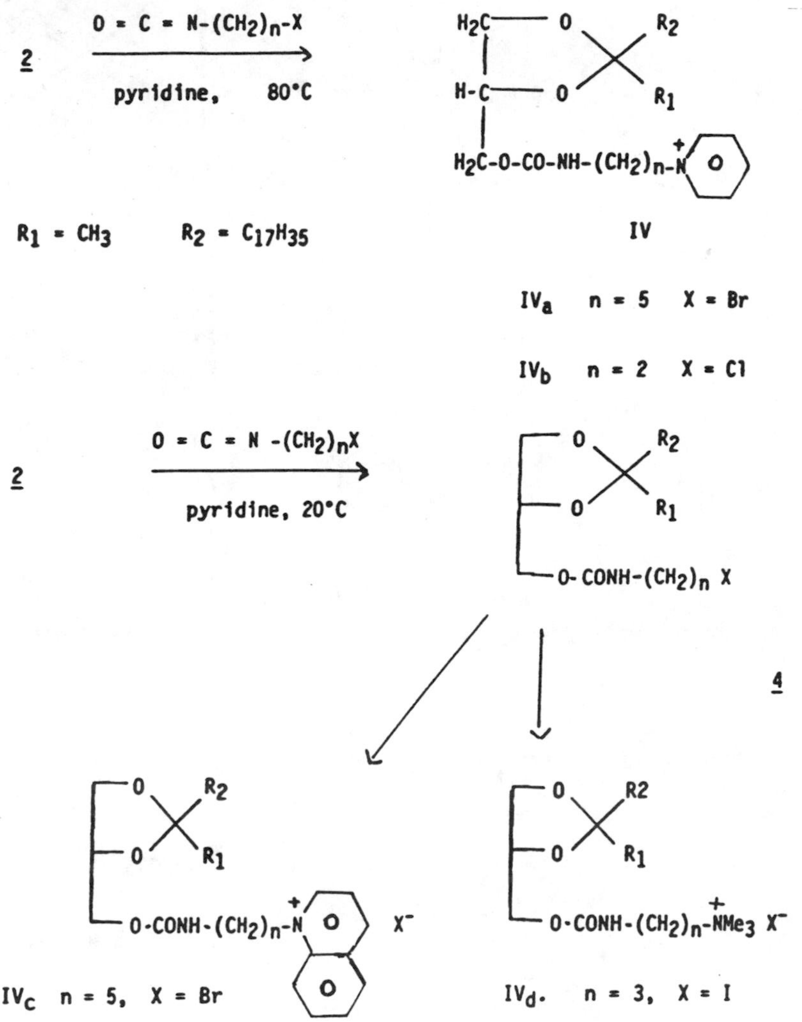

FIGURE 3.   General synthetic scheme of aminocarbamates of dioxalans (compounds IV).

Polymorphonuclear Leukocyte (PMN) Aggregation

PAF induces aggregation and degranulation of neutrophils. PAF (10^{-8} to 10^{-6} M) induced PMN activation as measured by aggregation is reduced by PAF antagonists. Polymorphonuclear leukocytes (PMN) were obtained as described by Ford-Hutchinson.[11]

Cell suspensions (>90% PMN) were prepared from peritoneal exudates obtained after a 5 ml i.p. injection of sodium caseinate 12% (W/V) to male Wistar rats. After centrifugation, cells were washed with Hanks and resuspended in MEM/Hepes 30 mM medium (pH = 7.4) at a concentration of 10^7 cells/ml.

Cytochalasin B was added 10 min before triggering aggregation to amplify the PMN-aggregation and the light transmittance through the cell suspension was measured. Drugs were added to the PMN suspension 2 min before PAF addition.

BN 52111 and BN 52115 dose dependently and significantly inhibit rat PMN activation induced by PAF (10^{-8} M). In comparison with BN 52021 and WEB 2086, BN 52111 seems to be the most effective (Figure 5).

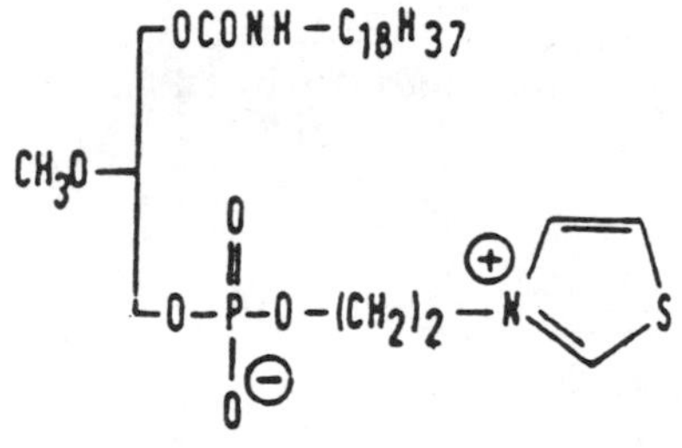

CV 3988

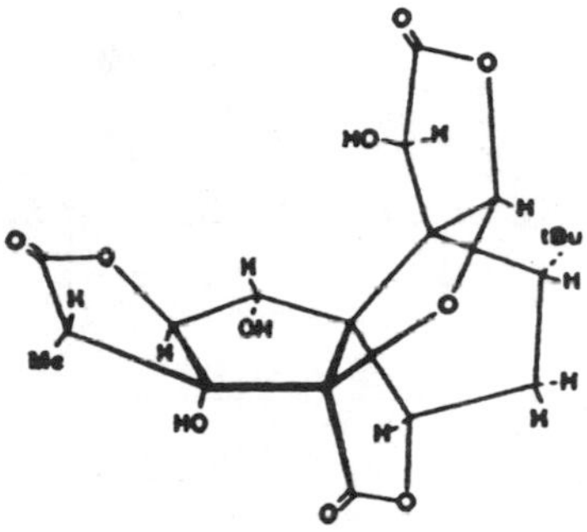

BN 52021

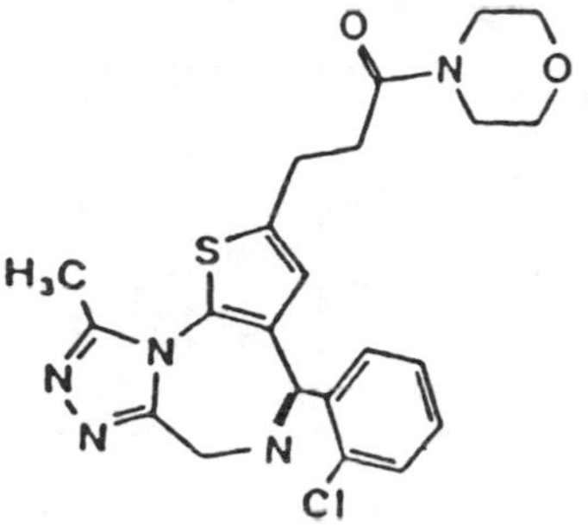

WEB 2086

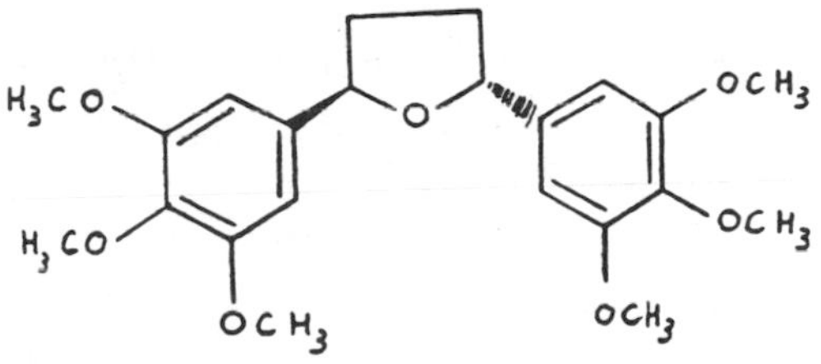

L 652 731

FIGURE 4. Chemical structure of other PAF antagonists used in present study.

Effects of BN 52111 and 52115 on PAF-Induced Calcium Mobilization in Washed Rabbit Platelets

PAF stimulates rapid shape-change, secretion of the contents of both dense and alpha granules and induces aggregation of platelets. The investigation of the stimulus-activity coupling processes has pointed out that the increase in cytoplasmic free calcium [Ca^{2+}] is a critical early event in platelet activation induced by PAF.

The use of fluorescent calcium indicator dye quin-2 has allowed the [Ca^{2+}] measurements in intact platelets at rest or during stimulation by agonists. PAF was shown to raise [Ca^{2+}] eight- to tenfold the basal level in a few seconds, as measured on platelets loaded with fluorescent probe.[12]

The inhibition by PAF antagonists on the quin-2 signal induced by PAF on washed and loaded rabbit platelet was carried according to Hallam.[12] BN 52021, 52111, and 52115

TABLE 1
Antagonistic Effect of Tested Compounds Against PAF-Induced Platelet Aggregation (PRP)

N°		R_1	R_2	n	$\overset{+}{N}$	X^-	$IC_{50}(M)$ *
BN 52101	I_a	$C_{17}H_{35}$	H	3	$\overset{+}{N}O$	Cl^-	$7.\ 10^{-6}$
BN 52102	I_b	$C_{17}H_{35}$	CH_3	3	''	•	$2.2\ 10^{-6}$
BN 52109	I_c	$C_{17}H_{35}$	C_3H_7	3	''	•	$3.04.\ 10^{-6}$
BN 52104		$C_{17}H_{35}$	CH_3	3	$\overset{+}{N}S$	•	$2.15\ 10^{-5}$
BN 52108	II_a	$C_{17}H_{35}$	H	3	$\overset{+}{N}O$	•	$3.1\ 10^{-6}$
BN 52105	II_b	$C_{17}H_{35}$	CH_3	3	''	•	$1.2\ 10^{-6}$
BN 52110	I_i	$(MeO)_3\ \Phi$	CH_3	3	$\overset{+}{N}O$	•	$1.13\ 10^{-5}$
BN 52107	I_d	$C_{17}H_{35}$	CH_3	4	''	•	$5.\ 10^{-6}$
BN 52111	I_e	$C_{17}H_{35}$	CH_3	5	$\overset{+}{N}O$	Br^-	$4.04\ 10^{-7}$

TABLE 1 (continued)
Antagonistic Effect of Tested Compounds Against PAF-Induced Platelet Aggregation
(PRP)

BN 52115 II$_e$	$C_{17}H_{35}$	CH_3	5	$\overset{+}{N}$ (bicyclic pyridinium structure)	•	$3.04 \ 10^{-7}$
BN 52113 I$_g$	$C_{17}H_{35}$	CH_3	10	$\overset{+}{N}$ (ring structure)	•	$3.12 \ 10^{-5}$
BN 52120 I$_n$	C_9H_{19}	CH_3	5	‖	•	$1.46 \ 10^{-6}$
BN 52121 I$_f$	$C_{17}H_{35}$	C_3H_7	5	‖	•	$1.73 \ 10^{-6}$
BN 52122	$C_{17}H_{35}$	CH_3	5	$NHCH_2$—(pyridine ring, N)	•	$- 39\% \ \text{à} \ 10^{-4}$
BN 52119	$C_{17}H_{35}$	CH_3	3	$CON(propyl)_2$	•	$- 13\% \ \text{à} \ 10^{-4}$
BN 52131 III$_e$	$C_{17}H_{35}$	CH_3	5	(quinolinium bicyclic structure, $\overset{-}{N}$)	Br^-	$1.21 \ 10^{-5}$

* PAF $2.5 \ 10^{-9} \ M$

added 5 min before PAF ($2 \times 10^{-9} \ M$) markedly antagonized the PAF induced [Ca^{2+}] mobilization. BN 52021 seems to be less active. The effect is dose dependent, totally abolished at $5.10^{-7} \ M$ for BN 52111 and 52115; it is reduced by 70% at $5.10^{-8} \ M$ for BN 52115 (Table 4).

Inhibition of the Binding of [^{3}H] PAF on Rabbit Platelet Membrane Preparation

Specific binding sites of PAF have been demonstrated in lysed or whole platelets of rabbit and human platelets[13-15] suggesting that platelet aggregation triggered by PAF may be induced via a receptor-mediated mechanism.

The binding of PAF is not only displaceable by PAF itself but also by PAF antagonists. We therefore examined the binding characterization vs. [^{3}H] PAF of different PAF antagonists on a rabbit platelet membrane preparation.

Binding Assay

Membrane proteins (100 to 150 μg) prepared according to Shen et al.[16] were added to a final volume of 1 ml in plastic tubes containing 1 nM [^{3}H]-PAF in Tris-HCl 10 mM pH 7 buffer containing 0.025% bovine serum albumin and incubated with or without unlabeled PAF or PAF antagonists. The incubation was carried out for 1.5 h at 0°C. After three washes

TABLE 2
Antagonistic Effect of Tested Compounds Against PAF-Induced Platelet Aggregates
(PRP)

N°		R$_1$	R$_2$	n	$\overset{+}{N}\lessgtr$	X$^-$	IC$_{50}$(M)*
IV$_c$	BN 52125	C$_{17}$H$_{35}$	CH$_3$	3	$\overset{+}{N}$(CH$_3$)$_3$	I$^-$	2.33 10^{-5}
IV$_b$	BN 52117	C$_{17}$H$_{35}$	CH$_3$	2	$\overset{+}{N}$◯O	Cl$^-$	1.7 10^{-5}
IV$_a$	BN 52132	C$_{17}$H$_{35}$	CH$_3$	5	$\overset{+}{N}$◯O	Br$^-$	6.45 10^{-7}
IV$_d$	BN 52133	C$_{17}$H$_{35}$	CH$_3$	5	$\overset{+}{N}$◯◯O O	Br$^-$	7 10^{-7}

* PAF 2.5 × 10^{-9} M

TABLE 3
***In Vitro* Agonistic Effect and Antagonistic Activities of Selected**
Compounds Against Other Inducers of Platelet Aggregation

Names	Agonistic effect (% aggregation at 10^{-3} M)	Antagonistic effects at 10^{-4} M % of variation from control DMSO		
		ADP (2.5 μM)	AA (0.5 mM)	A23187 (5 μM)
BN 52021	0	−28	−2	−5
BN 52102 (I$_b$)	0	−34	−10	−9
BN 52109 (I$_c$)	0	−28	−1	−5
BN 52107 (I$_d$)	0	−28	−2	−3
BN 52111 (I$_e$)	0	−24	−2	−2
BN 52121 (I$_f$)	0	−23	+3	+1
BN 52120 (I$_h$)	0	−8	+3	+3
BN 52105 (II$_b$)	0	−26	−4	−2
BN 52115 (II$_e$)	0	−27	−8	−6
BN 52132 (IV$_a$)	0	−12	+7	0

at 0°C, the bound [3H]-PAF was separated from free [^{3}H]-PAF by immediate filtration through Whatman GF/C glass fiber filters. The specific binding was calculated by subtracting nonspecific binding from the total binding. The inhibition by PAF antagonists on the specific [^{3}H]-PAF binding was normalized as the percent inhibition by the equation:

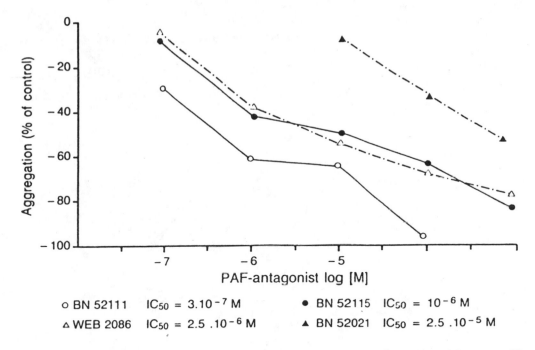

FIGURE 5. Dose dependent inhibition of [PAF (10^{-8} M) + cytochalasin (10^{-10} M)] induced Rat neutrophil aggregation.

TABLE 4
Percent Inhibition of PAF Induced [Ca^{2+}] Mobilization in Platelets
by PAF Antagonists

Doses Products	$5 \cdot 10^{-7}$ M	10^{-7} M	$5 \cdot 10^{-8}$ M
BN 52021	86 - 82	68 - 49	41 - 43
BN 52111	100	81 - 82	44
BN 52115	100	89 - 86	81 - 69

$$\% \text{ inhib.} = \frac{[^3H]\text{-PAF total bound } [^3H]\text{-PAF bound in presence of the product}}{[^3H]\text{-PAF specifically bound}} \times 100$$

Displacement of [^{3}H]-PAF (1 nM) binding in rabbit platelet membranes by several antagonists is shown in Figure 6.

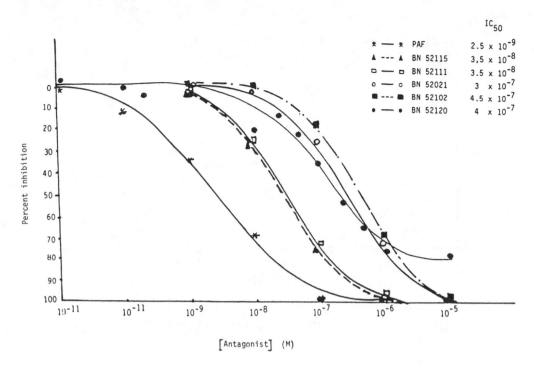

FIGURE 6.   Inhibition of [³H]-PAF (1 n*M*) specific binding to rabbit platelet membrane.

All these compounds inhibit [³H]-PAF binding dose dependently. The most potent inhibition is observed with BN 52111 and BN 52115 with an identical IC_{50} value of 3.5 10^{-8} *M*.

In comparison, the concentration required to inhibit the specific binding by 50% is 2.5 10^{-9} *M* for unlabeled PAF. Scatchard plot analysis of [³H]-PAF binding to its receptor or in presence of the most effective PAF antagonists, namely, BN 52111 and 52115, shows that these compounds alter, in dose-dependent manner, the PAF affinity for its receptor sites (K_d) without changing the total number of PAF sites.

This suggests that BN 52111 and BN 52115 act in a competitive manner on the inhibition of PAF binding. Morever, these substances differ from other competitive PAF inhibitors. As illustrated in Figures 7 and 8, after 30 min in the presence of PAF antagonists, the inhibition of [³H]-PAF binding cannot be reversed by repeated washing, whereas it is totally reversed in the case of L 65273 and partially in the case of CV 3988 (Figures 7 and 8). Although the mechanism of this effect has to be determined, this could explain the long lasting actions observed *in vivo* with BN 52111 and BN 52115.

Effect on Natural Killer Activity of BN 52111

Natural killer (NK) cells are a subset of lymphocytes that expresses cytotoxicity *in vitro* and *in vivo* against tumor cells and virus-infected cells. They exert cytotoxicity without prior sensitization and play an important role in the first line of defense against tumor cells and virus infections. NK cells are suspected to be involved in graft rejection of bone marrow transplants. PAF has been shown to be released by large granular lymphocytes, the cells involved in NK activity.[17]

PAF antagonists inhibit, in dose-dependent fashion, the cytotoxic activity of NK cells towards K562 (Figure 9). BN 52111 is effective at the concentration of 0.6 µ*M*, BN 52021 and WEB 2086 are less active. From this data, it seems reasonable to speculate that activated NK cells release PAF and/or its metabolic products.

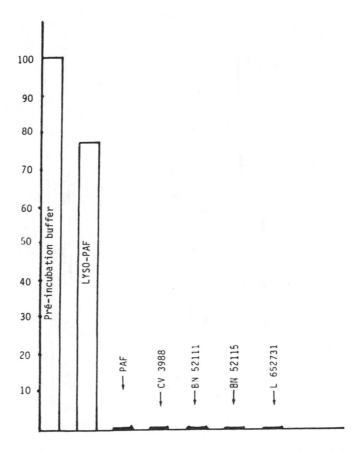

FIGURE 7.   Reversibility test [³H]-PAF binding after incubation period and without washing.

IN VIVO STUDIES
Action on the Bronchopulmonary Effect of PAF in the Guinea Pig

Intravenous administration of PAF to guinea pigs induces platelet dependent broncho-constriction, thrombopenia, and leukopenia.[18] The interaction between several PAF antag-onists of this series and the effects of PAF on bronchopulmonary system was studied.

Male Hartley guinea pigs (400 to 500 g) were anesthetized with ethyl carbamate and prepared for recording bronchoconstriction according to the Konzett and Rossler method.[19] Blood samples (200 μl) were obtained from the carotid artery 1 min before and after the administration of PAF for the determination of the platelet and leukocyte numbers with a Coulter Counter ZBI.

Different PAF antagonists (water solution) were injected (5, 1, 0.5, and 0.1 mg/kg) 5 min before PAF (60 ng/kg). BN 52021 and all selected antagonists, except BN 52120 (I_h), dose dependently reduced the bronchoconstriction induced by PAF. The most active were BN 52111 (70% inhibition at 0.5 mg/kg) and BN 52115 (72% at 0.5 mg/kg).

With respect to platelet aggregation *in vivo*, most of BN significantly inhibited the drop of circulating platelets following PAF injection in a dose-dependent fashion. BN 52111 and BN 52115 are active at 1 mg/kg (83 and 70% protection). However, only BN 52111 reduces significantly the concomitant leukopenia induced by PAF (91% at 1 mg/kg). General results are given in Table 5.

PAF-Induced Hypotension

Intravenous administration of PAF (0.25 to 1.0 μg/kg) elicited a dose-related decrease

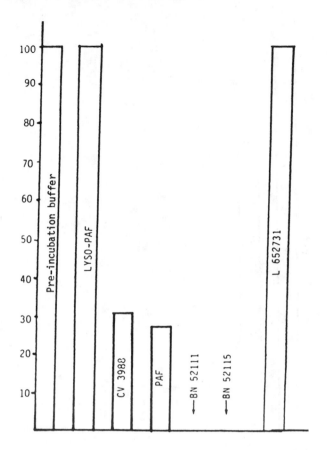

FIGURE 8.   Reversibility test [³H]-PAF binding after incubation period and several washings.

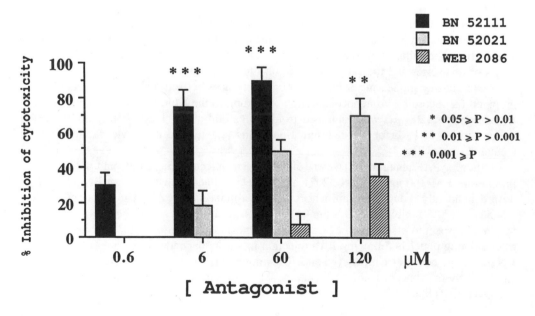

FIGURE 9.   Effect of PAF antagonists on NK cytotoxicity against K562 target cells. One hundred percent value was 37 ± 4.1% cytotoxicity.

TABLE 5

***In vivo* Antagonistic Effects of Selected Compounds Against Bronchoconstriction, Thrombocytopenia, and Leukopenia Induced by PAF**

Compounds	Dose (mg/kg) i.v.	Bronchoconstriction (% protection)	Thrombocytopenia (% protection)	Leukopenia (% protection)
BN 52021	3	94 ***	56.1 **	17.3 NS
	1	54 ***	9.4 NS	6.5 NS
BN 52102 (I$_b$)	5	94.9 ***	77.1 ***	58.6 *
	1	61.3 ***	43 *	NS
BN 52107 (I$_d$)	5	73.5 **	68 **	NS
BN 52111 (I$_e$)	5	95.6 ***	93.9 ***	59.6 *
	1	76.1 ***	83.2 ***	91.4 ***
	0.5	70.4 ***	71.9 ***	NS
	0.1	45.1 **	56.1 **	NS
BN 52121 (I$_f$)	1	83.5 ***	80.1 ***	87 **
	0.5	54 ***	65.5 ***	60.6 *
BN 52120 (I$_h$)	1	14.1 NS	No effect	No effect
BN 52105 (II$_b$)	5	86.8 ***	62 **	NS
BN 52115 (II$_e$)	1	91.1 ***	70.42 ***	41 *
	0.5	72.4 ***	59.9 **	58.9 *
	0.1	11.5 NS	NS	NS
BN 52132 (VI$_a$)	1	57 ***	62.8 ***	36 ***
	0.5	68 ***	45.2 ***	25.4 ***

[a]   PAF 60 ng.

[b]   n = 4—6 animals.

[c]   NS, nonsignificant. * $p < 0.05$, ** $p < 0.01$, *** $p < 0.001$.

in arterial blood pressure in anesthetized normotensive rats with an even greater fall in diastolic blood pressure.

Male Sprague-Dawley rats (250 g) were anesthetized with ethyl carbamate (1.2 mg/kg i.p.). Systolic and diastolic arterial blood pressures (PAS and PAD) were continuously measured in the left carotid artery via a P50 Gould transducer.

BN 52111 and BN 52115 dissolved in physiological serum were injected curatively 3 min after PAF (1 µg/kg).

BN 52115 was the most active to inhibit PAF induced hypotension on systolic and diastolic pressure (Figure 10).

Arterial Thrombosis

Application of an electrical current (5 mA, 1 min) on a segment of a branch of the guinea pig mesenteric artery followed by superfusion of PAF (10^{-7} *M in situ*) induces a continuous thromboformation even if superfusion is discontinued.[20] PAF is effective alone if superfused above 10^{-6} *M*.

The arterial thrombosis induced *in vivo* by PAF superfusion results in thrombosis due to the autogeneration of the autacoid within the vessel wall. BN 52021, BN 52111, and BN 52115 (10^{-5} *M*, superfused), specific PAF receptor antagonists, inhibit arterial thromboformation preventively. BN 52111 is the most active drug (Figure 11). Curatively, they significantly decrease the thrombus size.

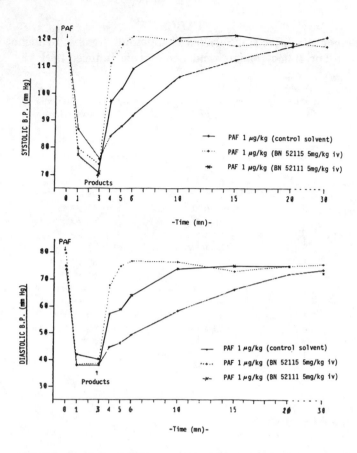

FIGURE 10.   Effect of BN 52111 and 52115 on PAF induced hypotension in the normotensive anesthetized rat (given curatively).

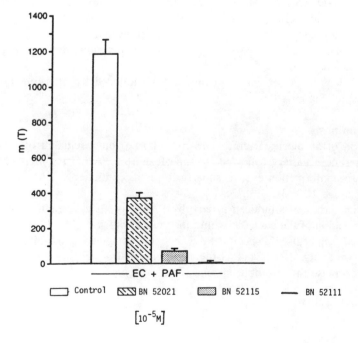

FIGURE 11.   Effect of PAF antagonists on, *in vivo*, electrical current (EC) and PAF mediated thrombosis.

REFERENCES

1. (a) **Winslow, C. M. and Lee, M. L.,** *New Horizons in Platelet-Activating-Factor Research,* Wiley, New York, 1987; (b) **Braquet, P., Touqui, L., Shen, T. Y., and Vargaftig, B. B.,** *Pharmacol. Rev.,* 39, 97, 1987.
2. **Vargaftig, B. B., Chignard, M., Benveniste, J., Lefort, J., and Wal, F.,** Background and present status of research on platelet-activating factor (PAF-acether), *Ann. N.Y. Acad. Sci.,* 370, 119, 1981.
3. **Braquet, P. and Vargaftig, B. B.,** Pharmacology of platelet-activating factor, *Transplant. Proc.,* 18, 10, 1986.
4. **Morley, J.,** Platelet-activating factor and asthma, *Agent Actions,* 19, 100, 1986.
5. **Snyder, F.,** Chemical and biochemical aspects of platelet-activating factor: a novel class of acetylated ether-linked choline phospholipids, *Med. Res. Rev.,* 5, 107, 1985.
6. **Terashita, Z., Tsushima, S., Yoshioka, Y., Nomura, H., Inada, Y., and Nishikawa, K.,** CV-3988, a specific antagonist of platelet-activating factor (PAF), *Life Sci.,* 32, 1975, 1983.
7. **Braquet, P. and Godfroid, J. J.,** PAF-acether binding sites. II. Design of specific antagonists, *Trends Pharmacol. Sci.,* 7, 397, 1986.
8. **Saunders, R. N. and Handley, D. A.,** Platelet-activating factor antagonists, *Annu. Rev. Pharmacol. Toxicol.,* 27, 237, 1987.
9. **Showler, A. J. and Darley, P. A.,** Condensation products of glycerol with aldehydes and ketones. 2-substituted m dioxan-5-ols and 1,3-dioxolane 4-methanols, *Chem. Rev.,* 57, 427, 1987.
10. **Kinlough-Rathbone, R., Cazenave, J. P., Packkam, M., and Mustard, F.,** Effect of inhibitors of the arachidonate pathway on the release of granule contents from rabbit platelets adherent to collagen, *Lab. Invest.,* 42, 28, 1980.
11. **Ford Hutchinson, A. W.,** Aggregation of rat neutrophils by nucleotide triphosphate, *Br. J. Pharmacol.,* 76, 371, 1982.
12. **Hallam, J. J. et al.,** Stimulus-response coupling in human platelets, *Biochem. J.,* 218, 819, 1984.
13. **Braquet, P. and Godfroid, J. J.,** Paf-acether specific binding sites, 2-design of specific antagonists, *TIPS,* 7, 397, 1986.
14. **Bussolino, F. et al.** Alkyl-ether phosphoglycerides influence calcium fluxes into human endothelial cells, *J. Immunol.,* 135, 2748, 1985.
15. **Casals-Stenzel, J. and Weber, K. H.,** Triazolo diazepines: dissociation of their PAF antagonistic and CNS activity, *Br. J. Pharmacol.,* 90, 139, 1987.
16. **Shen, T. Y. et al.** Characterization of a platelet-activating factor (PAF) receptor antagonist isolated from hainfenteng (piper futokadsura). Specific inhibition, of in vitro and in vivo, PAF induced effects, *Proc. Natl. Acad. Sci. U.S.A.,* 82, 672, 1985.
17. **Malvasi, F. et al.,** Fc receptor triggering induces expression of surface activation antigens and releases platelet-activating factor in large granular lymphocytes, *Proc. Natl. Acad. Sci. U.S.A.,* 83, 2443, 1986.
18. **Vargaftig, B. B., Lefort, J., Chignard, M., and Benveniste, J.,** Platelet-activating factor induces a platelet-dependent bronchoconstriction unrelated to the formation of prostaglandin derivatives, *Eur. J. Pharmacol.,* 65, 185, 1980.
19. **Konzett, H. and Rossler, R.,** *Naunym Schmiedebergs Arch. Exp. Pathol. Pharmakol.,* 195, 71, 1940.
20. **Bourgain, R. H., Maes, L., Braquet, P., Andries, R., Touqui, L., and Braquet, M.,** The effect of 1.0.alkyl 2.0.acetyl, sn glycerol 3.phosphorylcholine (PAF acether) on the arterial wall, *Prostaglandins,* 30, 185, 1985.

Chapter 6

GS 1065-180 AND RELATED PAF ANTAGONISTS: CHEMISTRY AND PHARMACOLOGY

Gunnar Grue-Sørensen and Christian Kaergaard Nielsen

ABBREVIATIONS

The following abbreviations are used: DCC = N,N'-dicyclohexylcarbodiimide, 4-DMAP = 4-(dimethylamino)pyridine, i.v. = intravenously, Ms = methanesulfonyl, PDC = pyridinium dichromate, p.o. = perorally, Tr = triphenylmethyl, and Ts = 4-toluenesulfonyl.

INTRODUCTION

Since the structure of a specific platelet activating factor (PAF) antagonist in 1983 was published for the first time[1] numerous substances with anti-PAF activity have become available. The purpose of producing PAF antagonists is two-fold: first, PAF antagonists are needed in the study of PAFs mode of action and, second, they are potentially useful as drugs in the treatment of diseases in which PAF takes part.

PAF (**92**) is a chiral compound and its enantiomer is essentially biologically inactive.[2,3] Surprisingly, it has been demonstrated that several analogs of PAF, chiral at C-2 of the 1,3-disubstituted glycerol backbone, are almost equipotent as PAF antagonists in either enantiomeric form.[4-9] Similarly, some *trans*-2,5-diaryltetrahydrofurans and their enantiomers are equiactive as PAF antagonists.[10] It has been pointed out that such equiactive enantiomers are unlikely to be optimal ligands for interference with PAF binding to its receptor, but represent a base line constellation of ''lead'' structures from which more active PAF antagonists can be invented.[10] A difference in activity between enantiomeric PAF antagonists has indeed been observed.[11] Thus the anti-PAF activity of the ($-$)-enantiomer of WEB 2170 is at least 20 times higher than that of the ($+$)-enantiomer and this is useful information in the design of still more active antagonists.

Generally, a racemate is more readily synthesized than its separate enantiomers, but in a chiral environment, like any biological system, enantiomers must be regarded as different compounds with different biological properties. Thus, any advantage gained by the synthesis of a racemate rather than a pure enantiomer might well be wasted by a complicated biological evaluation of the racemate, because the evaluation of a mixture of active compounds is much more delicate than the evaluation of a single compound.[12] Bearing this in mind we decided to determine some of the optimal structural requirements for PAF analogs to obtain good antagonist activity and we thought that the advantage of both a simple chemical synthesis and a simple biological evaluation could be achieved by compounds which are achiral analogs of PAF.

In our analysis we have divided PAF into six substructures: **A-B-C-D-E-F** (**A** = $CH_3(CH_2)_{15}$, **B** = O, **C** = $CH_2CH(OOCCH_3)CH_2$, **D** = $OP(O)(O^-)O$, **E** = $(CH_2)_2$, **F** = $^+N(CH_3)_3$) and we have investigated the anti-PAF activity of analogs of PAF in which the substructures **A** to **F** have been changed.

To obtain achiral analogs the glycerol subunit **C** was replaced with a unit which rendered achiral analogs. An sp^2 hybridized carbon atom was introduced at the position which mimicked C-2 of the glycerol moiety. Both compounds which had oxo and alkylidene substituents at the mimicked 2-position of glycerol were prepared and tested for anti-PAF and other biological activities. Some of the results from our investigation have been published,[13] others are reported here for the first time.

CHEMISTRY

All compounds reported in the following Section gave satisfactory spectroscopic data
(^{1}H NMR, IR), adequate for confirmation of identity. The reactions described are standard
reactions and gave as such the expected products in acceptable yields. All synthetic intermediates were isolated by standard techniques which, first of all, involved purification by
liquid chromatography on silica gel. Not all the yields have been optimized, because the
main objective with these preparations was to obtain sufficient material for an initial biological
evaluation of potential PAF antagonists.

The "2-oxo" analogs were prepared from (RS)-2,2-dimethyl-4-hydroxymethyl-1,3-
dioxolane (**93**) as outlined in Scheme 1. 1-O-Hexadecyl-*rac*-glycerol[14] (**94**) was esterified
with 1 equiv of 4-bromobutanoic acid and 6-bromohexanoic acid to give 1-O-hexadecyl-3-
O-*n*-bromoalkanoyl-*rac*-glycerol compounds **95** and **96**, respectively, (53 to 61%). Oxidation
with PDC yielded the 1,3-dihydroxyacetone derivatives **97** and **98** (33 to 40%) which upon
reaction with pyridine gave the desired analogs **33** and **34** in near quantitative yields. The
formation of the carbamate analog **91** took place through a similar series of compounds (**93**
→ **99**(7) → **100**(7) →**101** → **102** → **91**) in just 1% overall yield.

The "2-alkylidene" analogs of PAF were synthesized from the corresponding diols **103**
(13) and **153** (15) as outlined in Schemes 2 though 6. The first reactions of the diols **103**
and **153** with 1 equiv of derivatizing reagent gave, as expected, moderate yields (Schemes
2 though 4). The purification of the monoderivatized diols was, however, readily accomplished by liquid chromatography.

Long alkyl groups were linked to **103** (Scheme 2) by reaction with (1) hexadecyl bromide
in DMF in the presence of sodium hydride to give **104** (33%), (2) long chain isocyanates[16]
to give the carbamates **105**—**107** (ca. 40%), (3) hexadecanoic acid to give the ester **108**
(15%), (4) alkyl chloroformates (prepared in near quantitative yield by treatment of
$CH_3(CH_2)_xOH$ (x = 15, 17) with a tenfold excess phosgene (toxic!) in toluene at r.t. for 5
h followed by removal of the excess phosgene (led through dilute sodium hydroxide) and
solvent *in vacuo*) to give the carbonates **109** and **110** (ca. 40%), and (5) hexadecyl
isothiocyanate[17] to give the thiocarbamate **111** (9%).

Various subunits **D** and **E** to substitute for the OP(O) (O⁻)-OCH₂CH₂ moiety of PAF
were attached to the alcohols **104**—**111**. Reaction of **104** with $MsO(CH_2)_hOMs$ (h = 4 (18),
5 (19)) gave the diether compounds **112** and **113** (37—49%) and with $Cl_2P(O)O$-
$(CH_2)_2Br^{20}$/triethylamine followed by hydrolysis gave the phosphate **114** (96%). Condensation of **104** with the bromoalkyl isocyanates $OCN(CH_2)_mBr^{21}$ produced the carbamates
115 (m = 2) and **116** (m = 4) and reaction of **107** with $OCN(CH_2)_mBr^{21}$ gave the carbamates
117 (m = 2), **118** (m = 4), **119** (m = 5), and **120** (m = 7). All the alcohols **104**—**111**
were condensed with *n*-bromoalkanoic acids to give the esters **121**—**139**. Thus, the alcohol
104 was condensed with *n*-bromoalkanoic acids $HOOC(CH_2)_kBr$ to give the bromo esters
121 (k = 1), **122** (k = 3), **123** (k = 4), **124** (k = 5), and **125** (k = 10). The carbamate
alcohol **105** was esterified with 6-bromohexanoic acid to give **126**, and **106** was condensed
with 6-bromohexanoic and 8-bromooctanoic acid to give **127** (k = 5), and **128** (k = 7),
respectively. The last carbamate alcohol **107** was converted to the esters **129** (k = 3), **130**
(k = 4), **131** (k = 5), **132** (k = 6), and **133** (k = 7). The ester alcohol **108** was esterified
to give the diesters **134** (k = 5) and **135** (k = 7). The carbonate alcohol **109** was converted
to **136** (k = 5) and **137** (k = 7) and the carbonate alcohol **110** gave the ester **138** (k =
6). Finally, the thiocarbamate alcohol **111** was converted to the ester **139** (k = 5).

The last step in the preparation of PAF analogs as outlined in Scheme 2 was the alkylation
of various tertiary amines (and a single sulfide) with the compounds **112**—**139**. The alkylation
conditions are listed in Table 1 and the products are readily identified by the use of Table
2. The preparation of two of these compounds, **62** (GS 1065-180) and **68** (GS 1160-180),
has been described in detail.[13]

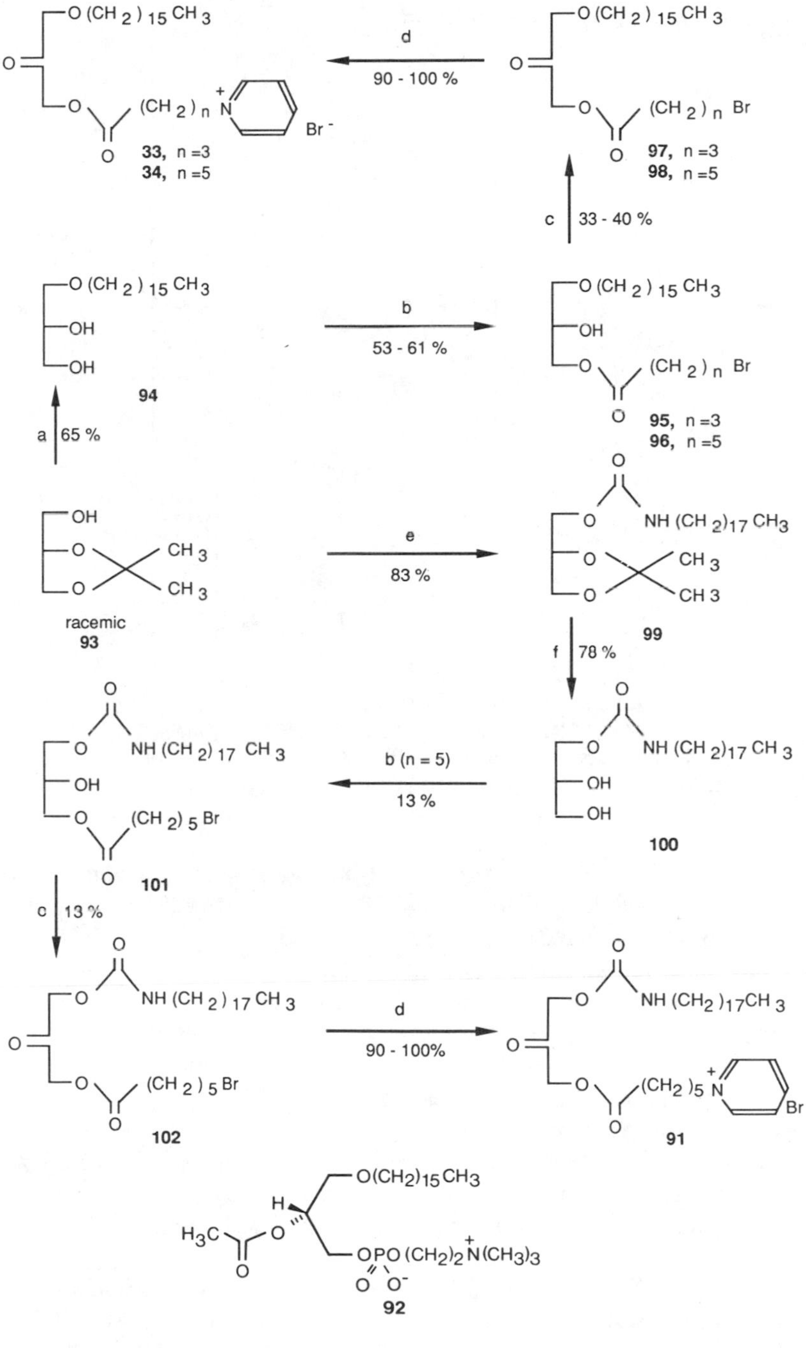

Scheme 1. (a) KOH/benzene/reflux/15 h, then Br(CH$_2$)$_{15}$CH$_3$/benzene/reflux/30 h, then CH$_3$OH/conc HCl/reflux/4 h. (b) DCC/0.1 equiv 4-DMAP/HOOC(CH$_2$)$_n$Br/CH$_2$Cl$_2$/r.t./1 h. (c) PDC/CH$_2$Cl$_2$/r.t./23 h. (d) Pyridine/60°C/23 h. (e) OCN(CH$_2$)$_{17}$CH$_3$/pyridine/r.t./17 h. (f) CH$_3$OH/conc HCl/reflux/1 h.

When the only ether oxygen in the PAF analog is positioned to replace the phosphate group (substructure ''D'') of PAF this ether bond was formed before the long alkyl group was attached to the other oxygen of 2-methylene-1,3-propanidiol (Scheme 3). Thus, **103** was alkylated with 6-trityloxy-1-chlorohexane (prepared in near quantitative yield from 6-chlorohexanol and triphenylmethyl chloride in CH$_2$Cl$_2$ in the presence of 5 equiv pyridine

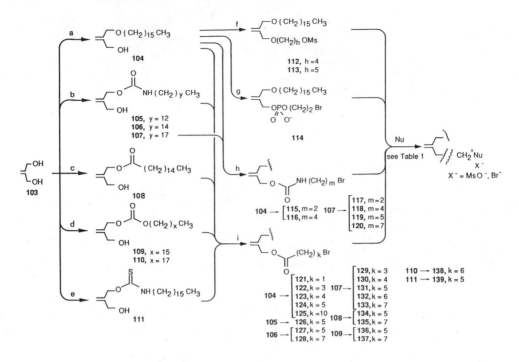

Scheme 2.   (a) Br(CH$_2$)$_{15}$CH$_3$/NaH/DMF/55°C/1 h/33%. (b) OCN(CH$_2$)$_y$CH$_3$/pyridine/r.t./24 h/ca. 40%. (c) HOOC(CH$_2$)$_{14}$CH$_3$/DCC/4-DMAP/CH$_2$Cl$_2$/r.t./24 h/15%. (d) ClCOO(CH$_2$)$_x$CH$_3$/pyridine/CH$_2$Cl$_2$/r.t./2.5 h/ca. 40%. (e) SCN(CH$_2$)$_{15}$CH$_3$/4-DMAP/pyridine/104°C/ 6.5 h/9%. (f) MsO(CH$_2$)$_h$OMs/NaH/DMF/54°C/23 h/37—49%. (g) Cl$_2$P(O)O(CH$_2$)$_2$Br/Et$_3$N/CHCl$_3$/r.t./5 h/H$_2$O/96%. (h) OCN(CH$_2$)$_m$Br/4-DMAP/Et$_2$O/r.t./23 h/47—61%. (i) HOOC(CH$_2$)$_k$Br/DCC/4-DMAP/Et$_2$O/r.t./16 h/70—100%.

and 0.1 equiv 4-DMAP at r.t. for 4 h) to give **140**. The long chain carbonates **141** (x = 15) and **142** (x = 17) and the carbamates **143** (z = 14) and **144** (z = 17) were prepared as described above (cf. Scheme 2). Detritylation (→ **145** (x = 15), **146** (x = 17), **147** (z = 14), and **148** (z = 15)), followed by methanesulfonation (→ **149** (x = 15), **150** (x = 17), **151** (z = 14), and **152** (z = 17)) and the reaction with thiazole or pyridine gave the PAF analogs, **5**, **6,**, **35**, **36**, **43**, **44**, **47**, and **48** (see Tables 1 and 2).

2-Isopropylidene-1,3-propanediol **153** (Scheme 4) was the starting compound for a series of eight PAF analogs prepared through intermediates **154—159** and the reaction conditions are described above (cf. Scheme 2).

The *n*-bromoalkanoates **119** and **120** were reacted with a number of "special" nucleofiles (Scheme 5). Mono-alkylation of *N,N,N',N'*-tetramethylethylenediamine gave the PAF analogs **57** (n = 5) and **73** (n = 7) and further alkylation with methyl iodide gave the bis quaternary ammonium salts **58** and **74**.

119 and **120** were also reacted with imidazole to give the N-substituted imidazoles **60** and **76**. Quaternization with methyl iodide gave the imidazolium salts **61** and **77**.

The zwitterionic PAF analogs **66** and **67** were prepared from **119** by alkylation of the sodium salts of 3-sulfopyridine and of N-(2-sulfoethyl)nicotinamide (prepared by acylation of taurine with nicotinoyl chloride[22] in pyridine at 0°C followed by stirring at r.t. overnight, 70%).

Nicotinic acid and iso-nicotinic acid were alkylated first with **119** to give the esters **160** and **161** and second with methyl iodide to give the pyridinium salts **64** and **65**, respectively.

The carbamate alcohol **107** (Scheme 6) was esterified with nicotinic acid, iso-nicotinic acid and 4-(4-pyridyl)butyric acid[23] to give **162**, **49**, and **163**, respectively. Methylation produced the pyridinium salts **51**, **50**, and **52**.

TABLE 1
Quaternization of Various Nucleophiles

R = H or CH$_3$
X = MsO$^-$ or Br$^-$

Nu	Solvent	Temp. (°C)	Time (h)	Product (see Table 2)	Scheme	Yield (%)
N(CH$_3$)$_3$	EtOH	56	4	15, 21, 23, 25, 27, 29, 31, 53, 56, 79, 81	2	70—100
(thiazole)	none	100	7	2, 7, 9, 16, 37, 39, 41, 45, 54, 59, 68, 75, 83, 85	2	70—100
				5, 35, 43, 47	3	
				11, 13, 87, 89	4	
(thiazole-OH)	none	56	130	17	2	79
(pyridine)	none	100	7	1, 3, 4, 8, 10, 18, 19, 20, 24, 26, 28, 30, 32, 38, 40, 42, 46, 55, 62, 69, 78, 80, 82, 84, 86	2	70—100
				6, 36, 44, 48	3	
				12, 14, 88, 90	4	
(pyridazine)	toluene	64	95	63	2	75
(quinoline)	none	110	9	70	2	17
(pyridine-CONH$_2$)	toluene	110	8	71	2	40
(nicotinamide)	none	110	7	72	2	33
S(CH$_3$)$_2$	CH$_3$CN AgOMs	60	120	22	2	58

PHARMACOLOGY

The measurement of platelet aggregation is a simple procedure and well suited for the primary screening of PAF antagonists.[24] Further evaluation of the anti-PAF compounds includes the PAF receptors in respiratory and cardiovascular systems.[25] Some pharmacological results from such tests with compounds 1—91 will be presented in the following. Results with two of the compounds 62 (GS 1065-180) and 68 (GS 1160-180), have previously been described.[13]

TABLE 2
Compounds Tested for Inhibition of PAF- and Collagen-Induced Platelet Aggregation[a] Structure A-B-C-D-E-F X−

Compound	A	B	C	D	E	F	X−	−log EC$_{50}$ PAF[b]	−log EC$_{50}$ Collagen
1	CH$_3$(CH$_2$)$_{12}$	NHC(O)O	CH$_2$C(CH$_2$)CH$_2$	OC(O)	(CH$_2$)$_5$		Br−	4.8	
2	CH$_3$(CH$_2$)$_{14}$	C(O)O						5.3	
3								5.2	
4					(CH$_2$)$_7$			5.3	
5		NHC(O)O		O	(CH$_2$)$_6$		MsO−	5.3	
6								5.1	
7				OC(O)	(CH$_2$)$_5$		Br−	6.0	
8								6.0	
9					(CH$_2$)$_7$			7.0	
10								5.5	
11			CH$_2$C(C(CH$_3$)$_2$)CH$_2$		(CH$_2$)$_5$			6.1 Ag	
12								6.1	
13					(CH$_2$)$_7$			6.6	4.7
14								5.6	

Compound	A	B	C	D	E	F	X⁻	−log EC$_{50}$ PAF[b]	−log EC$_{50}$ Collagen
15	$CH_3(CH_2)_{15}$	O	$CH_2C(CH_2)CH_2$	O	$(CH_2-)_4$	$^+N(CH_3)_3$ (thiazole)	MsO⁻	4.6	4.3
16					$(CH_2)_5$	—OH (thiazole/phenyl)		5.3	
17				OC(O)	CH_2		Br⁻	4.5	
18					$(CH_2)_3$			4.3	
19					$(CH_2)_4$			5.3 Ag	
20					$(CH_2)_5$			4.6	
21						$^+N(CH_3)_3$		4.1	
22						$^+S(CH_3)_2$		< 4	
23						$^+N(CH_3)_3$		5.0	
24						(pyridinium)		5.6	4.7
25					$(CH_2)_{10}$	$^+N(CH_3)_3$		4.3	
26						^+N (pyridinium)		4.3	
27				OC(O)NH	$(CH_2)_2$	$^+N(CH_3)_3$		< 4	4.1
28						(pyridinium)		4.4	4.1

Table 2. contd.

Compound	A	B	C	D	E	F	X⁻	−log EC$_{50}$ PAF[b]	−log EC$_{50}$ Collagen
29					$(CH_2)_4$	$^+N(CH_3)_3$ / pyridinium		4.7	5.0
30						$^+N(CH_3)_3$ / pyridinium		5.1	4.4
31				$OP(O)(O^-)O$	$(CH_2)_2$		−	5.0 Ag	
32								< 4	
33			$CH_2C(O)CH_2$	$OC(O)$	$(CH_2)_3$		Br^-	4.0	
34					$(CH_2)_5$			5.0	
35		$OC(O)O$	$CH_2C(CH_2)CH_2$	O	$(CH_2)_6$	thiazolium/pyridinium	MsO^-	5.5 Ag	
36						thiazolium/pyridinium		5.1	
37				$OC(O)$	$(CH_2)_5$	thiazolium/pyridinium	Br^-	6.6	
38						thiazolium/pyridinium		6.7	
39					$(CH_2)_7$	thiazolium/pyridinium		6.8	
40						thiazolium/pyridinium		6.1	
41		$NHC(S)O$				thiazolium/pyridinium		6.0	
42					$(CH_2)_5$	pyridinium		5.4	4.1

Compound	A	B	C	D	E	F	X^-	−log EC_{50}	
								PAF[b]	Collagen
43	$CH_3(CH_2)_{17}$	OC(O)O		O	$(CH_2)_6$	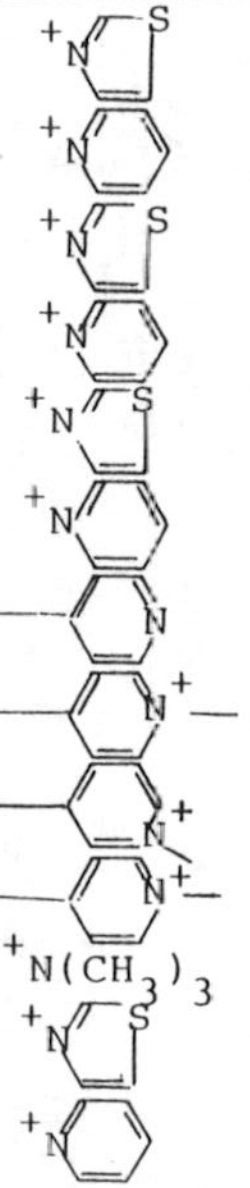	MsO^-	5.3	
44								5.3	
45				OC(O)			Br^-	6.3 Ag	
46								5.7	
47		NHC(O)O		O			MsO^-	5.1	
48								5.0	
49				OC(O)			–	< 4	
50							I^-	4.6	
51								5.1	
52					$(CH_2)_3$			5.8	
53					$(CH_2)_4$	$^{+}N(CH_3)_3$	Br^-	5.0	5.0
54								5.6	
55								5.6	
56					$(CH_2)_5$	$^{+}N(CH_3)_3$		5.3	

Table 2. contd.

Compound	A	B	C	D	E	F	X^-	$-\log EC_{50}$ PAF[b]	$-\log EC_{50}$ Collagen
57					$(CH_2)_5$	$^+N(CH_3)_2(CH_2)_2N(CH_3)_2$	$Br^-\ I^-$	5.3	
58						$^+N(CH_3)_2(CH_2)_2{}^+N(CH_3)_3$		4.6	
59							Br^-	6.4	4.1
60							I^-	< 4	
61							I^-	5.7	
62							Br^-	6.0	4.1
63								5.6	
64								4.3 Ag	
65							I^-	5.0 Ag	
66							I^-	< 4	
67								< 4	
68							Br^-	6.6	
69					$(CH_2)_6$			6.0 Ag	
70								< 4	

Compound	A	B	C	D	E	F	X⁻	$-\log EC_{50}$ PAF[b]	$-\log EC_{50}$ Collagen
71						C(O)NH₂ (pyridinium)		5.0 Ag	
72						C(O)NH₂ (pyridinium)		5.0 Ag	
73					$(CH_2)_7$	$^+N(CH_3)_2(CH_2)_2N(CH_3)_2$		6.0	
74						$^+N(CH_3)_2(CH_2)_2{}^+N(CH_3)_3$	Br⁻I⁻	4.1	
75							Br⁻	6.5	
76							–	< 4	
77							I⁻	5.4	
78							Br⁻	6.1	
79				OC(O)NH	$(CH_2)_2$	$^+N(CH_3)_3$		4.3	4.1
80								5.0	
81					$(CH_2)_4$	$^+N(CH_3)_3$		5.1	4.3
82								5.5	
83					$(CH_2)_5$			7.0 Ag	
84								6.6	4.1

Table 2. contd.

Compound	A	B	C	D	E	F	X⁻	-log EC_{50} PAF^b	-log EC_{50} Collagen
85					$(CH_2)_7$			6.6 Ag	
86								6.1	4.5
87			$CH_2C(C(CH_3)_2)_2CH_2$	$OC(O)$	$(CH_2)_5$			6.4	
88								6.4	4.3
89					$(CH_2)_7$			6.1	
90								6.0 Ag	
91			$CH_2C(O)CH_2$		$(CH_2)_5$			5.5	
CV 3988								4.7	
WEB 2080								6.2	

[a] Experimental procedure described in Section on Pharmacology, Subsection - Platelet Aggregation.
[b] Ag denotes proaggregating properties.

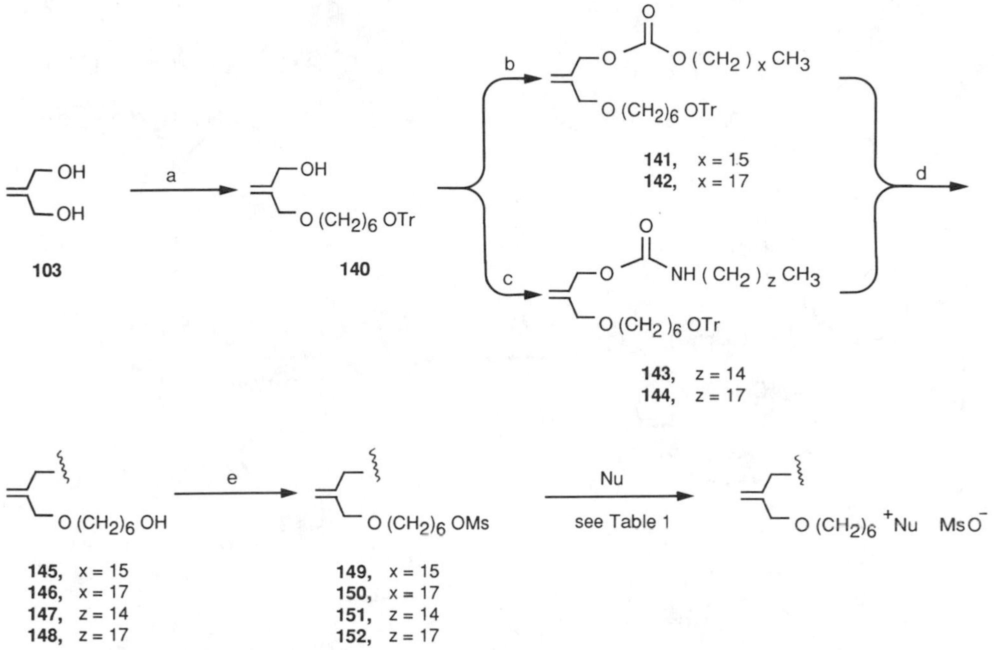

141, x = 15
142, x = 17

143, z = 14
144, z = 17

103

140

b

c

d

O(CH₂)ₓCH₃

O(CH₂)₆OTr

NH(CH₂)ₓCH₃

O(CH₂)₆OTr

e

Nu

see Table 1

O(CH₂)₆OH

O(CH₂)₆OMs

O(CH₂)₆⁺Nu   MsO⁻

145, x = 15
146, x = 17
147, z = 14
148, z = 17

149, x = 15
150, x = 17
151, z = 14
152, z = 17

Scheme 3. (a) Cl(CH₂)₆OTr/NaH/DMF/85°C/3 h/26%. (b) ClCOO(CH₂)ₓCH₃/pyridine/CH₂Cl₂/r.t./5 h/59—82%. (c) OCN(CH₂)ₓCH₃/4-DMAP/CH₂Cl₂/r.t./5 h/53—57%. (d) TsOH/H₂O/CH₂Cl₂/r.t./20 h/40—45%. (e) MsCl/pyridine/CH₂Cl₂/r.t./2 h/ca. 95%.

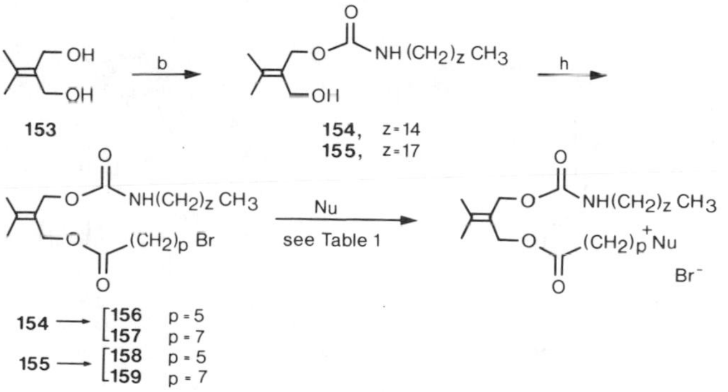

153

b

h

Nu

see Table 1

NH(CH₂)z CH₃

OH

154, z=14
155, z=17

154 → [**156** p=5 / **157** p=7]
155 → [**158** p=5 / **159** p=7]

(CH₂)p Br

(CH₂)p⁺Nu

Br⁻

Scheme 4. Reaction conditions, see Scheme 2 (b) and (h).

PLATELET AGGREGATION

All the compounds listed in Table 2 have been tested *in vitro* for their ability to inhibit platelet aggregation caused by PAF or collagen in platelet rich plasma from rabbits.[13] The compounds to be tested were added 3 min before racemic C_{16}-PAF (0.06 μM) or collagen (60 $\mu g/ml$) and the concentration (EC_{50}) required to reduce the aggregation by 50% was determined. The PAF-EC_{50} values are listed in Table 2. ''Ag'' denotes that the compound exhibited aggregating properties. Most of the compounds showed no antagonist activity towards collagen induced platelet aggregation at concentrations smaller than 10^{-4} M and those remaining few compounds which did show collagen antagonist activity (from 10^{-5} to 10^{-4} M) are listed in Table 2. For comparison we have also included the well-known PAF antagonists CV-3988[1] and WEB 2086,[26] in the platelet aggregation test.

The data listed in Table 2 can be used to obtain knowledge about the structure/activity

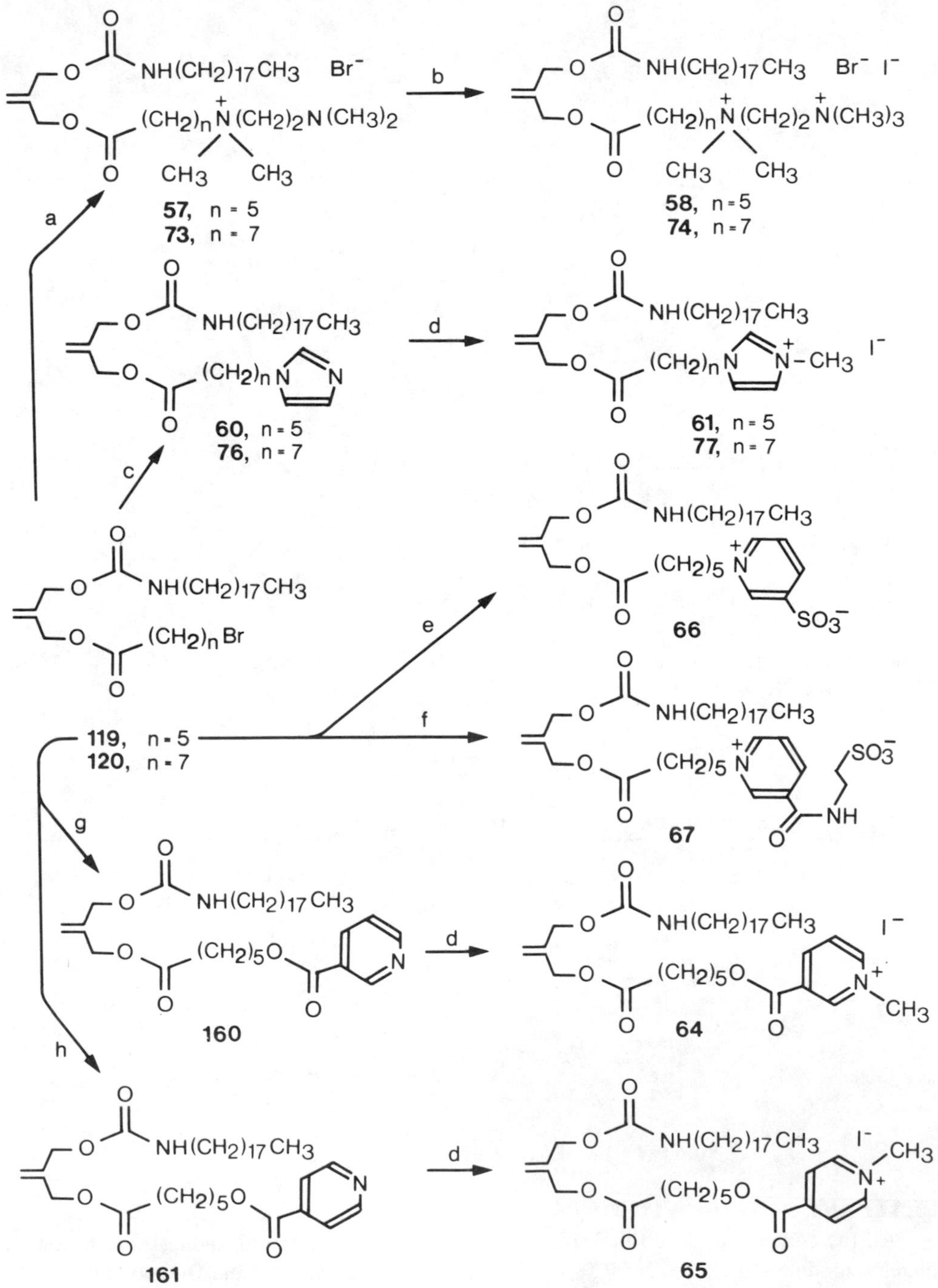

Scheme 5.   (a) $(CH_3)_2N(CH_2)_2N(CH_3)_2/112°C/6$ h/ca. 90%. (b) $CH_3I/CH_2Cl_2/r.t./5$ h/90%. (c) imidazole/toluene/104°C/8 h/68—84%. (d) $CH_3I/CHCl_3/r.t./19$ h/ca. 90%. (e) 3-sulfopyridine, Na salt/DMF/ 140°C/13 h/37%. (f) N-(2-sulfoethyl)nicotinamide, Na salt/DMF/ 140°C/23 h/40%. (g) Potassium nicotinate/DMF/66°C/16 h/78%. (h) Potassium isonicotinate/DMF/66°C/16 h/72%.

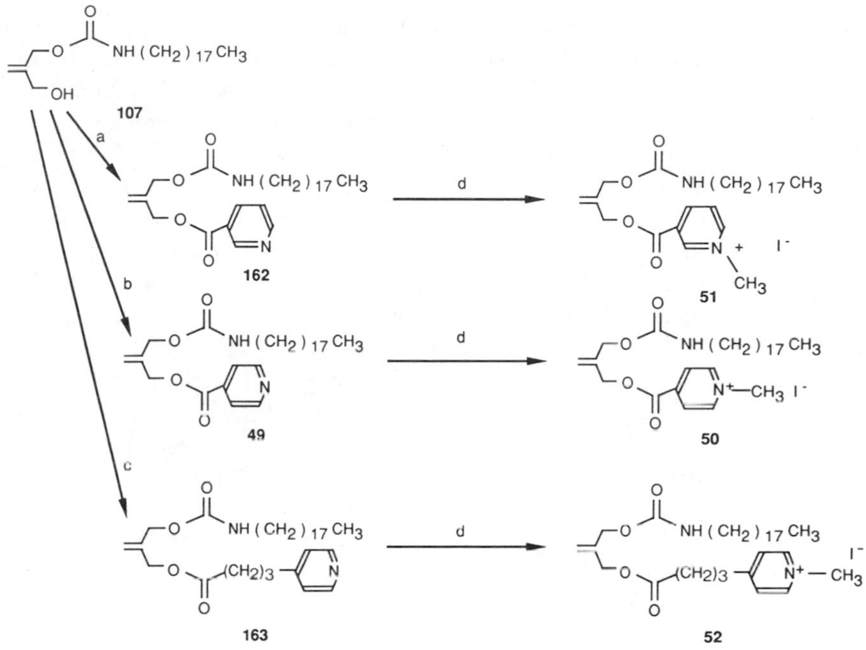

Scheme 6.   (a) Nicotinic acid/DCC/4-DMAP/CH₂Cl₂/r.t./23 h/ca. 90%. (b) Isonicotinic acid/DCC/4-DMAP/CH₂Cl₂/r.t./23 h/72%. (c) 4-(4-pyridyl)butyric acid, HCl/DCC/4-DMAP/pyridine/r.t./24 h/67%, (d) CH₃I/CH₂Cl₂/r.t./24 h/ca. 90%.

relationship of this type of achiral PAF antagonist analogs. The essence will be highlighted in the following.

The substructures **A** to **F** seem to be independently variable.

A lipophilic chain, **A**, of 13 carbon atoms was out of the optimal range which in these studies included compounds with 15, 16, and 18 carbon atoms. Longer carbon chains were not tested. The optimal length of the alkyl chain is the same as found for agonist analogs.[27]

The best substructure **B** to replace the ether oxygen of PAF was either carbonate or carbamate although an ether, ester or thiocarbamate function makes the PAF antagonists no more than ten times less active. Other potent antagonists with ether or carbamate as substructure **B** have been described.[9,24,28,29]

Three achiral substitutes, **C**, for the glycerol moiety are reported in this chapter. Only three compounds, **33, 34,** and **91**, with a keto group in the mimicked 2-position of glycerol were tested, but they appeared less active (although less than ten times) than the corresponding 2-alkylidene analogs. No distinction in activity could be made between compounds with a 2-methylene and a 2-isopropylidene group.

Besides the "natural" phosphate group three other substructures **D** were evaluated. The phosphate analog **31**, which is very closely related to PAF, showed weak agonistic activity in platelet aggregation whereas the other phosphate analog **32** was inactive. Compounds with an ether linkage appeared less active than those with an ester linkage and these seemed to be only slightly less active than those compounds with a carbamate group as substructure **D**. Other compounds with anti-PAF activity with phosphate, ether, ester or carbamate substructures **D** have been described.[9,28,29]

The length of the alkylidene chain $(CH_2)_n$ = substructure **E** was optimal for n = 5, 6, or 7 and the activity decreased with increasing deviation from these values.

Two non-charged substructures **F** were tested in compounds **49, 60,** and **76** and neither of these compounds exhibited any activity. The superior group **F** was the thiazolium ion followed by the pyridinium ion. Somewhat inferior were the N-methyl-imidazolium and pyrimidinium ions, but the antagonist activity of compounds with the "natural" trimethyl-ammonium ion was even lower. Compounds with a quinolinium or dimethylsulfonium ion were inactive, just like the betaines **66** and **67**. The only compound (**17**) with the thiazolium ion derived from thiamin was less active than the corresponding compound **16** with the unsubstituted thiazolium ion. Compounds **57** and **73** in which one methyl group of the trimethylammonium group has been replaced by a 2-(dimethylamino)-ethyl group were quite active, but the corresponding compounds **58** and **74** in which the dimethylamino group has been quaternized to give substructure **F** with two quaternary ammonium ions were almost inactive. Compounds **71** and **72** produced by quaternization of isonicotinamide or nicotin-amide were moderately active, but they both showed agonist platelet aggregating properties. The same properties can be ascribed to compounds **64** and **65** in which the pentamethylene chain is linked with an ester bond to *N*-methylnicotinate and *N*-methylisonicotinate. Other compounds **50**, **51**, and **52** with "turned around" pyridinium ions showed moderate antag-onist activity.

As already mentioned, some of the compounds listed in Table 2 have proaggregating properties, but the structural features which give rise to this activity are not obvious.

The lack or almost lack of antagonist activity towards collagen induced platelet aggre-gation demonstrates that the most active of the PAF antagonists in Table 2 are specific to PAF. Compounds **62** and **68** were tested and shown not to be antagonists in platelet aggre-gation induced by ADP.[13]

BRONCHOCONSTRICTION

The effectiveness of the inhibition of PAF induced bronchoconstriction in the guinea pig by PAF antagonists is well investigated.[24,30-32] Potent PAF antagonists listed in Table 2 were also tested for their ability to inhibit PAF induced bronchoconstriction in guinea pigs.[13] The antagonists were dosed i.v. to anesthetized guinea pigs 3 min before PAF (30 ng/kg) and the doses (ED_{50}) required to reduce the bronchoconstriction caused by PAF by 50% were determined (see Table 3).

Any precise conclusions from Table 3 regarding the structure activity relationship cannot be drawn. However, the more potent antagonists in the platelet aggregation test appeared to be among the strongest antagonists in the bronchoconstriction experiments as well. The ED_{50} values (0.1—1.0 mg/kg) of the most potent compounds were in between the ED_{50} values of the known PAF antagonists CV-3988 (3.5 mg/kg) and WEB 2086 (0.01 mg/kg).

Interestingly, compounds (**11**, **19**, and **83**) which appeared as PAF agonists in the platelet aggregation test were among the most potent compounds to inhibit PAF-induced broncho-constriction.

BLOOD PRESSURE

The hypotensive effect of PAF and its inhibition by anti-PAF compounds has been extensively covered in the literature.[1,6,24-26,31,33]

Most of the compounds listed in Table 2 were tested for their ability to inhibit PAF-induced hypotension in rats. The antagonists were dosed i.v. to anesthetized rats 10 min before PAF (25 ng/kg) and the doses (ED_{50}) required to reduce the arterial blood pressure fall caused by PAF by 50% were determined (see Table 3).

The ED_{50} values of the most active PAF antagonists in this test had ED_{50} values in the range 0.1 to 1 mg/kg, and there was a reasonable, but not perfect, correlation between the PAF antagonist potencies in the platelet aggregation, bronchoconstriction, and blood pressure tests. Compound **62** (GS 1065-180) had an ED_{50} of 2 mg/kg i.v. when PAF was administered 1 h after **62**, compared with an ED_{50} of 0.5 mg/kg i.v. when PAF was given 10 min after **62**, thus indicating a reasonable duration of action for **62** in the rat.

TABLE 3
PAF Antagonist Activities[a]

Compound	Bronchoconstriction ED$_{50}$ (mg/kg i.v.)	Blood pressure ED$_{50}$ (mg/kg i.v.)	Compound	Bronchoconstriction ED$_{50}$ (mg/kg i.v.)	Blood pressure ED$_{50}$ (mg/kg i.v.)
2	0.2	1	39	0.3	0.6
3	>1	1	40	0.6	5
4	>1	>5	54	>1	0.8
7	>1	2	55	1	2
8	>1	0.8	56		1
9	>1	0.2	59	0.2	0.3
10	0.5	0.8	62	0.2	0.5
11	0.3	1	68	0.1	0.5
12	>0.3	0.3	69	0.8	>1
13	0.5	0.8	73		3
17		5	75	0.2	0.3
18	>5		78	0.8	3
19	0.7	3	81	1	5
20		3	82	0.5	1
21		>5	83	0.25	0.1
23		0.5	84	0.3	0.25
24		1	85		0.3
25		>5	86	>1	1
26		5	87	0.2	1
30	>3	0.8	88	0.1	0.2
31		>1	89	0.6	0.6
32		>5	91	1	0.5
33		5	CV-3988	3.5	1.0
34	>5	1	WEB 2086	0.01	
37	0.8	0.8			
38	0.3	0.4			

[a] Experimental procedures described in section on Pharmacology, Subsections Bronchoconstriction and Blood Pressure.

FURTHER PHARMACOLOGY OF GS 1065-180

Because GS 1065-180 (**62**) was the first of the more potent PAF antagonists synthesized at Leo this compound was taken through further evaluation in pharmacological tests.

Ovalbumin Induced Asthma

The exact role of PAF in lung pathophysiology is not clear, but the inhibition of antigen-induced lung anaphylaxis by PAF antagonistic compounds has been demonstrated.[32,34]

Guinea pigs were sensitized with an intraperitoneal injection of 10 mg ovalbumin. One month later the animals were anesthetized with urethane and prepared for artificial respiration in a modified Konzett-Rössler system.[13] The animals were dosed i.v. with GS 1065-180, 7 min later with suxamethonium chloride (1.2 mg/kg i.v.) and then 3 min later with ovalbumin (0.3 mg/kg i.v.). The reduction in airway obstruction was measured as percentage of maximum obtainable bronchoconstriction. This reduction with doses of GS 1065-180 of 0.1, 0.3, and 1 mg/kg was 27, 64, and 86%, respectively.

In comparison, we found that WEB 2086 at 1 mg/kg i.v. given 1 min before the ovalbumin challenge reduced the airway obstruction by 43%.

When GS 1065-180 was given orally at doses of 1 mg/kg/day or 10 mg/kg/day for 21 days no effect was observed upon challenge with ovalbumin.

Anti-Hypertensive Effect

Six spontaneously hypertensive female rats were dosed orally 1 mg/kg or 10 mg/kg of GS 1065-180 and the animals were placed in a box at 38°C for 30 min immediately before the indirect measurement of the systolic blood pressure on the tail arteries with a blood pressure recorder. The blood pressure and the heart rate were unaffected by the administration of GS 1065-180.

Passive Cutaneous Anaphylaxis

Several different provocators, such as immune complexes, can induce endogenous release of PAF, known to be one of the most potent inducers of increased endothelial permeability.[5]

To evaluate the potential of GS 1065-180 in this context LEW/Mol inbred female rats were passively immunized in the dorsal skin with an antiserum to ovalbumin raised in BN rats. Ovalbumin and Evan's Blue were injected intravenously 24 h later and the antigen reaction with the antiserum causing plasma leakage, was visualized by the presence of Evan's Blue. After 30 min more the rats were killed, the dorsal skin inverted, and two diameters of each reaction spot measured. GS 1065-180 (1 mg/kg i.v.) given simultaneously with ovalbumin and Evan's Blue gave no inhibition. Similar results with other PAF antagonists have been observed.[5]

Carrageenin Edema

PAF is recognized as a mediator in inflammatory disorders.[35] In order to investigate the potential of PAF antagonists in inflammatory diseases GS 1065-180 was tested in the carrageenin induced rat paw edema.

SD/Mol female outbred rats were fasted for 18 h. Carrageenin (1.5%, 0.1 ml, Wiscarin 402, Marine Colloids, USA) was injected into the right hindpaw of each rat, causing an acute inflammatory edema. Paw volumes were measured after 3 and 5 h. When GS 1065-180 was dosed (10 mg/kg i.v.) 1 h before carrageenin injection no change in effect was observed. A similar result has been obtained by others.[36]

Stomach Ulcer

PAF plays a role as an endogenous mediator in the severe acute gastric damage associated with septic shock.[37]

When GS 1065-180 was dosed (10 mg/kg i.v.) to Sprague Dawley rats 10 min before PAF (10 μg/min/kg for 10 min) a highly significant reduction in the gastric ulceration was observed. Interestingly, when GS 1065-180 (10 mg/kg) was dosed orally no reduction of the ulceration was observed.

CELLULAR ACTIVITIES
Anti-Tumor Activity

Compounds that inhibit the growth of tumor cells may be useful as anticancer drugs. It is well established that a number of ether lipids exhibit anti-tumor activity[38-40] and a screening of the PAF analogs in Table 2 thus seemed particularly warranted.

Yoshida Sarcoma cells, originally derived from rat hepatic tumors induced by the carcinogen o-amino-azo-toluene, were cultured *in vitro* for 24 h in the presence of the drug under investigation. DNA synthesis was measured by incorporation of ^{3}H-thymidine into DNA and cell survival was assessed microscopically by the exclusion of the dye Eosin Y. The results were calculated as the concentration (IC_{50}) resulting in 50% inhibition of the control response.

The IC_{50} values were determined for the compounds **1—4, 7—26, 28—31, 33—34, 37—42, 49—65, 67—69**, and **73—91** (cf. Table 2). Most active were the compounds that were ether lipids, **15, 16, 18**, and **19**, and the bis-carbamates **81** and **82**, with IC_{50} values of 0.4, 0.6, 0.6, 0.8, 0.7, and 1.0 μM, respectively. In comparison, the IC_{50} value for **62** (GS 1065-180) was 8.8 μM.

Lymphocyte Transformation

Compounds that suppress the immunological reactivity are potentially useful in the treatment of autoimmune diseases and in patients undergoing transplantation procedures. In this context, ether lipids have demonstrated interesting properties.[40]

The lymphocyte transformation test was used to detect compounds that interfered with the reactivity of the immune system. Rat lymphocytes were activated *in vitro* with the plant-derived stimulator (mitogen) concanavalin A. After culture for 48 h cellular DNA synthesis was assessed by the incorporation of ^{3}H-thymidine into the DNA. The results were calculated as the concentration (IC_{50}) resulting in 50% decrease of the control response.

The IC_{50} values were determined for compounds **1—4, 7—20, 22—30, 33—34, 37—42, 49—51, 53—65, 68—69**, and **73—91** (cf. Table 2). Compounds with IC_{50} values below 1 μM are listed together with **62** (GS 1065-180) in Table 4. Most active were the ether lipids **15—19** and **29—30** and the bis-carbamates **80—82**.

CONCLUSIONS

A series of achiral PAF analogs, **1—91**, has been prepared by straightforward chemical synthesis. All compounds were tested as PAF antagonists in the rabbit platelet aggregation assay and it appeared that each substructure **A** to **F** (Table 2) could be optimized for PAF antagonist activity more or less independently

Some of the most potent anti-PAF compounds from the platelet aggregation test were also highly active *in vivo*. PAF-induced bronchoconstriction in the guinea pig and hypotension in the rat were effectively inhibited by some of the compounds in Table 3 ($ED_{50} = 0.1$ to 1.0 mg/kg i.v.).

A further investigation of GS 1065-180 (**62**) demonstrated that ovalbumin induced asthma was inhibited by low doses (0.1— 1.0 mg/kg/i.v.) of GS 1065-180. Oral administration of GS 1065-180 to hypertensive rats had no effect on blood pressure and heart rate. GS 1065-180 was ineffective to inhibit ovalbumin provoked passive cutaneous anaphylaxis or acute carrageenin edema in the rat. However, PAF-induced gastric damage was reduced by GS 1065-180, dosed intravenously.

TABLE 4
Lymphocyte
Transformation[a]

Compound	IC_{50} (μM)
15	0.5
16	0.8
17	0.2
18	0.6
19	0.4
29	0.3
30	0.9
53	0.9
62	9.8
80	0.3
81	0.2
82	0.2

[a] Experimental procedure described in Section on Pharmacology, Subsection Lymphocyte Transformation.

Of a series of PAF analogs tested for direct activity on tumor cells and on cells from the immune system a few compounds were found to be active in concentrations below 1 μM. It is interesting to note that the ether lipids **15**, **16**, **18**, and **19** and the bis-carbamates **81** and **82** were among the most active compounds in both tests. Besides the obvious potential of PAF-analogs to interfere with PAF mediated inflammatory reactions some of these compounds possess additional value as potential immuno inhibitory or anti-tumor agents. Whether these reactivities are linked to the PAF structure, to the surface-active properties of these compounds or to other features remains to be assessed.

ACKNOWLEDGMENTS

A generous gift from Takeda of CV-3988 and from Boehringer Ingelheim of WEB 2086 is greatly acknowledged. Skillful help from our colleagues I.M. Nielsen (chemical synthesis), N. Rastrup Andersen (spectral data), E. Bramm (passive cutaneous anaphylaxis and carrageenin edema), Dr. L. Binderup (cellular activities), L. Pridal, H. Selvig, and L. Frøjk (technical assistance), B. Tellefsen (typing of the manuscript), and J. Gramkow (drawing of figures) is greatly appreciated.

REFERENCES

1. **Terashita, Z., Tsushima, S., Yoshioka, Y., Nomura, H., Inada, Y., and Nishikawa, K.,** CV-3988 — a specific antagonist of platelet activating factor (PAF), *Life Sci.,* 32, 1975, 1983.
2. **Wykle, R. L., Miller, C. H., Lewis, J. C., Schmitt, J. D., Smith, J. A., Surles, J. R., Piantadosi, C., and O'Flaherty, J. T.,** Stereospecific activity of 1-O-alkyl-2-O-acetyl-sn-glycero-3-phosphocholine and comparison of analogs in the degranulation of platelets and neutrophils, *Biochem. Biophys. Res. Commun.,* 100, 1651, 1981.
3. **Heymans, F., Michel, E., Borrel, M.-C., Wichrowski, B., Godfroid, J.-J., Convert, O., Coeffier, E., Tence, M., and Benveniste, J.,** New total synthesis and high resolution ^{1}H nmr spectrum of platelet-activating factor, its enantiomer and racemic mixtures, *Biochim. Biophys. Acta,* 666, 230, 1981.

4. **Barner, R., Hadvary, P., Burri, K., Hirth, G., Cassal, J.-M., and Müller, K.,** Glycerol derivatives, Eur. Patent 147,768, 1985.

5. **Handley, D. A., Anderson, R. C., and Saunders, R. N.,** Inhibition by SRI 63-072 and SRI 63-119 of PAF-acether and immune complex effects in the guinea pig, *Eur. J. Pharmacol.,* 141, 409, 1987.

6. **Takatani, M., Yoshioka, Y., Tasaka, A., Terashita, Z., Nishikawa, K., and Tsushima, S.,** Platelet activating factor (PAF) antagonists: development of the potent PAF antagonist, CV-6209, *J. Pharm. Sci.,* 76, S174, 1987.

7. **Wichrowski, B., Jouquey, S., Broquet, C., Heymans, F., Godfroid, J.-J., Fichelle, J., and Worcel, M.,** Structure-activity relationship in PAF-acether. IV. Synthesis and biological activities of carboxylate isosteres, *J. Med. Chem.,* 31, 410, 1988.

8. **Tomesch, J., Koletar, J., Prashad, M., Handley, D., Larson, D., and Winslow, C.,** PAF antagonists SDZ 63-441 and SDZ 63-675. Synthesis of and pharmacological characterization of the individual enantiomers, *Prostaglandins,* 35, 845, 1988.

9. **Takatani, M., Yoshioka, Y., Tasaka, A., Terashita, Z., Imura, Y., Nishikawa, K., and Tsushima, S.,** Platelet activating factor antagonists: synthesis and structure-activity studies of novel PAF analogues modified in the phosphorylcholine moiety, *J. Med. Chem.,* 32, 56, 1989.

10. **Corey, E. J., Chen, C.-P., and Parry, M. J.,** Dual binding modes to the receptor for platelet activating factor (PAF) of anti-PAF *trans*-2,5-diarylfurans, *Tetrahedron Lett.,* 29, 2899, 1988.

11. **Heuer, H., Birke, F., Brandt, K., Muacevic, G., and Weber, K.-H.,** Biological characterization of the enantiomeric hetrazepines of the PAF-antagonist WEB 2170, *Prostaglandins,* 35, 847, 1988.

12. **Williams, K. and Lee, E.,** Importance of drug enantiomers in clinical pharmacology, *Drugs,* 30, 333, 1985.

13. **Grue-Sørensen, G., Nielsen, I. M., and Nielsen, C. K.,** Derivatives of 2-methylenepropane-1,3-diol as new antagonists of platelet activating factor, *J. Med. Chem.,* 31, 1174, 1988.

14. **Baumann, W. J. and Mangold, H. K.,** Reactions of aliphatic methanesulfonates. I. Synthesis of long-chain glyceryl-(1) ethers, *J. Org. Chem.,* 29, 3055, 1964.

15. **Marshall, J. A. and Warne, T. M., Jr.,** The total synthesis of (±)-isonootkatone. Stereochemical studies of the Robinson annelation reaction with 3-penten-2-one, *J. Org. Chem.,* 36, 178, 1971.

16. **MacKay, K. D., Rogier, E. R., and Kreevoy, M. M.,** Verfahren zur Herstellung organischer Isocyanate, German Patent 2,245,611, 1974.

17. **Schmidt, E. and Fehr, L.,** Zur Kenntnis aliphatischer Carbodiimide. XI. Darstellung höherer n-Alkyl-isothiocyanate, *Liebigs Ann. Chem.,* 621, 1, 1959.

18. **Haggis, G. A. and Owen, L. N.,** Alicyclic glycols. VIII. 1:2-Bishydroxymethylcyclohexane, *J. Chem. Soc.,* 389, 1953.

19. **Laaksu, T. M. and Reynolds, D. D.,** Preparation of N,N,N′,N′-tetrasubstituted diamines, *J. Am. Chem. Soc.,* 73, 3518, 1951.

20. **Hirt, R. and Berchtold, R.,** Zur Synthese der Phosphatide. Eine neue Synthese der Lechitine, *Pharm. Acta Helv.,* 33, 349, 1958.

21. **Kricheldorf, H. R.,** Ringöffnung von Lactonen und cyclischen Carbonaten mit Brom- oder Iodtrimethyl-silan, *Angew. Chem.,* 91, 749, 1979.

22. **Ford, M. C. and Mackay, D.,** Decomposition reactions of heterocyclic diacyl peroxides. IV. Nicotinoyl peroxide, *J. Chem. Soc.,* 1294, 1958.

23. **Mikhlina, E. E. and Rubtsov, M. V.,** Synthesis of 1-azabicyclo [3.2.2]nonane-2-carboxylic acid, *Zh. Obshch. Khim.,* 32, 2177, 1962. *Chem. Abstr.,* 58, 1924g, 1963.

24. **Saunders, R. N. and Handley, D. A.,** Platelet-activating factor antagonists, *Annu. Rev. Pharmacol. Toxicol.,* 27, 237, 1987.

25. **Casals-Stenzel, J. and Heuer, H.,** Pharmacology of PAF antagonists, *Prog. Biochem. Pharmacol.,* 22, 58, 1988.

26. **Casals-Stenzel, J., Muacevic, G., and Weber, K.-H.,** WEB 2086, a new and specific antagonist of platelet activating factor (PAF) in vitro and in vivo, *Naunyn-Schmiedeb. Arch. Pharmacol.,* 334 (Suppl.), R44, 1986.

27. **Godfroid, J.-J., Broquet, C., Jouquey, S., Lebbar, M., Heymans, F., Redeuilh, C., Steiner, E., Michel, E., Coeffier, E., Fichelle, J., and Worcel, M.,** Structure-activity relationship in PAF-acether. III. Hydrophopic contribution to agonistic activity, *J. Med. Chem.,* 30, 792, 1987.

28. **Braquet, P., Mencia-Huerta, J. M., Chabrier, P. E., Touqui, L., and Vargaftig, B. B.,** The promise of platelet-activating factor, *ISI Atlas of Science: Pharmacology,* 187, 1987.

29. **Godfroid, J.-J. and Heymans, F.,** Chemistry of PAF antagonists, *Prog. Biochem. Pharmacol.,* 22, 25, 1988.

30. **Coëffier, E., Borrel, M.-C., Lefort, J., Chignard, M., Broquet, C., Heymans, F., Godfroid, J.-J., and Vargaftig, B. B.,** Effects of PAF-acether and structural analogues on platelet activation and broncho-constriction in guinea-pigs, *Eur. J. Pharmacol.,* 131, 179, 1986.

31. **Casals-Stenzel, J., Muacevic, G., and Weber, K.-H.,** Pharmacological actions of WEB 2086, a new specific antagonist of platelet activating factor, *J. Pharmacol. Exp. Ther.,* 241, 974, 1987.
32. **Lagente, V., Desquand, S., Hadvary, P., Cirino, M., Lellouch-Tubiana, A., Lefort, J., and Vargaftig, B. B.,** Interference of the Paf antagonist Ro 19-3704 with Paf and antigen-induced bronchoconstriction in the guinea-pig, *Br. J. Pharmacol.,* 94, 27, 1988.
33. **Handley, D. A., Valen, R. G. V., Melden, M. K., Flury, S., Lee, M. L., and Saunders, R. N.,** Inhibition and reversal of endotoxin-, aggregated IgG- and paf-induced hypotension in the rat by SRI 63-072, a paf receptor antagonist, *Immunopharmacology,* 12, 11, 1986.
34. **Touvay, C., Etienne, A., and Braquet, P.,** Inhibition of antigen-induced lung anaphylaxis in the guinea-pig by BN 52021 a new specific paf-acether receptor antagonist isolated from Ginkgo biloba, *Agents Actions,* 17, 371, 1985.
35. **Page, C. P., Archer, C. B., Paul, W., and Morley, J.,** Paf-acether: a mediator of inflammation and asthma, *Trends Pharmacol. Sci.,* 5, 239, 1984.
36. **Hwang, S.-B., Lam, M.-H., Li, C.-L., and Shen, T.-Y.,** Release of platelet activating factor and its involvement in the first phase of carrageenin-induced rat foot edema, *Eur. J. Pharmacol.,* 120, 33, 1986.
37. **Rosam, A.-C., Wallace, J. L., and Whittle, B. J. R.,** Potent ulcerogenic actions of platelet-activating factor on the stomach, *Nature,* 319, 54, 1986.
38. **Andreesen, R.,** Ether lipids in the therapy of cancer, *Prog. Biochem. Pharmacol.,* 22, 118, 1988.
39. **Hallgren, B.,** Therapeutic effects of ether lipids, in *Ether Lipids, Biochemical and Biomedical Aspects,* Mangold, H. K. and Paltauf, F., Eds., Academic Press, New York, 1983, chap. 15.
40. **Weltzien, H. U. and Munder, P. G.,** Synthetic alkyl analogs of lysophosphatidylcholine: membrane activity, metabolic stability, and effects on immune response and tumor growth, in *Ether Lipids, Biochemical and Biomedical Aspects,* Mangold, H. K. and Paltauf, F., Eds., Academic Press, New York, 1983, chap. 16.

Chapter 7

STRUCTURE ACTIVITY RELATIONSHIPS IN CYCLIC ANALOGS OF PAF WITH PAF ANTAGONIST PROPERTIES

William J. Houlihan

INTRODUCTION

The structure of natural platelet-activating factor (PAF) was established in 1979 by three independent research groups[1-3] to be a mixture of 1-hexadecyl and 1-octadecyl-2-acetyl-*sn*-glycero-3-phosphocholine. Subsequent work by Godfroid[4] determined that the absolute configuration of natural PAF as the R-enantiomer (Figure 1).

The search for compounds that could antagonize the effects of PAF has focused on the synthesis of analogs of PAF, screening of natural products, and the evaluation of a variety of synthetic compounds, some having known pharmacological activity. Several reviews on PAF antagonists have recently been published.[5-13]

PAF ANTAGONISTS

ASSAYS FOR PAF ANTAGONISTS

The ease of measuring PAF-induced human or rabbit platelet aggregation has led to the use of this assay as a primary laboratory screen for detecting potential PAF antagonists.[14,15] The ability to displace or compete with [³H]PAF for the high affinity binding sites on isolated human[14] or rabbit[15] platelets can then be used to classify a compound as a specific PAF receptor antagonist.

The physiological responses of PAF that are used by most laboratories for evaluating potential PAF antagonists are the hypotensive responses in rats,[2,16] hemoconcentration effects in the guinea pig[17] or rabbit,[18] and the bronchoconstriction in the rabbit or guinea pig.[20]

CYCLIC PAF ANTAGONISTS

The initial attempts to find antagonists of PAF focused on the open-chain analogs of PAF.[7-13] The structure activity findings in the open-chain PAF antagonists served as a basis for the design of most of the reported cyclic PAF antagonists. A summary of the open-chain modifications of the PAF molecule that gave rise to PAF receptor antagonist activity is given in Figure 2.

The structural relationship of the cyclic analogs of PAF reported in this chapter to the glycerol framework of PAF is shown in Figures 3 and 4.

In Figure 3 the 2,2-disubstituted tetrahydrofuran, II.B.1.a, is formed by joining the C-2 and β-O of glycerol into a five-membered ring while the II.B.1b analog results from the linkage of the β-oxygen atom with the C-1 carbon. The 2,5-disubstituted tetrahydrofuran, II.B.1.c, can be looked on as a dimer of glycerol where the two C-3 positions are linked and the ring is completed by one β-oxygen atom. The tetrahydropyran, II.B.2, results from linkage of the C-1 and β-O atoms by a three carbon unit. Two 1,3-dioxa derivatives, II.B.3 and II.B.5, are both formed by joining the α- and β-O atoms with a one and two carbon linking unit, respectively. The six-membered derivatives, II.B.4 and II.B.7, are obtained by linking the α- and γ-O atoms with a carbon and phosphorous atom, respectively. The oxabicyclo system, II.B.9, is formed by joining the C-2 and C-2′ atoms of II.B.1.c with two carbon atoms.

The piperidine and the 1,3,2-oxaphospholidine ring systems, II.B.8 and II.B.6, given

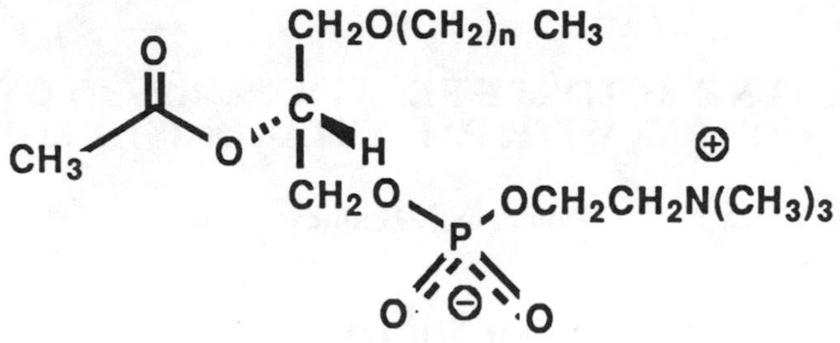

R - Enantiomer   n = 15, 17

FIGURE 1.   Absolute configuration of natural PAF.

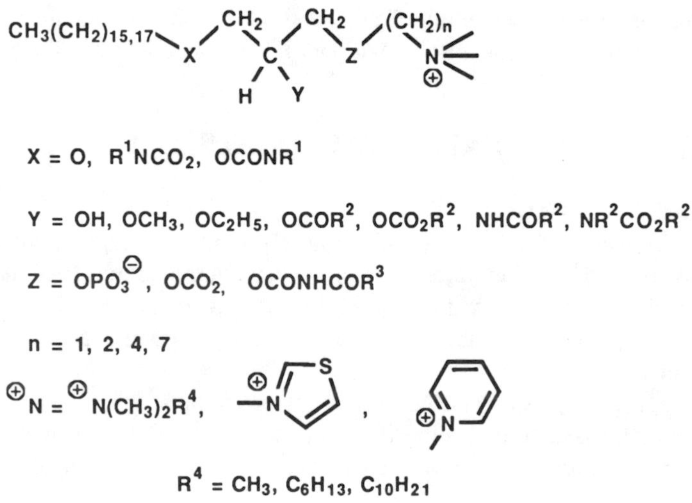

X = O, R^1NCO_2, $OCONR^1$

Y = OH, OCH_3, OC_2H_5, $OCOR^2$, OCO_2R^2, $NHCOR^2$, $NR^2CO_2R^2$

Z = $OPO_3^{\ominus}$, OCO_2, $OCONHCOR^3$

n = 1, 2, 4, 7

$^{\oplus}N =$ $^{\oplus}N(CH_3)_2R^4$,

R^4 = CH_3, C_6H_{13}, $C_{10}H_{21}$

FIGURE 2.   Modifications of the PAF molecule leading to useful PAF receptor antagonists.

in Figure 4 can be regarded as N-PAF or aza-glycerol derivatives. The piperidine system, II.B.8, is formed by a linkage of the α-N and the C-2 while II.B.6 is formed by linking the α-N and β-O with a phosphorous atom.

Tetrahydrofurans

2,2-Disubstituted

The 2,2-bis-hydroxymethyltetrahydrofuran derivative, SRI 63-072, (**1**) is the only member of the 2,2-disubstituted tetrahydrofurans (II.B.1.a; Figure 3) analog of PAF that has been reported.[21-23]

SRI 63-072 inhibited PAF-induced aggregation of human, guinea pig, rabbit, dog, and baboon platelets with IC_{50} = 22.3, 1.4, 4.7, <100, and 19 μM, respectively.[24] Significant inhibition of PAF-induced degranulation of human neutrophils was seen at 50 μM.[25] Racemic SRI 63-072 inhibited PAF receptor binding on human platelets (IC_{50} 1.44 μM) in the same range as the (+)- (IC_{50} 0.86 μM) and (−)- (IC_{50} 0.42 μM) enantiomers.[26] The high affinity PAF binding sites and PAF-induced elastase release from human polymorphonuclear leukocytes were both blocked by SRI 63-072.[27] PAF-induced hemoconcentration in the guinea pig[26,28,29] and *Cebus apella*[30-32] primate was inhibited by SRI 63-072 with ED_{50} = 0.4

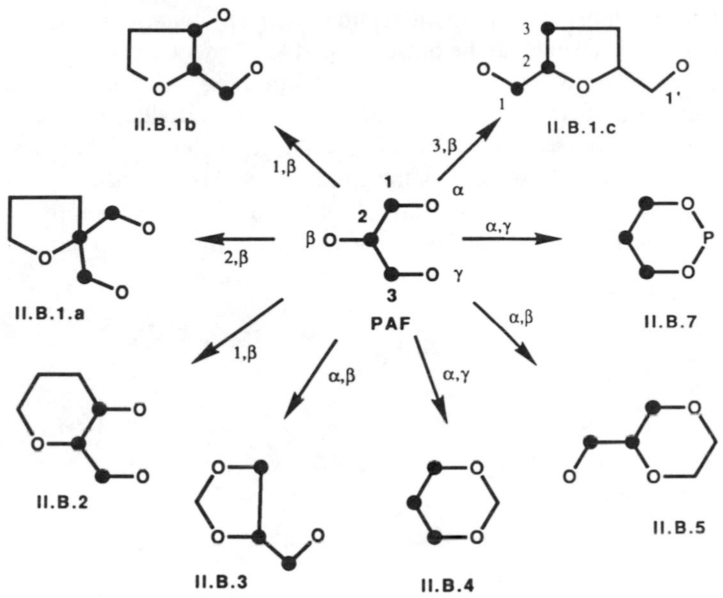

FIGURE 3. Structural relationship of cyclic analogs of PAF to the glycerol framework of PAF.

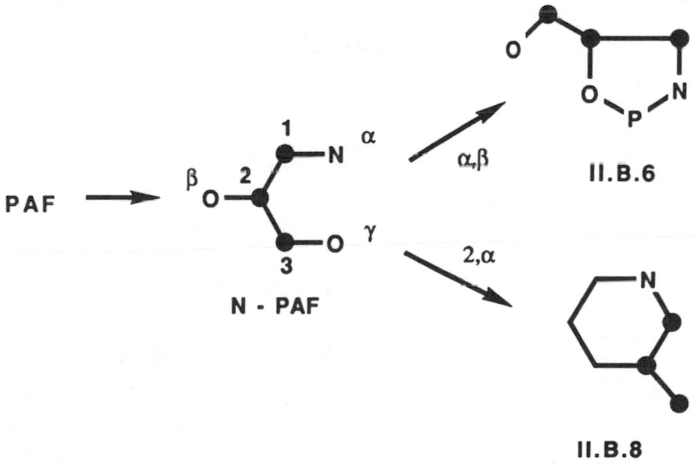

FIGURE 4. Structural relationship of cyclic analogs of PAF to aza-glycerol.

mg/kg i.a. and 0.95 mg/kg i.v., respectively. The PAF, *E. coli* endotoxin, and human heat aggregated IgG-induced hypotension in the rat was inhibited with ED_{50} = 0.16 mg/kg, 1.0 mg/kg, and 0.05 mg/kg i.v., respectively.[33-36] SRI 63-072 at 5 mg/kg i.v. partially blocked the hypotension induced by *E. coli* toxin in rabbits[37] and PAF in dogs.[38] In the perfused rabbit heart SRI 63-072 at 0.6 mg/kg reversed by 70% the reduction in coronary flow.[39] PAF-induced bronchoconstriction in the guinea pig was inhibited by SRI 63-072 (ED_{50} 0.4 mg/kg i.a.),[26,28,29] and the lung response, but not vasoconstriction induced by PAF in perfused isolated rabbit lungs, was prevented.[40] In addition, SRI 63-072, aerosolized at a concentration of 1 mg/ml inhibited PAF aerosol-induced airways response in the rhesus monkey,[41] but had little or no effect on the airway constrictive response seen in guinea pigs after exposure to an aerosol of A23187.[42] Pretreatment with 3 mg/kg i.v. of SRI 63-072 significantly improved initial hypotension, hematocrit, white blood cell count, and extent of bowel perfusion and microscopic changes in the bowel in a rat PAF-endotoxin induced ischemic bowel necrosis model.[43] When SRI 63-072 was co-administered i.d. with PAF it blocked the cutaneous reactivity of PAF in the rhesus monkey[41] and partially reversed dermal plasma leakage in the reverse, passive Arthus reaction in the guinea pig.[26,44] At a dose of 25 mg/kg i.p. the compound reduced the severity of the glomerulonephritis induced by *in situ* deposition of immune complexes in the rat.[45] A mixture of SRI 63-072 and a nonsteroidal anti-inflammatory is claimed to be useful in accelerating wound healing in deep dermal burns.[46]

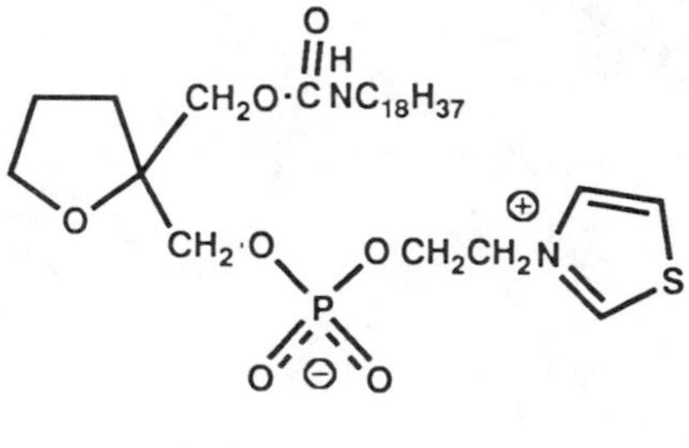

1

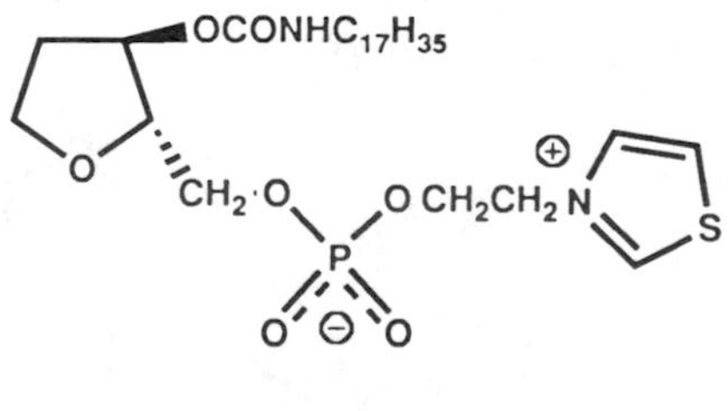

2

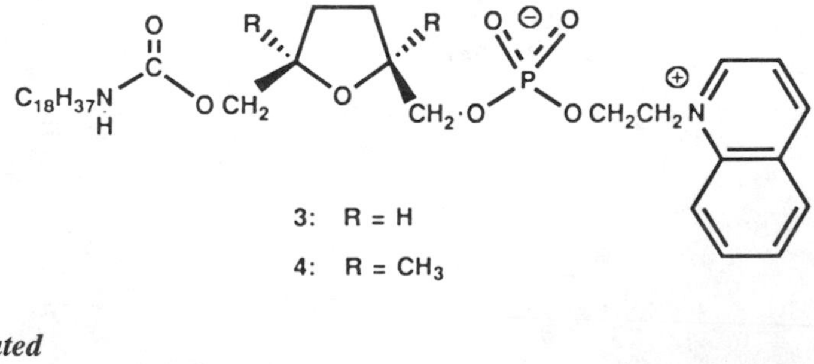

3: R = H

4: R = CH₃

2,3-Disubstituted

The 2,3-disubstituted tetrahydrofuran (II.B.1.b, Figure 3) derivative compound (**2**) is reported to inhibit PAF-induced rabbit platelet aggregation (IC_{50} 21 μM) and PAF-induced hypotension in the rat (ED_{50} 0.4 mg/kg i.v.).[47]

2,5-Disubstituted

The 2,5-disubstituted tetrahydrofuran analogs (II.B.1.b; Figure 3) are represented by 2,5-bis-hydroxymethyl- and 2-substituted-5-oxyalkylene quaternary salts of tetrahydrofuran.

SRI 63-441 (**3**) the cis-2,5-disubstituted analog of SRI 63-072 (**1**) antagonized PAF-induced human, guinea pig, rabbit, baboon, and dog platelet aggregation (IC_{50} = 3.3, 0.3, 0.8, 0.3, and 10.2 μM, respectively), and PAF receptor binding to human platelets (IC_{50} 0.35 μM).[48] It inhibited PAF stimulated phospholipase activity in rabbit platelets (IC_{50} 0.78

μM)[49] and elastase release in human polymorphonuclear leukocytes (IC$_{50}$ 2.3 μM).[27] Enhanced TXA$_2$ synthesis and PGI$_2$ production was seen when equine peritoneal macrophages were treated with SRI 63-441 (50 μM).[50] SRI 63-441 also inhibited PAF-induced hypotensive responses in the rat[51,52] and dog[53] (ED$_{50}$ 0.15 mg/kg and 0.20 mg/kg i.v., respectively); hemoconcentration in the dog and primate (ED$_{50}$ 0.18 and 0.11 mg/kg i.v., respectively); and the hemoconcentration and bronchoconstriction responses in the guinea pig (ED$_{50}$ 0.012 mg/kg and 0.035 mg/kg i.a., respectively).[51]

PAF-induced increase in airways responsiveness and platelet accumulation in the thorax could be inhibited by SRI 63-441 at 1.0—2.5 mg/kg i.v. given pre-PAF challenge in the normal guinea pig,[54,55] but at 10 mg/kg i.v., i.p., or inhaled the compound failed to block the acute increase in airway hyperreactivity caused by PAF in ovalbumin sensitized animals.[56] In aerosolized form, SRI 63-441 (10 mg/ml) blocked the acute airway response to aerosolized PAF in healthy adult rhesus monkeys, but failed to block the acute IgE-mediated airways response to *Ascaris suum* in sensitized monkeys.[57] SRI 63-441 also failed to block the allergic reaction in *Ascaris suum* allergic dogs when given at 5 mg/kg i.v. and 10 mg/ml by inhalation 1 h before allergen challenge.[58]

A single dose of SRI 63-441 (15 mg/kg i.v.) given 4 min prior to revascularization in the rat-to-rabbit orthotopic renal xenograft and the heterotopic cardiac transplant model in presensitized inbred rats caused significant increase in survival rates compared to controls.[59] SRI 63-441 alone failed to prolong renal xenograft survival and function in a pig-to-dog heterotransplantation model.[60] However, the combination of SRI 63-441 given at 5 mg/kg i.v. bolus 5 min before and 5 min after revascularization and given every 15 min thereafter, together with either prostacyclin (PGI$_2$) or PGI$_1$ continuous infusion demonstrated significant synergism and resulted in a six- to ninefold increase in kidney survival and a 3- to 20-fold increase in urine output.[59] Isolated livers from male rats that had been treated 5 min before harvesting with SRI 63-441 (20 mg/kg i.v.) produced significantly more bile than untreated livers.[61,62]

Early ischemic arrhythmias and ventricular fibrillation in greyhounds with occluded left anterior descending coronary artery were reduced or modified by SRI 63-441 at 10 mg/kg i.v.[63] At 3 μM SRI 63-441 improved PAF-induced decrease in coronary flow and alleviates arrhythmias during cardiac anaphylaxis in an *in vitro* guinea pig model[64] and at 0.01 μM caused a marked decrease in PAF-induced negative inotropic effects in non-coronary perfused human right atrial pectinate muscle.[65]

SRI 63-441 at 20 to 50 mg/kg i.p. effectively inhibited a variety of endotoxin-induced effects in rats, such as acute lung damage and neutropenia caused by *S. enteriditis*[66,67] and the arterial pressure decrease, hyperglycemia and hyperlactacidemia,[68] and changes in plasma glutathione[69] induced by *E. coli*. In *E. coli* endotoxin treated sheep, SRI 63-441 given at 20 mg/kg/h i.v. blocked the resultant pulmonary pressor response, hypoxemia, and reduced cardiac output[70,71] but had minimal effects on lung mechanics and lung fluid and solute exchange.[72] In the rabbit, SRI 63-441 at 20 mg/kg i.v. inhibited alterations in ocular vascular permeability induced by *E. coli*[73,74] or anterior chamber paracentesis.[75]

In a study designed to determine the effect of PAF in establishing pregnancy, a total of 20 μg of SRI 63-441 given i.p. per mouse over 4 days caused a 90% reduction in embryos due to implantation failure.[76,77]

SRI 63-441 has also been shown to block PAF stimulated events such as phosphorylation in washed rabbit platelets,[78] increase in complement (C3bi and C3b) receptor expression,[79] and actin filament assembly[80] in human neutrophils.

SRI 63-675 (**4**), the cis-2,5-dimethyl analog of SRI 63-441 (**3**), has a similar *in vitro* and *in vivo* profile of activity against PAF-induced events, such as platelet aggregation (IC$_{50}$ = 3.42, 0.25 and 0.97 μM against human, guinea pig, and rabbit platelets, respectively) and human platelet receptors (IC$_{50}$ 0.37 μM).[81] The compound inhibited PAF-induced hypotension in the rat (ED$_{50}$ 32 μg/kg i.v.); hemoconcentration in the guinea pig (ED$_{50}$ 1.7μg/

TABLE 1

Inhibition of PAF-Induced Platelet Aggregation, PAF Receptor Binding, and PAF-Induced Hemoconcentration and Bronchoconstriction Changes in the Guinea Pig by the Enantiomeric and Geometric Isomers of Compounds 2 and 3[80,81]

Compound no.	Isomer	Human platelets		Guinea pig	
		PAF-induced aggregation	PAF receptor	Hemoconc.[a]	Broncho.[b]
		IC_{50}, μM		ED$_{50}$ mg/kg i.a. or (% inhibition at 0.06 mg/kg)	
2	(±)-cis	2.7	0.56	(61)	(45)
2	2S,5R-cis	3.5	0.43	(71)	(45)
2	2R,5S-cis	6.5	0.44	(46)	(43)
2	(±)-trans	11.4	1.19	(60)	(40)
3	(±)-cis	0.52	0.31	0.017	0.025
3	(+)-cis	6.1	0.89	0.045	0.070
3	(−)-cis	0.12	0.14	0.013	0.016

[a] Hemoconcentration.
[b] Bronchoconstriction.

kg i.v.) and primate (ED$_{50}$ 28 μg/kg i.v.); and bronchoconstriction in the guinea pig (ED$_{50}$ 2.4 μg/kg i.v.).[81] SRI 63-675 at 1.0 mg/kg i.v. significantly reduced PAF-induced changes in mean arterial pressure in the pithed[82] and normal[83] rat at doses of 1.0 mg/kg i.v. and 10 mg/kg i.p., respectively. In ovalbumin sensitized rats, SRI 63-675 (1.2 mg/kg i.v.) increased the survival rate, reduced the vascular collapse and suppressed the hemoconcentration changes induced by i.v. injection of PAF.[84] In spontaneous hypertensive rats it blocked PAF and PAG (1-palmitoyl-2-acetyl-glycerol), but not nitroprusside-induced changes in blood pressure and mesenteric flow/resistance.[85] In the domestic pig it prevented PAF-induced increases in mean pulmonary arterial, systemic arterial, and peak tracheal pressure.[86] At doses of 0.1 mg/kg i.v. and greater, SRI 63-675 prevented PAF-induced airway microvascular leakage of colloidal carbon in the tracheobronchial region of conscious guinea pigs,[87] but failed to prevent PAF-induced contractions in isolated peripheral lung strips and trachea from guinea pigs.[88] At a dose of 50 μg/kg/min i.v. it completely reversed the effects of PAF on gastric bleeding from an induced gastric mucosal wound in rats.[89] Partial inhibition (45%) of edema formation in rabbit skin induced by intradermal injections of PAF plus PGI$_2$ resulted when SRI 63-675 was given i.d. (0.01 μM) but not i.v. (to 10 mg/kg).[90]

Several studies have been reported on attempts to increase the potency or biological half-life of compounds **3** and **4**. Separation of the enantiomers[91] of **3** and **4** and preparation of the trans-isomer[92] of **3** gave compounds that showed some potency differences *in vitro* but not *in vivo* as inhibition of PAF-induced hemoconcentration and bronchoconstriction in the guinea pig appears to be similar (Table 1).

Substitution of the alkyl nitrogen atom of compound **3** by N-methylation (**5**) to decrease the rate of hydrolysis of the carbamate group and modification of the linearity of the alkyl chain by a terminal t-butyl (**6**) or trimethylsilyl (**7**) group to prevent ω-1 metabolism resulted in compounds with a three- to fivefold increase in duration of biological activity and potency similar to **3** against PAF-induced bronchoconstriction in the guinea pig.[93,94] Replacement of the carbamoyl side chain in **3** by an alkyl ether (**8**) or the PO$_3^-$ moiety by a two carbon unit (**9**) gave substances with similar potency and duration of action.[93,94]

	n	R^1	R^2
5	17	CH_3	CH_3
6	14	$(CH_3)_3C$	H
7	14	$(CH_3)_3Si$	H

	R	X
8	$C_{18}H_{37}$	$PO_3^{\ominus}CH_2CH_2$
9	$C_{18}H_{37}NHCO$	$CH_2CH_2CH_2CH_2$

A series of 2-substituted tetrahydrofuran-5-yloxy-alkylene quaternary salts, exemplified by **10**,[95] inhibited PAF-induced rabbit platelet aggregation and myotropic activity in the guinea pig parenchymal strip and at 10 mg/kg i.p. showed a significant reduction in PAF-induced thrombocytopenia and leukopenia in the rabbit.[96]

Tetrahydropyrans

A number of tetrahydropyrans (II.B.2., Figure 3) of cis- and trans-3-hydroxy or 3-mercapto-2-hydroxymethyl phosphate[97] and carbamate[98] quaternary salts (**11**) have been reported to have PAF antagonist activity. A listing of the more potent analogs and enantiomers of this class of compounds is given in Table 2. Maximum *in vitro* and *in vivo* PAF inhibition for the racemic 3-hydroxy 2-phosphate derivatives was found in the trans-series where n = 5 or 6 and R is a $C_{17}H_{35}$ group in formula **11** (Table 2; **11a—e**). The racemic cis-3-mercapto-2-phosphate series showed the same trend (Table 2; **11k—j, m**). In each pair of enantiomers evaluated, the 3-*S* enantiomer (Table 2; **11f, 11l, 12b**) was more potent than the 3-R enantiomer as a PAF antagonist both *in vitro* and *in vivo*. Interestingly, the racemic analogs (Table 2, **11e, 11j, 12a**) were similar in activity to the 3-S enantiomers.[46,49]

The cis- and trans-isomers of lactone **13** (X = O) failed to show any PAF-like activities at the doses tested while the ether analogs (**13** X = H$_2$) gave weak PAF-like activity.[46]

1,3-Dioxolanes

The 1,3-dioxolane (II.B.3, Figure 3) derivative BN 52110 (**14**) is reported to inhibit the PAF-induced amplification of superoxide O_2^- in human neutrophils.[100]

TABLE 2

Inhibition of PAF-Induced Platelet Aggregation and PAF-Induced Hypotension in the Rat by Analogs and Enantiomers of Compounds 11 and 12[46,99]

Compound no.	X	n	R	Isomer	Rabbit platelets PAF-induced aggregation (IC_{50} μM)	Rat hypotension (ID_{50}, mg/kg, i.v.)
11a	O	2	$C_{18}H_{37}$	RS-cis	9.6	0.09
11b	O	2	$C_{18}H_{37}$	RS-trans	3.8	0.46
11c	O	2	$C_{17}H_{35}$	RS-trans	1.5	0.57
11d	O	5	$C_{17}H_{35}$	RS-trans	0.55	0.044
11e	O	6	$C_{17}H_{35}$	RS-trans	0.55	0.046
11f	O	6	$C_{17}H_{35}$	2R, 3S-trans	0.59	0.054
11g	O	6	$C_{17}H_{35}$	2S, 3R-trans	4.7	0.30
11h	S	2	$C_{17}H_{35}$	RS-cis	3.1	0.22
11i	S	4	$C_{17}H_{35}$	RS-cis	1.1	0.24
11j	S	5	$C_{17}H_{35}$	RS-cis	0.57	0.076
11k	S	5	$C_{17}H_{35}$	2R, 3R-cis	1.10	0.92
11l	S	5	$C_{17}H_{35}$	2S, 3S-cis	0.27	0.064
11m	S	6	$C_{17}H_{35}$	RS-cis	0.78	0.19
12a	—	—	—	RS-	0.24	0.034
12b	—	—	—	2R, 3S-	0.20	0.032
12c	—	—	—	2S, 3R-	2.20	0.21

1,3-Dioxanes

The 1,3-dioxane (II.B.4, Figure 3) derivative SDZ 63-754 (**15**) failed to give any protection against PAF-induced human platelet aggregation at doses up to 100 μM.[101]

1,4-Dioxanes

PAF-antagonist inhibition against rabbit platelets has been reported for a series of 1,4-dioxanes (II.B.5, Figure 3) of which **16** is a representative.[102]

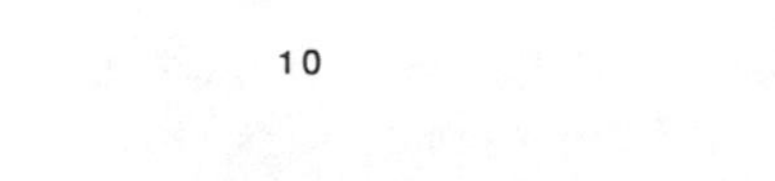

10

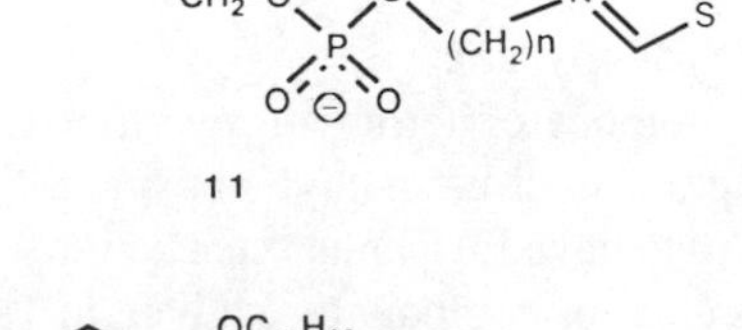

11

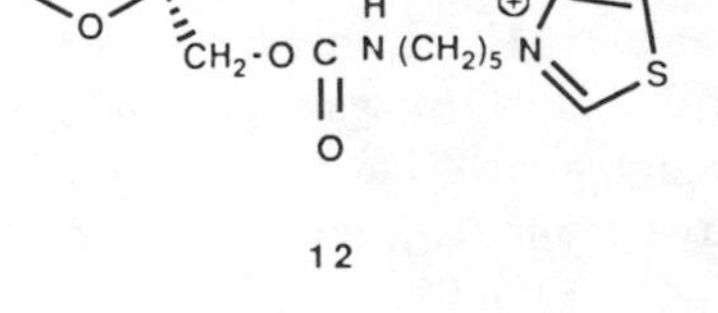

12

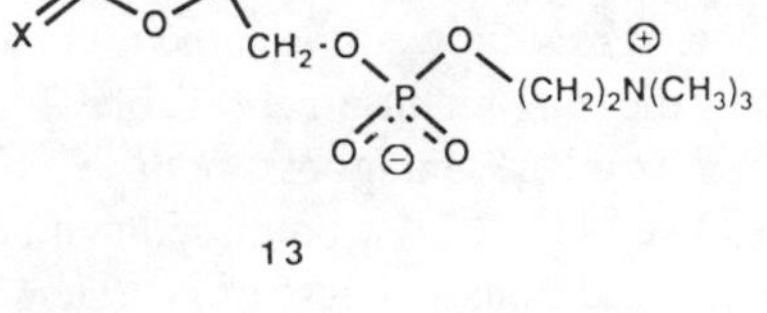

13

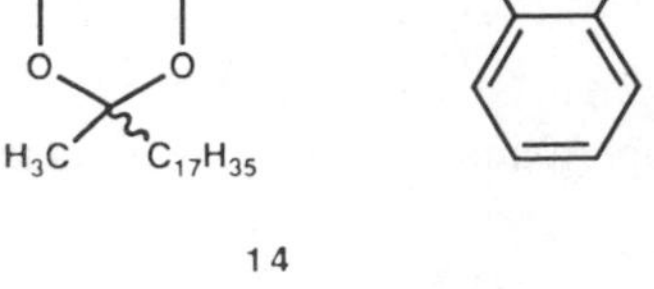

14

2-Oxo-1,3,2-oxazaphospholidines

No PAF antagonist activity against PAF-induced rabbit platelet aggregation at doses up to 30 μM was found in a series of 2-oxo-1,3,2-oxazaphospholidines (II.B.6, Figure 3) with phosphorodiamidic quaternary salts, such as compound **17**.[103]

2-Oxo-1,3,2-dioxaphosphorinanes

A series of compounds where the phosphate group is conformationally restricted by being incorporated into a 1,3,2-dioxaphosphorinane ring system (II.B.7, Figure 3) have been reported.[103] In the cyclic phosphates and phosphoramidates, compounds with an equatorial side chain are significantly better PAF antagonists than the axial diastereoisomers. The most active analogs, **18a** and **18b**, had IC$_{50}$ values of 2.1 and 3.2 μM, respectively, against PAF-induced rabbit platelet aggregation.

Piperidines

The novel piperidine (II.B.8, Figure 4) derivative SRI 63-073 (**19**) which has a thiamine moiety as a polar head showed unusual selectivity in inhibiting PAF-induced aggregation of human and guinea pig platelets with IC$_{50}$ values of 37.7 and 0.015 μM respectively, and PAF receptor binding to human platelets (IC$_{50}$ 3.4 μM).[104] At doses of 0.55 to 3.1 mg/kg i.a., the compound gave a dose-dependent inhibition of PAF-induced hemoconcentration and bronchoconstriction in the guinea pig.

Oxabicyclo[2.2.1]heptanes

The oxabicyclo[2.2.1]heptane (II.B.9) SDZ 63-880 (**20**), which is an ethylene bridged analog of SRI 63-441 (**3**), inhibited PAF receptor binding to human platelets (IC$_{50}$ 0.34 μM) in the same range as **3** (IC$_{50}$ 0.35 μM) but is ca. tenfold weaker when evaluated i.v. against PAF-induced bronchoconstriction in the guinea pig.[92]

19

20

ACKNOWLEDGMENTS

The assistance of Mrs. Ellen Brennan in typing and Dr. Charles Jewell in preparing the artwork for this chapter is greatly appreciated.

REFERENCES

1. **Demopoulous, C. A., Pinckard, R. N., and Hanahan, D. J.,** Platelet-activating factor. Evidence for 1-O-alkyl-2-acetyl-sn-glyceryl-3-phosphorylcholine as the active component (a new class of lipid chemical mediators), *J. Biol. Chem.,* 254, 9355, 1979.
2. **Blank, M. L., Snyder, F., Byers, L. W., Brooks, B., and Muirhead, E. E.,** Antihypertensive activity of an alkyl ether analog of phosphatidylcholine, *Biochem. Biophys. Res. Commun.,* 90, 1194, 1979.
3. **Benveniste, J., Tencé, M., Varenne, P., Bidault, J., Boullet, C., and Polonsky, J.,** Semi-synthesis and proposed structure of platelet-activating factor (PAF): PAF-acether an alkyl ether analog of lysophosphatidylcholine, *C. R. Hebd. Seances Acad. Sci. Ser. D,* 289, 1037, 1979.
4. **Godfroid, J. J., Heymans, F., Michel, E., Redeuilh, C., Steiner, E., and Benveniste, J.,** Platelet activating factor (PAF-acether): total synthesis of 1-octadecyl-2-O-acetyl-sn-glycero-3-phosphorylcholine, *FEBS Lett.,* 116, 161, 1980.
5. **Saunders, R. N. and Handley, D. A.,** Platelet-activating factor antagonists, *Annu. Rev. Pharmacol. Toxicol.,* 27, 237, 1987.
6. **Hanahan, D. J. and Kumar, R.,** Platelet activating factor; chemical and biochemical characteristics, *Prog. Lipid Res.,* 26, 1, 1987.
7. **Braquet, P. and Godfroid, J. J.,** Conformational properties of the PAF-acether receptor on platelets based on structure-activity studies, in *Platelet-Activating Factor and Related Lipid Mediators,* Snyder, F., Ed., Plenum Press, New York, 1987, 191.
8. **Shen, T. Y., Hwang, S.-B., Doebber, T. W., and Robbins, J. C.,** The chemical and biological properties of PAF agonists, antagonists and biosynthetic inhibitors, in *Platelet-Activating Factor and Related Lipid Mediators,* Snyder, F., Ed., Plenum Press, New York, 1987, 153.
9. **Piwinski, J. J., Kreutner, W., and Green, M. J.,** Pulmonary and antiallergy agents, *Annu. Rep. Med. Chem.,* 22, 73, 1987.
10. **Godfroid, J. J. and Braquet, P.,** PAF-acether specific binding sites. I. Quantitative SAR study of PAF-acether isosteres, *Trends Pharmacol. Sci.,* 7, 368, 1986.
11. **Handley, D. A.,** Development and therapeutic indications for PAF antagonists, *Drugs Future,* 13, 137, 1988.
12. **Chang, M. N.,** PAF and PAF antagonists, *Drugs Future,* 11, 867, 1986.
13. **Houlihan, W. J.,** Platelet activating factor antagonists, in *Platelet Activating Factor in Endotoxin and Immune Disease,* Handley, D., Houlihan, W. J., Saunders, R., and Tomesch, J., Eds., Marcel Dekker, New York, 1990, 31.
14. **Valone, F. H., Coles, E., Reinhold, V. R., and Goetzl, E. J.,** Specific binding of phospholipid platelet-activating factor by human platelets, *J. Immunol.,* 129, 1637, 1982.
15. **Hwang, S-B., Lee, C. S., Cheah, M. J., and Shen, T. Y.,** Specific receptor sites of 1-O-alkyl-2-O-sn-glycero-3-phosphocholine (platelet activating factor) on rabbit platelet and guinea pig smooth muscle membranes, *Biochemistry,* 22, 4756, 1983.
16. **Tanaka, S., Kasuya, Y., Masuda, Y., and Shigenobu, K.,** Studies on the hypotensive effects of platelet activating factor (PAF, 1-O-alkyl-2-acetyl-sn-glyceryl-3-phosphorylcholine) in rats, guinea pigs, rabbits, and dogs, *J. Pharmacol. Dyn.,* 6, 866, 1983.

17. **Handley, D. A., VanValen, R. G., Melden, M. K., and Saunders, R. N.,** Evaluation of dose and route effects of platelet activating factor-induced extravasation in the guinea pig, *Thromb. Haemost.,* 52, 34, 1984.

18. **McManus, L. M., Hanahan, D. M., Demopoulos, C. A., and Pinckard, R. N.,** Pathobiology of the intravenous infusion of acetyl glyceryl ether phosphorylcholine (AGEPC), a synthetic platelet activating factor (PAF), in the rabbit, *J. Immunol.,* 124, 2919, 1980.

19. **Stimler, N. P., Bloor, C. M., Hugli, T. E., Wykle, R. L., McCall, C. E., and O'Flaherty, J. T.,** Anaphylactic actions of platelet-activating factor, *Am. J. Pathol.,* 105, 64, 1981.

20. **Lefort, J., Wal, F., Chignard, M., Medeiros, M. C., and Vargaftig, B. B.,** Pharmacological properties of PAF-acether in guinea pigs: platelet dependent and independent reactions, *Agents Actions,* 12, 723, 1982.

21. **Saunders, R., Anderson, R., Handley, D., Houlihan, W., Lee, M., Tomesch, J., and Winslow, C.,** The biological activity of SRI 63-072, *2nd Int. Conf. on Platelet-Activating Factor and Structurally Related Alkyl Ether Lipids,* Gatlinburg, TN, October 26—29, 1986, abstr. p 33.

22. **Houlihan, W. J. and Saunders, R. N.,** Platelet activating factor (PAF): a biologically active ether phospholipid, *Triangle,* 25, 97, 1986.

23. **Handley, D. A. and Saunders, R. N.,** Platelet activating factor and inflammation in atherogenesis: targets for drug development, *Drug. Dev. Res.,* 7, 361, 1986.

24. **Winslow, C. M., Anderson, R. C., D'Aries, F. J., Frisch, G. E., DeLillo, A. K., Lee, M. L., and Saunders, R. N.,** Toward understanding the mechanism of action of platelet activating factor receptor antagonists, in *New Horizons in Platelet Activating Factor Research,* Winslow, C. M. and Lee, M. L., Eds., John Wiley & Sons, New York, 1987, 153.

25. **Hunt, D. A. and Barefoot, S. T.,** Effect of various platelet activating factor (PAF) antagonists on neutrophil degranulation, *Clin. Res.,* 35, 478A, 1987.

26. **Handley, D. A., Anderson, R. C., and Saunders, R. N.,** Inhibition by SRI 63-072 and SRI 63-119 of PAF-acether and immune complex effects in the guinea pig, *Eur. J. Pharmacol.,* 141, 409, 1987.

27. **Marquis, O., Robaut, C., and Cavero, I.,** Evidence for the existence and ionic modulation of platelet-activating factor receptors mediating degranulatory responses in human polymorphonuclear leukocytes, *J. Pharmacol. Exp. Ther.,* 250, 293, 1989.

28. **Deacon, R. W., Melden, M. K., Van Valen, R. G., Farley, C., Anderson, R. C., Lee, M. L., Saunders, R. N., and Handley, D. A.,** Pharmacological inhibitory profiles of SRI 63-072 and SRI 63-119 in PAF-induced hemoconcentration and bronchoconstriction in the guinea pig, *New Horizons in Platelet Activating Factor Research,* Hilton Head Island, October 15—18, 1985, abstr. 65.

29. **Farley, C., Melden, M. K., Van Valen, R. G., Deacon, R. W., Anderson, R. C., Lee, M. L., Saunders, R. N., and Handley, D. A.,** *In vivo* inhibition by SRI 63-072 and SRI 63-119 in PAF-induced hemoconcentration and bronchoconstriction in the guinea pig, *Fed. Proc.,* 45, 855, 1986.

30. **Handley, D. A., VanValen, R. G., and Saunders, R. N.,** Vascular responses of platelet-activating factor in the *Cebus apella* primate and inhibitory profiles of antagonists SRI 63-072 and 63-119, *Immunopharmacology,* 11, 175, 1986.

31. **Handley, D. A., VanValen, R. G., and Saunders, R. N.,** *Cebus apella* primate responses to platelet activating factor and inhibition by PAF antagonist SRI 63-072, in *New Horizons in Platelet Activating Factor Research,* Winslow, C. M. and Lee, M. L., Eds., John Wiley & Sons, Chichester, 1987, 335.

32. **Handley, D. A., VanValen, R. G., Lee, M. L., and Saunders, R. N.,** Inhibition of PAF-induced vascular responses in the *Cebus apella* primate by SRI 63-072, *New Horizons in Platelet Activating Factor Res.,* Hilton Head Island, October 15—18, 1985, abstr. 24.

33. **Handley, D. A., VanValen, R. G., Melden, M. K., Flury, S., Lee, M. L., and Saunders, R. N.,** Inhibition and reversal of endotoxin-, aggregated IgG and PAF-induced hypotension in the rat by SRI 63-072, a PAF receptor antagonist, *Immunopharmacology,* 12, 11, 1986.

34. **VanValen, R. G., Saunders, R. N., and Handley, D. A.,** Reversal by SRI 63-072 of endotoxin and immune aggregate-induced hypotension in the rat, in *New Horizons in Platelet Activating Factor Research,* Winslow, C. M. and Lee, M. L., Eds., John Wiley & Sons, Chichester, 1987, 123.

35. **VanValen, R. G., Melden, M. K., Lee, M. L., Saunders, R. N., and Handley, D. A.,** Reversal by SRI 63-072 of endotoxin and immune aggregate-induced hypotension in the rat, *New Horizons in Platelet Activating Factor Research,* Hilton Head Island, October 15—18, 1985, abstr. 8.

36. **Melden, M. K., Flury, S., Saunders, R. N., and Handley, D. A.,** Inhibition and reversal by SRI 63-072 and SRI 63-119 of PAF-induced hypotension in the rat, *Fed. Proc.,* 45, 856, 1986.

37. **Smallbone, B. W., de Kergommeaux, B. D., and McDonald, J. W. D.,** Effects of indomethacin and SRI 63-072 on endotoxin-induced hypotension, *FASEB J.,* 2, A976, 1988.

38. **Toth, P., VanCamp, J., Mikulaschek, A., and Demeter, R.,** The effects of CV-3988 and SDZ 63-072 on PAF-induced hypotension in dogs, *Circ. Shock,* 21, 297, 1987.

39. **Camussi, G., Niesen, N., Saunders, R. N., and Milgrom, F.,** Release of platelet-activating factor from rabbit heart perfused *in vitro* by sera with transplantation alloantibodies, *Transplant,* 44, 113, 1987.

40. **Arnoux, B. and Gillis, C. N.**, Are platelets required for platelet-activating factor-induced pulmonary smooth muscle contraction?, *2nd Int. Conf. Platelet Activating Factor*, Gatlinburg, TN, October 26—29, 1986, 70.

41. **Patterson, R., Harris, K. E., Lee, M. L., and Houlihan, W. J.**, Inhibition of rhesus monkey airway and cutaneous responses to platelet activating factor (PAF) (AGEPC) with the anti-PAF agent SRI 63-072, *Int. Arch. Allergy Appl. Immunol.*, 81, 265, 1986.

42. **Stengel, P. and Silbaugh, S. A.**, Reversal of A23187-induced airway constriction in the guinea pig, *J. Pharmacol. Exp. Ther.*, 248, 1084 (1989).

43. **Hsueh, W., Gonzalez-Crussi, F., Arroyave, J. L., Anderson, R. C., Lee, M. L., and Houlihan, W. J.**, Platelet activating factor-induced ischemic bowel necrosis: the effect of PAF antagonists, *Eur. J. Pharmacol.*, 123, 79, 1986.

44. **Deacon, R. W., Melden, M. K., Saunders, R. N., and Handley, D. A.**, PAF involvement in dermal extravasation in reverse passive arthus reaction, *Fed. Proc.*, 45, abstr. 995, 1986.

45. **Camussi, G., Pawlowski, I., Saunders, R., Brentjens, J., and Andres, G.**, Receptor antagonist of platelet activating factor inhibits inflammatory injury induced by *in situ* formation of immune complexes in renal glomeruli and in the skin, *J. Lab. Clin. Med.*, 11, 196, 1987.

46. **Bauer, J.**, Combination preparation for treatment of inflammation, German Patent 3,808,039, March 10, 1988.

47. **Miyazaki, H., Ohkawa, N., Nakamura, N., Ito, T., Sada, T., Oshima, T., and Koike, H.**, Lactone and cyclic ether analogues of platelet-activating factor. Synthesis and biological activities, *Chem. Pharm. Bull.*, 37, 2379 (1989).

48. **Winslow, C. M., Gubler, H. U., DeLillo, A. K., D'Aries, F. J., Tomesch, J. C., and Saunders, R. N.**, Inhibition of PAF-induced ulcer formation by the specific PAF receptor antagonist, SRI 63-441, *2nd Int. Conf. on Platelet-Activating Factor and Structurally Related Alkyl Ether Lipids*, Gatlinburg, TN, Oct. 26—29, 1986, abstr. p. 33.

49. **Morrison, W. J. and Shivendra, D.**, Antagonism of platelet activating factor receptor binding and stimulated phosphoinositide-specific phospholipase C in rabbit platelets, *J. Pharmacol. Exp. Ther.*, 250, 831, 1989.

50. **Morris, D. D. and Moore, J. N.**, Equine peritoneal macrophage production of thromboxane and prostacyclin in response to platelet activating factor and its receptor antagonist SRI 63-441, *Circ. Shock*, 28, 149, 1989.

51. **Handley, D. A., Tomesch, J. C., and Saunders, R. N.**, Inhibition of PAF-induced responses in the rat, guinea pig, dog and primate by the receptor antagonist, SRI 63-441, *Thromb. Haemost.*, 56, 40, 1986.

52. **Siren, A. L. and Feuerstein, G.**, Effects of PAF and BN 52021 on cardiac function and regional blood flow in conscious rats, *Am. J. Physiol.*, 257, H25, 1989.

53. **Handley, D. A., VanValen, R. G., Tomesch, J. C., Melden, M. K., Jaffe, J. M., Ballard, F. H., and Saunders, R. N.**, Biological properties of the antagonist SRI 63-441 in the PAF and endotoxin models of hypotension in the rat and dog, *Immunopharmacology*, 13, 125, 1987.

54. **Anderson, G. P. and Fennessy, M. R.**, Lipoxygenase metabolites mediate increased airways responsiveness to histamine after acute platelet activating factor exposure in the guinea pig, *Agents Actions*, 24, 8, 1988.

55. **Smith, D., Sanjar, S., and Morley, J.**, The effect of prophylactic anti-asthma drugs on PAF-induced platelet accumulation in the thorax of the guinea pig, *Jpn. J. Pharmacol.*, 51, 161, 1989.

56. **Boubekeur, K. and Morley, L.**, Use of PAF antagonists to assess the role of PAF in allergen-induced responses of the guinea-pig airway, *Prostaglandins*, 35, 799, 1988.

57. **Patterson, R., Harris, K. E., Handley, D. A., and Saunders, R. N.**, Evaluation of the effect of a platelet antagonist on platelet activating factor and *Ascaris* antigen-induced airway response in rhesus monkeys, *J. Lab. Clin. Med.*, 110, 606, 1987.

58. **Stenzel, H., Hümmer, B., and Hahn, H. L.**, Effect of the PAF-antagonist SRI 63-441 on the allergic reaction in awake dogs with natural asthma, *Agents Actions (Suppl.)*, 21, 253, 1987.

59. **Makowka, L., Chapman, F., Mazzaferro, V., Qian, S., Enriches, F., Olivero, G., Zerbe, A., Saunders, R., and Starzl, T.**, The role of a PAF-antagonist in experimental hyperacute rejection (HAR), *Prostaglandins*, 35, 806, 1988.

60. **Makowka, L., Miller, C., Chapchap, P., Podesta, L., Pan, C., Pressley, D., Mazzaferro, V., Esquivel, C. O., Todo, S., Banner, B., et al.**, Prolongation of pig-to-dog renal xenograft survival by modification of the inflammatory mediator response, *Ann. Surg.*, 206, 482, 1987.

61. **Ontell, S. J., Makowka, L., Ove, P., and Starzl, T.**, Improved hepatic function in the 24-hour preserved rat liver with UW-lactobionate solution and SRI 63-441, *Gastroenterology*, 95, 1617, 1988.

62. **Wainwright, C. L., Chang, S. W., and Voelkel, N. F.**, Platelet activating factor decreases vascular reactivity in rat lungs, *Fed. Proc.*, 46, 1112, 1987.

63. **Wainwright, C. L., Bigaud, M., Parratt, J. R., and Stoclet, G. C.**, Effects of PAF antagonists on platelet behavior and arrhythmias during myocardial ischemia, *Prostaglandins*, 35, 809, 1988.

64. **Robertson, D. A., Levi, R., McManus, L. M., and Pinckard, R. N.,** The PAF antagonist SRI 63-441 alleviates arrhythmias and improper coronary flow during cardiac anaphylaxis, *2nd Int. Conf. on Platelet Activating Factor and Structurally Related Alkyl Ether Lipids,* Gatlingburg, TN, October 26—29, 1986, 35.

65. **Robertson, D. A., Genovese, A., and Levi, R.,** Negative inotropic effect of platelet-activating factor on human myocardium: a pharmacological study, *J. Pharmacol. Exp. Ther.,* 243, 834, 1987.

66. **Chang, S.-W., Feddersen, C. O., Henson, P. M., and Voelkel, N. F.,** Platelet-activating factor mediates hemodynamic changes and lung injury in endotoxin-treated rats, *J. Clin. Invest.,* 79, 1498, 1987.

67. **Chang, S. and Voelkel, N. F.,** SRI 63-441, a PAF antagonist, attenuates endotoxin-induced lung injury in rats, *2nd Int. Conf. on Platelet-Activating Factor and Structurally Related Alkyl Ether Lipids,* Gatlinburg, TN, October 26—29, 1986, 108.

68. **Lang, C. H., Dobrescu, C., Hargrove, D. M., Bagby, G. J., and Spitzer, J. J.,** Attenuation of endotoxin-induced increase in glucose metabolism by platelet-activating factor antagonist, *Circ. Shock,* 23, 179, 1987.

69. **Chang, S. W., Lauterberg, B. H., and Voelkel, N. F.,** Endotoxin-induced oxidative stress in rats: role of neutrophils and platelet activating factor, *J. Clin. Invest.,* submitted.

70. **Christman, B. W., Parker, R. E., Lefferts, P. L., Arnold, T. G., and Snapper, J. R.,** Thromboxane does not mediate the initial rise in pulmonary artery pressure following bolus PAF in awake sheep, *2nd Int. Conf. on Platelet-Activating Factor and Structurally Related Alkyl Ether Lipids,* Gatlinburg, TN, October 26—29, 1986, 131.

71. **Sessler, C. N., Glauser, F. L., Sigal, B., Davis, D., and Fowler, A. A.,** SRI 63-441, a platelet-activating factor antagonist, prevents endotoxin induced pulmonary hypertension and hypoxemia in anesthetized sheep, *Clin. Res.,* 35, 30A, 1987.

72. **Christman, B. W., Lefferts, P. L., and Snapper, J. R.,** Effect of a platelet-activating factor receptor antagonist (SRI 63-441) on the sheep's response to endotoxin, *Am. Rev. Respir. Dis.,* 135, A82, 1987.

73. **Rubin, R. M., Samples, J. R., and Rosenbaum, J. R.,** Inhibition of prostaglandin-mediated ocular vascular permeability by the platelet activating factor antagonist SRI 63-441, *Invest. Ophthalmol.* 28, 99, 1987.

74. **Rubin, R. M., Samples, J. R., and Rosenbaum, J. T.,** Inhibition of endotoxin induced ocular vascular permeability by the platelet-activating factor antagonist SRI 63-441, *Fed. Proc.,* 46, 1454, 1987.

75. **Rubin, R. M., Samples, J. R., and Rosenbaum, J. T.,** Prostaglandin-independent inhibition of ocular vascular permeability by a platelet-activating factor antagonist, *Arch. Ophthalmol.,* 106, 1116, 1988.

76. **Spinks, N. R. and O'Neill, C. O.,** Embryo-derived platelet-activating factor is essential for establishing pregnancy in the mouse, *Lancet,* 106, 1987.

77. **O'Neill, C.,** Composition and methods for fertility control using platelet-activating factor, its analogs and antagonists, Eur. Pat. Appl. 261798, March 30, 1988.

78. **Shukla, S. D., Morrison, W. J., and Carter, M.,** Phosphorylation of proteins in platelets by platelet activating factor: studies with receptor antagonists and desensitized platelets, *FASEB J.,* 2, abstr. 682, 1988.

79. **Shalit, M., VonAllmen, C., Atkins, P. C., and Zweiman, B.,** Platelet activating factor increases expression of complement receptors on human neutrophils, *J. Leukocyte Biol.,* 44, 212, 1988.

80. **Shalit, M., Dabiri, G. A., and Southwick, F. S.,** Platelet-activating factor both stimulates and "primes" human polymorphonuclear leukocytes action filament assembly, *Blood,* 70, 1921, 1987.

81. **Handley, D. A., VanValen, R. G., Winslow, C. M., Tomesch, J. C., and Saunders, R. N.,** *In vitro* and *in vivo* pharmacological profiles of the PAF receptor antagonist SRI 63-675, *Thromb. Haemost.,* 57, 187, 1987.

82. **English, J. and Toth, P. D.,** The effects of different platelet activating factor (PAF) antagonists on PAF induced hypotension in the pithed rat, *Prostaglandins,* 35, 825, 1988.

83. **Haynes, J., Chang, S. W., and Voekel, N. F.,** Chronic administration of a platelet activating factor antagonist does not produce pulmonary hypertension in the rat, *FASEB J.,* 2, abstr. 2482, 1988.

84. **Damas, J.,** Involvement of Paf-acether in the anaphylactic shock in the rat, *J. Lipid Mediators,* 1, 161, 1989.

85. **Ma, Y.-H., and Dunham, E. W.,** Antagonism of the vasodilator effects of a platelet activating factor precursor in anesthetized spontaneously hypertensive rats, *Eur. J. Pharmacol.,* 145, 153, 1988.

86. **Olson, N. C., Anderson, D. L., and Joyce, P. B.,** SRI 63-675 and indomethacin block cardiopulmonary responses to exogenous infusion of platelet activating factor in anesthetized pigs, *Am. Rev. Respir. Disease,* 137, 100, 1988.

87. **Jones, S. L., O'Donnell, S. R., and Barnett, D. J. K.,** A new potent, and specific PAF-antagonist drug, SRI 63-675, *Clin. Exp., Pharmacol. Physiol. Suppl.,* 13, 6, 1988.

88. **O'Donnell, S. R., Greaves, C. A., and Zeng, X. P.,** Effects of platelet activating factor (PAF) antagonists on isolated preparations of lung and trachea from guinea-pigs, *Clin. Exp. Pharmacol. Physiol. Suppl.,* 12, 8, 1988.

89. **Berstad, A., Almodovar, K., Weatherstone, R. G., and Hirschowitz, B. I.,** Effect of platelet-activating factor and its receptor antagonist, SRI 63-675, on gastric bleeding in rats, *Scand. J. Gastroenterol.,* 23, 738, 1988.

90. **Hellewell, P. G. and Williams, T. J.,** Antagonism of PAF-induced edema formation in rabbit skin: a comparison of different antagonists, *Br. J. Pharmacol.,* 97, 171, 1989.

91. **Tomesch, J., Koletar, J., Prashad, M., Handley, D., Larson, D., and Winslow, C.,** PAF antagonists SDZ 63-441 and SDZ 63-675, synthesis and pharmacological characterization of the individual enantiomers, *Prostaglandins,* 35, 845, 1988.

92. **Tomesch, J. C., Winslow, C. M., Handley, D. A., Koletar, J. M., and Prashad, M.,** SRI 63-441, Structure-activity relationship of variations in the central portion of the molecule, *2nd Int. Conf. on Platelet Activating Factor,* Gatlinburg, TN, October 26—29, 1986, 115.

93. **Handley, D. A., Houlihan, W. J., Tomesch, J., Farley, C., Deacon, R., Prashad, M., Hughes, J. Jaeggi, C., and Koletar, J.,** Chemistry and pharmacology of PAF antagonists with sustained duration of biological activity, *Taipei Conference on Prostaglandin and Leukotriene Research,* Taipei, Taiwan, R.O.C., abstr. p. 78, 1988.

94. **Handley, D. A., Houlihan, W. J., Tomesch, J. C., Farley, C., Deacon, R. W., Koletar, J. M., Prashad, M., Hughes, J. W., and Jaeggi, C.,** Chemistry and pharmacology of PAF antagonists, evaluation of changes at potential metabolism sites on activity and duration of activity, *Adv. Prostaglandin, Thromboxane, and Leukotriene Research,* 19, 367, 1988.

95. **Heymans, F., Redeuilh, C., Massicot, F., Wichrowski, B., Favre, E., Spinewyn, B., Blavet, N., Braquet, P., and Godfroid, J. J.,** Tetrahydrofuran derivatives as PAF-acether antagonists-structure-activity relationship, *Prostaglandins,* 35, 845, 1988.

96. **Godfroid, J. J., Heymans, F., and Braquet, P.,** U.K. Patent Appl. 2,200,634A, 1988.

97. **Nakamura, N., Ookawa, N., Koike, H., Sada, T., Oshima, T., and Iizuka, Y.,** Phosphate ester derivatives, their preparation and their therapeutic use, Eur. Pat. 210804-A1, February 4, 1987.

98. **Nakamura, N., Miyazaki, H., Kolke, H., and Oshima, T.,** New cyclic ether derivatives, Eur. Pat. Appl. 0215827, January 1, 1988.

99. **Miyazaki, H., Nakamura, N., Ito, T., Sada, T., Oshima, T., and Koike, H.,** Synthesis and antagonistic activities of enantiomers of cyclic platelet-activating factor analogues, *Chem. Pharm. Bull.,* 37, 2371, 1989.

100. **Paubert-Braquet, M., Lonchampt, M.-O., Klotz, P., and Guilbaud,** Tumor Necrosis Factor (TNF) primes platelet activating factor (PAF)-induced superoxide generation by human neutrophils (PMN): consequences in promoting PMN-mediated endothelial cell (EC) damages, *Prostaglandins,* 35, 803, 1988.

101. **Houlihan, W. J., Lee, M. L., Winslow, C. M., Cheon, S. H., D'Aries, F. J., Kowal-DeLillo, A., Jaeggi, C. S., Mason, R., and Parrino, V.,** Cyclic oxygen analogs of ET-18-OCH$_3$, antitumor and platelet activating factor inhibitory activity, *1st Int. Symp. on Ether Lipids in Oncology,* Göttingen, FRG, December 5, 1986.

102. **Burri, K., Barner, R., Cassal, J. M., Hadváry, P., Hirth, G., and Mueller, K.,** PAF: from agonists to antagonists by synthesis, *Prostaglandins,* 30, 691, 1985.

103. **Hadváry, P. and Weller, T.,** Conformationally restricted analogs of platelet-activating factor (PAF), *Helv. Chim. Acta,* 69, 1862, 1986.

104. **Lee, M. L., Winslow, C. M., Jaeggi, Ch., D'Aries, F., Frisch, G., and Farley, C.,** Inhibition of platelet activating factor: synthesis and biological activity of SRI 63-073, a new phospholipid PAF-acether antagonist, *Prostaglandins,* 30, 690, 1985.

Chapter 8

PHARMACOLOGY OF HETRAZEPINES AS PAF-ANTAGONISTS

Hubert O. Heuer

INTRODUCTION

Current antagonists of platelet activating factor (PAF) can be classified into three types: (1) PAF analogues, e.g., CV 3988 and Ro 19-3704, (2) natural products or their derivatives, e.g., ginkgolide B and L 652,731, and (3) synthetic compounds, e.g., 48740 RP, 52770 RP and the hetrazepines (WEB 2086 and others); for review see Reference 1. This contribution will focus on the preclinical and clinical pharmacology of the latter group of synthetic compounds: hetrazepines.

Hetrazepines are defined as oxazepines (X = O), thiazepines (X = S) and diazepines (X = N) with two annelated 5-membered heterocycles (2; Figure 1).

When Casals-Stenzel started the screening for leads with PAF-antagonistic activity in 1982 he discovered that both the *benzo*-triazolo-diazepines, alprazolam and triazolam and the *thieno*-triazolo-diazepine brotizolam, inhibited PAF-induced platelet aggregation *in vitro* and furthermore that they were also active against PAF-effects *in vivo*.[3-5] Kornecki et al. also described similar results with these compounds.[6]

The hetrazepine brotizolam was found by Casals-Stenzel to be 20 to 30 times more effective as a specific PAF-antagonist than the benzoderivatives alprazolam and triazolam.[3,4] In contrast other 1,4-benzodiazepines like diazepam,[5] flunitrazepam[5] and the peripheral type benzodiazepine (BDZ) receptor ligand Ro 5-4864[5] exhibited only weak activity against PAF-induced platelet aggregation.[5]

Once brotizolam had been discovered as a lead for a potent antagonist of PAF the requirement for a dissociation of the CNS-sedative effects from the retained PAF-antagonistic properties was evident. First a pharmacological approach for the separation was made, by combination of brotizolam with a strong BDZ receptor antagonist, Ro 15-1788, which is less potent as a PAF-antagonist.[5] This BDZ-receptor antagonist in combination with brotizolam did not affect the PAF-antagonism of brotizolam but clearly blocked the hypnotic effect of brotizolam in guinea pigs.[5] These results opened the possibility to dissociate the PAF- and hypnogenic activities of brotizolam. Furthermore this result triggered the synthesis of new and potent PAF-antagonists in this series of structures, which are lacking sedative effects. WEB 2086, WEB 2170, and WEB 2347 (Figure 2) are the outstanding examples of a series of new and potent antagonists of PAF which are lacking any sedative or hypnogenic action but which belong to the most potent antagonists of PAF known so far.[7]

Aspects of the chemistry and structure activity relationship in this series of hetrazepinoic PAF-antagonists have been reviewed elsewhere.[8,9]

The following will review preclinical and clinical aspects of the pharmacology of PAF-antagonists from the hetrazepine series. *In vitro* and *in vivo* data against alterations induced by exogenously introduced PAF or by PAF which is endogenously released in disease-related models are summarized. In addition, the hetrazepines WEB 2086 (apafant), WEB 2170 (INN: bepafant), and WEB 2347 are compared with special attention to kinetic (duration of action), and orally to intravenously effective doses in different species. Particular attention is paid to WEB 2086, the so far most widely studied PAF-antagonist of the hetrazepine series.

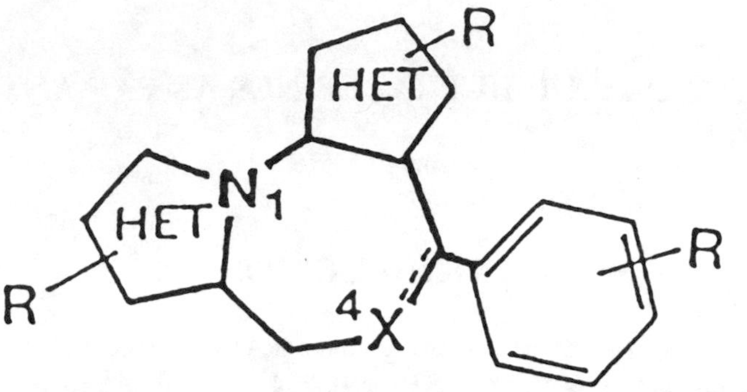

FIGURE 1.   General chemical structure of hetrazepines (oxazepines X =O; thiazepines X = S; diazepines X = N).

PRECLINICAL CHARACTERISTICS AND PHARMACOLOGY OF HETRAZEPINES (WEB 2086, WEB 2170, WEB 2347 ETC.)

PAF-ANTAGONISM *IN VITRO*
Inhibition of PAF Effects at the Cellular Level
Binding to the PAF Receptor

WEB 2086 has been shown to *bind to the PAF-receptor* of platelets of several sources and species[10-12] (K_i = 15 nM) (K_B = 8.3 nM). When compared to hetrazepine, unrelated PAF-antagonists WEB 2086 turned out to be one of the most potent antagonists in terms of its ability to compete with ^{3}H PAF at the PAF-receptor site.[10-13] The interaction of WEB 2086 with the PAF-receptor on platelets is competitive.[10,11] This is in accordance with the reported competitive inhibition of the binding of PAF to human platelets by the structurally related triazolo-benzodiazepines alprazolam and triazolam.[14]

PAF-Induced Platelet Aggregation

Antagonism of PAF-induced aggregation in platelet-rich plasma (PRP), whole blood, and washed platelets has been shown for WEB 2086 on platelets of different sources and species.[15-19] Table 1 outlines the inhibition characteristics obtained for WEB 2086 in different laboratories. These are comparable no matter which platelet source and species was tested. When comparing the results with hetrazepine-unrelated PAF-antagonists in the same laboratory, WEB 2086 was always one of the most potent substances to antagonize PAF-induced platelet aggregation.[7,12,13,15-19] This is also evident from Table 6 comparing ED_{50} values *in vivo* with inhibition parameters against PAF-induced changes in *vitro* for several types of PAF-antagonists including WEB 2086 (Table 6).

WEB 2086 has been shown to counteract PAF-induced platelet aggregation in a competitive manner. Schild plot slopes were not significantly different from unity and WEB 2086 shifted PAF-induced aggregation to the right in a parallel and concentration-dependent manner using platelets from various sources.[17-19] The hetrazepines WEB 2170 and WEB 2347 showed inhibition of PAF-induced human platelet aggregation in PRP, at least at the same magnitude as shown for WEB 2086 (IC_{50}-values 0.3 μM).[20-22] In PRP from rabbits WEB 2347 inhibited the PAF-induced (1 × 10^{-8} M) platelet aggregation with an IC_{50} of 0.08 μM (WEB 2086: IC_{50} = 0.70 μM; WEB 2170: IC_{50} = 0.55 μM).[22,23] The hetrazepine etizolam inhibited PAF-induced platelet aggregation (IC_{50} = 3.8 μM in PRP from the rabbit) and displaced ^{3}H PAF from the PAF-receptor site on washed rabbit platelets.[24] Thus the latter study confirmed the higher PAF-antagonistic potency of the hetrazepine etizolam, a thienotriazolodiazepine, compared to the benzodiazepine triazolam used in the same study.[24] (Casals-Stenzel, unpublished).

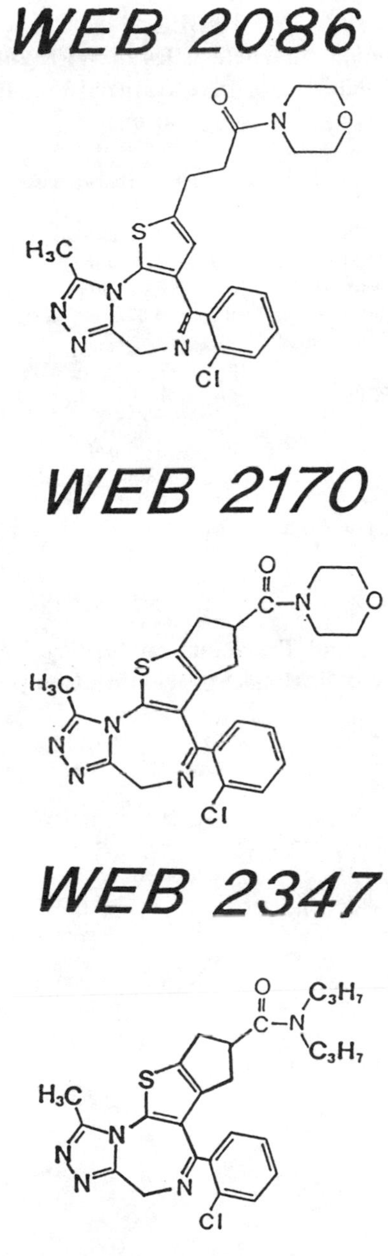

WEB 2086

WEB 2170

WEB 2347

FIGURE 2.   Chemical structure of WEB 2086, WEB 2170, and WEB 2347.

PAF-Induced Alterations on Leukocytes

With respect to PAF-induced alterations on leukocytes, the hetrazepines brotizolam, WEB 2086 and WEB 2170 also antagonized the PAF-induced aggregation of purified human leukocytes.[3,15] Table 2 summarizes the IC_{50} values for inhibition of PAF-induced human leukocyte aggregation. Inhibition was selective because aggregation of human leukocytes induced by Con A, FMLP or LTB_4 was not significantly inhibited by these antagonists of PAF.[3,15]

WEB 2086 counteracted competitively the PAF-induced aggregation of PMNLs from the rabbit.[18] The pA_2 value for WEB 2086 was not significantly different from that obtained

TABLE 1
Inhibition Characteristics of WEB 2086 for
Inhibition of PAF-Induced Platelet
Aggregation

Platelet source	Inhibition characteristic	Ref.
Human (PRP)	$IC_{50} = 0.17 \ \mu M$	15
Human (PRP)	$IC_{50} = 0.12 \ \mu M$	58
Human (washed)	$IC_{50} = 0.021 \ \mu M$	34
Human (PRP)	$IC_{50} = 0.072 \ \mu M$	16
Human (whole blood)	$ED_{50} = 0.39 \ \mu M$	19
	$pA_2 = 7.74$	
Rabbit (PRP)	$pA_2 = 7.31$	17
	$pK_B = 7.63$	
Rabbit (PRP)	$IC_{50} = 0.70 \ \mu M$	22, 23
Rabbit (washed)	$IC_{50} = 28 \ nM$	75
Rabbit (washed)	$pA_2 = 7.58$	18
Guinea pig (washed)	$pA_2 = 7.69$	18
Dog	$IC_{50} = 0.15 \ \mu M$	12

TABLE 2
Effects of Hetrazepines and Triazolam on *In Vitro* Neutrophil Aggregation
Induced Various Aggregating Compounds

Aggregating agent (μM)	PAF (0.05)	Con A[a]	FMLP[b] (0.1)	A 23187 (50)	LTB$_4$ (0.01)
Triazolam	6.6	≥1000	≥1000	n.d.[c]	374
	(4.4—12.4)				(263—498)
Brotizolam	0.21	≥1000	≥1000	≥1000	628
	(0.14—0.27)				(386—1409)
WEB 2086 BS	0.37	≥1000	≥1000	555	≥1000
	(0.26—0.54)			(348—1064)	
WEB 2170 BS	0.83	≥1000	≥1000	n.d.	265
	(0.57—1.20)				(. . . ⁻ . . .)**

Note: IC_{50} (μM) with 95% confidence limits, n = 4.

[a]   35 $\mu g/ml$.
[b]   f-met-leu-phe.
[c]   n.d. = not determined.

on the platelets.[18] Thus the latter study supports that the receptors on the platelets and PMNLs of the rabbit are similar.

Both brotizolam and WEB 2086 have been described to inhibit, in a similar and concentration-dependent way, both the production of oxygen radicals and intracellular accumulation of calcium on human PMNLs induced by PAF.[25] The inhibition was selective for both hetrazepines since they were inactive against FMLP-induced activation.[25]

WEB 2086 has been reported to inhibit the PAF ($3 \times 10^{-8} \ M$) chemotaxis of leukocytes in a concentration-dependent manner ($IC_{50} = 5 \times 10^{-8} \ M$).[26]

Effects on Eosinophils

Eosinophils deserve particular attention since they are one of the most prominent cells in the pathophysiology of asthma and PAF is a potent chemotactic factor for eosinophils. When eosinophils from primate (*Macaca fascicularis*) were purified and adhered *in vitro* to protein-coated wells of microtiter plates, the PAF-induced adhesion of eosinophils was inhibited by WEB 2086 with an IC_{50} of 2.1 μg/ml (Craig Wegner, Boehringer Ingelheim, unpublished). WEB 2170 and STY 2108 could also inhibit PAF-induced eosinophil adhesion but were at least one log-step more potent (IC_{50}s = 0.09 and 0.087 μg/ml, respectively, C. Wegner, Boehringer Ingelheim, personal communication). These differences in activity between WEB 2086, and both WEB 2170 and STY 2108, in the eosinophil adherence test contrasts with the similar IC_{50}-values observed in PAF-induced aggregation studies on platelets. This might suggest that there are distinct PAF receptor subtypes on platelets and eosinophils. Interestingly specific binding of ^{3}H WEB 2086 to PAF-receptors on purified human eosinophils (K_B = 18 nM) has recently been demonstrated.[27] On purified eosinophils from the guinea pig WEB 2086 shifted the dose response curves for PAF-induced degranulation with enzyme release and the intracellular calcium accumulation to the right, indicating a competitive antagonism (K_B = 7.5 nM for degranulation; K_B = 12.6 for calcium accumulation;[28]). Also the induction of hypodense eosinophils by PAF *in vitro* is inhibited by the PAF antagonist WEB 2086.[29] The PAF (3 $\times$ 10^{-8} M) induced chemotaxis of human eosiniphils was inhibited by WEB 2086 in a concentration-dependent manner (IC_{50} = 6.6 $\times$ 10^{-7} M).[26] WEB 2086 was about 17 times less potent than CV 6209 in inhibiting the PAF-induced chemotaxis of eosinophils; with respect to neutrophils this was just the other way around: WEB 2086 was about 13 times more potent than CV 6209 in inhibiting the chemotaxis of neutrophils.[26] This result may support the existence of PAF receptor subtypes on human eosinophils and neutrophils.[26]

PAF-activated eosinophils have been shown to disrupt the guinea pig ciliated tracheal epithelium and to reduce the ciliation of the tracheal circumference by 94%.[30] The PAF-antagonist WEB 2086 at 1 μM inhibited the reduction of the ciliation by PAF-activated eosinophils significantly.[30]

PAF Effects on Other Cells

In the resident peritoneal macrophages of the guinea pig, WEB 2086 was about one log-step less potent at inhibiting the PAF-induced generation of 6-oxo-PGF$_{1\alpha}$ than at blocking PAF-induced platelet aggregation in the same species.[18] Since this discrepancy of potencies at the PAF-receptor between platelets and macrophages was even more pronounced for two other PAF-antagonists (L-652.731 and BN 52021), the authors speculate on the presence of PAF receptor-subtypes on platelets and PMNLs on one side and macrophages on the other side.[18] On the other hand WEB 2086 did not influence the A 23187-stimulated generation of 6-oxo-PGF$_{1\alpha}$. The latter finding supports a specific antagonism of PAF-induced effects on macrophages[18] by WEB 2086.

WEB 2086 inhibited PAF-induced calcium mobilization in a human premonocytic cell line (U 937) with an IC_{50} of 48 nM.[31] This effect was specific since LTB$_4$- and ionomycin-induced calcium mobilization was not affected. Both in macrophages and monocytes, WEB 2086 belonged to the most potent antagonists of PAF yet described.[18,31]

With respect to lymphocytes the results for WEB 2086 are divergent. WEB 2086 at concentrations up to 10 μM had no effect on mitogen or IL-2-induced proliferation of human T-lymphocytes.[32] The same was true for another specific PAF-antagonist (BN 52021). In contrast three other selective PAF-antagonists inhibited the T-lymphocyte proliferation induced by these ligands in a concentration dependent manner.[32] The authors of the paper describing these results suggest the existence of a PAF receptor on lymphocytes with different structural requirements as compared to those receptors present on platelets. In addition, PAF at concentrations as low as 10^{-13} to 10^{-11} M enhanced the natural killer (NK) activity of human lymphocytes which could, surprisingly in view of the results with lymphocyte proliferation be further increased by WEB 2086 as well as BN 52 021.[33]

WEB 2086 inhibited the ^{3}H-PAF binding to confluent human endothelial cells *in vitro* in a concentration-dependent manner.[34,35] This points also to a specific interaction of WEB 2086 with the PAF-receptor on this cell type.[34,35]

In smooth muscle cells grown on glass coverslips, WEB 2086 at 10 μM blocked the PAF-induced increase of cytosolic calcium.[36]

Inhibition of PAF Effects at the Organ Level
Inhibition of In Vitro PAF-Induced Effects in the Lung

Isolated lung or lung strips may permit the complex action of mediators like PAF *in vivo* to be dissected and thus shed more light on the mechanism and the sequence of events involved.

The first pieces of evidence for an interaction between WEB 2086 and a PAF receptor in the peripheral lung arose from guinea pig lung tissue.[37] WEB 2086 displaced ^{3}H-PAF from guinea pig lung membranes with a $K_{0.5}$ of 86 nM.[37] This showed that WEB 2086 interacts with specific PAF-binding sites in the peripheral lung with relative high affinity.[37] In another study ^{3}H-WEB 2086 binding was displaced from guinea pig as well as human lung membranes by unlabeled WEB 2086 (K_i = 19.4 and 20.1 nM, respectively) and PAF.[38] Specific binding of ^{3}H WEB 2086 was also shown on guinea pig and human peripheral lung, vessels, and parenchyma but not on human segmental airways.[38]

Isolated lung parenchymal strips can be contracted by PAF in a concentration dependent manner.[39] When guinea pig parenchymal strips were contracted by, e.g., 50 nM PAF, WEB 2086 prevented PAF-induced contractions in a concentration-dependent manner with an IC_{50} of 1.6 μM. This suggests a receptor-mediated mechanism.[39] WEB 2086 also reversed the sustained contraction produced by 1 μM PAF ($-\log EC_{50}$ = 5.97) in a concentration-dependent manner when applied after the response to PAF had reached a plateau.[39] Similar inhibitory action of both brotizolam and WEB 2086 could also be shown by other authors.[40] In addition on human isolated bronchial smooth muscle WEB 2086 blocked not only the contraction induced by PAF but also the hyperresponsiveness to histamine induced by 10^{-7} M PAF.[41] Although PAF does not contract the trachea (PAF even relaxes the trachea) PAF enhances the contractile reactivity to K^+ of tracheal strips.[42] This PAF-induced enhanced reactivity of the isolated tracheal smooth muscle to K^+ was abolished by WEB 2086 at a concentration of 10 nM.[42]

On the other hand it has to be considered that the contraction of the isolated guinea pig parenchymal lung strip is not always very reproducible, but is long lasting. Thus, whole lung preparations or *in vivo* models may be better suited in this respect. In isolated lung of the rat, PAF increases the pulmonary artery perfusion pressure and bronchial inflation pressure as well as the wet-to-dry lung weight ratio.[43] When these alterations were produced by a bolus of 20 μg PAF, a concentration-related inhibition by WEB 2086 was obtained.[43] These results have recently been confirmed by another study in the rat: WEB 2086 at 10 μM prevented PAF (0.1—10 nmol)-induced increase in perfusion pressure, lung weight, and leukotriene release.[44]

The bronchoconstriction caused by 10 or 30 ng PAF was suppressed when the isolated guinea pig lung was perfused with WEB 2086 (0.1 μM).[45] In contrast, bronchoconstriction induced by arachidonic acid was unaffected, thus confirming the selective inhibition of PAF-induced alterations.[45] In addition, WEB 2086 inhibited the production of thromboxane B_2 (TXB_2) provoked by 10, 30, or 100 ng PAF in a dose-dependent manner, but again TXB_2 release induced by arachidonic acid was not affected.[45]

On the other hand, in the isolated lungs from actively sensitized guinea pigs, WEB 2086 like BN 52021 failed to inhibit the bronchoconstriction and mediator release (histamine, LTC_4-like material) evoked by intrapulmonary instilled PAF.[46] Irrespective of the failure of WEB 2086 to interact with the bronchoconstriction and mediator release induced by PAF, the edema formation as measured by the increase in lung wet weight induced by PAF was still inhibited.[46]

Inhibition of Effects of PAF in the Heart and Circulation In Vitro

In the autoperfused rat hindlimb, dose response curves for the vasodilating effect of bolus doses of PAF were shifted to the right by increasing concentration of WEB 2086.[47] In contrast, the vasodilating response to acetylcholine was not affected. This points to specificity in this respect.[47]

When guinea pig hearts were perfused with PAF, the resulting coronary vasoconstriction was reversed by WEB 2086 at 0.1 to 1 μM.[48]

WEB 2086 (0.03 to 1 μM) antagonized the sustained increase of coronary perfusion pressure and decrease of cardiac developed tension elicited by a bolus injection of PAF at 50 pmol.[49] In addition, the same concentration range of WEB 2086 also markedly reduced the release of LTC_4-like material and TXB_2 induced by PAF.[49] Selectivity of WEB 2086 in this respect was shown since it did not inhibit the changes induced by LTC_4 or the TXA_2-mimetic U 46619.[49]

Inhibition of PAF in the Gastrointestinal System In Vitro

The pro-diarrheal colonic secretagogue action of PAF was investigated on muscle-stripped rat colon, measuring transepithelial potential difference and short circuit current.[51] PAF increased both parameters, suggesting that PAF may be a powerful pro-diarrheal secretagory agent.[51] In contrast, several PAF-antagonists including WEB 2086 failed to block this response which suggested that this effect of PAF is not mediated by PAF-receptors, or that there is a PAF-receptor of a type distinct from that inhibited by usual PAF-antagonists in the gastrointestinal system.[51]

ANTAGONISM OF PAF *IN VIVO*
Platelet Aggregation *In Vivo*

Intravenous PAF induces platelet aggregation and thrombocytopenia as well as leukopenia or leukocytosis *in vivo*.[52] Particularly, the bronchoconstriction by intravenous PAF is a platelet-dependent reaction.[53]

The infusion of PAF (e.g., 30 ng $\times$ kg^{-1} $\times$ min^{-1}) to guinea pigs results in intrathoracic accumulation of platelets which can be indicated by following the increase of gamma-radiation in the thoracic region of ^{111}In-labeled platelets.[15] Peroral (60 min prior to PAF) or intravenous (10 min prior to PAF) administration of hetrazepinoic PAF-antagonists (brotizolam, WEB 2086, WEB 2170, STY 2108;[3,4,15,21,54]) or the hetrazepine related PAF-antagonists triazolam[3,4] inhibited the PAF-induced accumulation of platelets in a dose-dependent manner. Figure 3 illustrates the effect of i.v. STY 2108 and Table 3 summarizes the respective ED_{50}-values of intravenous or peroral PAF-antagonists to inhibit the PAF-induced increase of gamma radiation.

Although when added to the test system *in vitro*, WEB 2086 and WEB 2170 were equi-effective at inhibiting aggregation of rabbit (or human) platelets, *in vivo* in a rabbit model WEB 2170 was considerably more effective. The oral dose of WEB 2170 required to render the platelets (tested in plasma) unable to respond to PAF was 0.5 mg/kg with some effect even at 0.01 mg/kg, whereas WEB 2086 had to be dosed to the rabbits between 0.3 and 30 mg/kg to give the same effect (Figure 4[23]).

Bronchoconstriction and Lung Alterations *In Vivo*

Although bronchoconstriction in response to PAF may not be the main contribution of the mediator in an acute asthmatic attack, PAF-induced bronchoconstriction in animals has been the most convenient approach to characterize PAF-antagonists in regard to PAF-induced alterations in the lung.

Continuous intravenous infusion of PAF at 30 ng $\times$ kg^{-1} $\times$ min^{-1} in guinea pigs produced a continuous decrease of respiratory flow and concomitant decrease of mean arterial

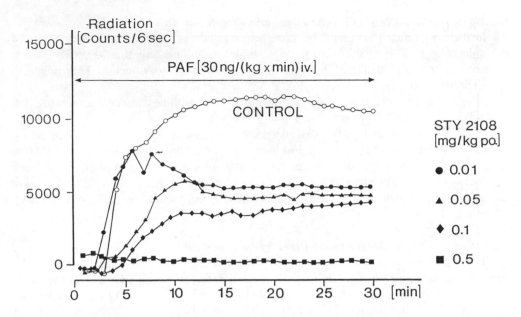

FIGURE 3.   Inhibition of PAF (30 ng × kg⁻¹ × min⁻¹) induced accumulation of ¹¹¹In labeled platelets in the lung of anesthetized guinea pigs by oral STY 2108 (each plot constitutes a representative time-response curve of an individual guinea pig).

TABLE 3
Inhibition of PAF-Induced Accumulation of ¹¹¹In-Labeled Platelets in the Thoracic Region of Guinea Pigs by Oral or i.v. WEB 2086, WEB 2170, or STY 2108

	ED_{50} mg/kg i.v.	ED_{50} mg/kg p.o.
	(95% confidence limits)	
WEB 2170	0.018	0.027
	(0.014—0.024)	(0.017—0.040)
STY 2108	0.008	0.14
	(0.004—0.015)	(0.09—0.21)
WEB 2086	0.060	0.84
	(0.020—0.25)	(0.58—1.31)

Note: ED_{50} values indicated for the inhibition of the plateau of gamma radiation at 30 min or death after infusion of PAF at 30 ng × kg⁻¹ × min⁻¹. 95% confidence limits are shown in brackets.

blood pressure which ended with death at about 15 to 20 min after start of PAF infusion.[3,4,15,21,54]

Oral (60 min prior to PAF), intravenous or intratracheal (10 min prior to PAF) treatment with hetrazepines like triazolam,[3,4] brotizolam,[3,4] WEB 2086,[15] WEB 2170,[21] STY 2108,[21] WEB 2347,[22] and other hetrazepines prevented these effects in a dose-dependent manner.

Inhalation of WEB 2086 for 3 min at 0.25 to 0.5 mg/ml 5 min before infusion of PAF (30 ng × kg⁻¹ × min⁻¹), slowed down the decrease of respiratory flow and mean arterial blood pressure (ED_{50} = 0.32 and 0.21 mg/ml inh., in each case[15]). The simultaneously occurring inhibition of decrease of MAP by WEB 2086 may point to a good systemic absorption from the lung when this antagonist is inhaled.[15]

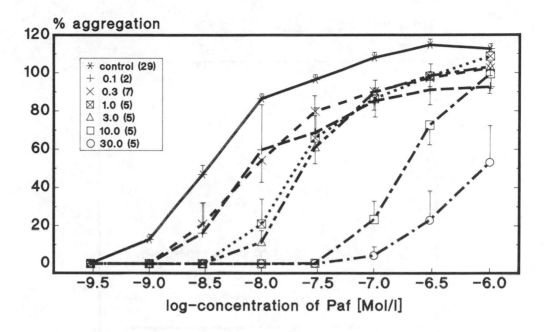

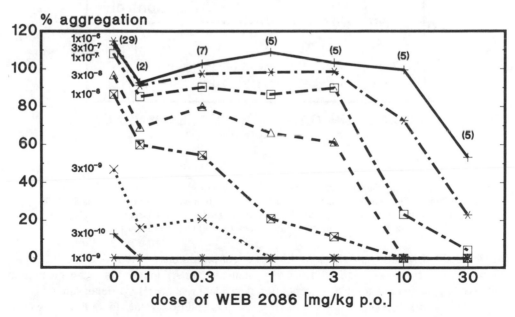

FIGURE 4. Aggregation of rabbit platelets in PRP *ex vivo* induced by different concentrations of PAF before (control) and 2 h after oral administration of different doses of WEB 2086; number of animals in brackets. Above: concentration-response curves for PAF are shifted to the right by various doses of WEB 2086 (indicated by differing symbols; mean ± SEM); below: aggregation induced by increasing concentrations of PAF (indicated by symbols) is inhibited by increasing doses of peroral WEB 2086.

When bronchoconstriction in the guinea pig is induced by a bolus of PAF at 100 ng/kg i.v., all the changes in pulmonary function associated with severe bronchoconstriction occur. Peroral (60 min before PAF) and i.v. (10 min before PAF) pretreatment with the PAF-antagonists WEB 2086, WEB 2170,[21,54] STY 2108,[21,54] and other hetrazepines inhibited the bronchoconstriction as well as the initial increase of blood pressure with subsequent drop. Using the Buxco device for monitoring pulmonary function, it has been possible to show

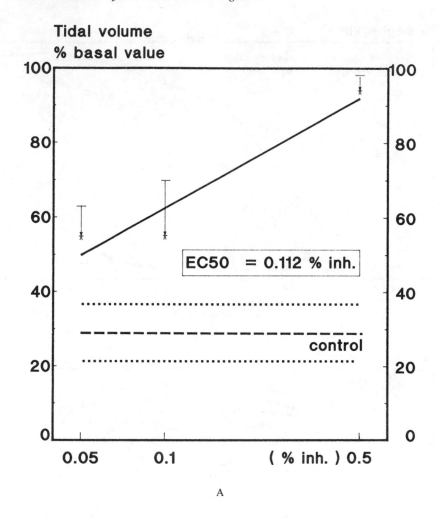

A

FIGURE 5.   Inhibition of paf (100 ng/kg i.v.)-induced bronchoconstriction (decrease in tidal volume and dynamic compliance) by inhaled WEB 2086 in the guinea pig. Mean ± SEM; n = 5/dose group. Pulmonary function parameters were followed and analyzed on a breath to breath basis by a pulmonary function analyzer (Buxco Electronics, model 6).

that inhaled WEB 2086 as well as WEB 2170 at concentrations of 0.05, 0.1, and 0.5% (for 3 min 10 min prior to 100 ng/PAF i.v.) also counteracted PAF-induced bronchoconstriction and blood pressure changes in a concentration-dependent manner (H.O. Heuer, unpublished; see Figure 5 and Table 4). Table 4 summarizes the ED_{50} and EC_{50} values for oral, intravenous, or inhaled WEB 2086 and WEB 2170, respectively, for antagonism of PAF-induced changes of several pulmonary function parameters. Antagonism by WEB 2086, not only of PAF-induced bronchoconstriction but also the drop in platelet and leukocyte count and the lethal effects of PAF has been confirmed by a number of other authors.[45] Also, etizolam dose dependently antagonized PAF (0.3 µg/kg i.v.) -induced bronchoconstriction in the guinea pig at doses of 0.01 to 0.03 mg/kg i.v. dose dependently.[55]

In contrast, *bronchoconstriction by intratracheal PAF* is a platelet-independent phenomenon.[56] Intratracheal administration of PAF at 300 µg/kg or 100 µg/kg to guinea pigs induced not only a continuous decrease of respiratory flow but had also systemic effects as expressed by the initial increase with subsequent drop of mean arterial blood pressure.[15,23,57] Figure 6 illustrates the effect of oral WEB 2086 in antagonizing the decrease of respiratory flow (bronchoconstriction) and blood pressure (hypotension) induced by intratracheal PAF

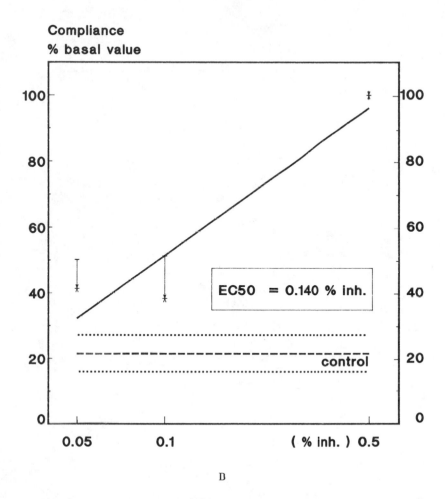

Compliance
% basal value

EC50 = 0.140 % inh.

control

(% inh.) 0.5

0.05   0.1

D

(100 µg/kg). Table 5 compares the ED_{50}s of oral, intravenous, and intratracheal WEB 2086 with those of WEB 2170 to antagonize intratracheal PAF. In comparison with WEB 2086, WEB 2170 was approximately ten times more potent when administered orally and was about two to five times more potent when administered intravenously or via the tracheal route (in the guinea pig!).

Aerosolized PAF at 1000 µg/ml for 3 min produced in conscious guinea pigs broncho-constriction. Oral (0.1—10 mg/kg) or inhaled (0.1—1.0 mg/ml) WEB 2086 inhibited this bronchoconstriction in a dose- or concentration-dependent manner (Craig Wegner, Boeh-ringer Ingelheim, personal communication).

With respect to PAF-associated contribution to *inflammation of the airways and edema formation in vivo* WEB 2086 has been shown to inhibit PAF-induced microvascular leakage in the guinea pig in a dose-dependent manner, as measured by the extravasation of i.v. administered Evans blue dye in the airways (main bronchi, trachea, nasal mucosa, and central and peripheral airways).[58] WEB 2086 showed maximal and complete inhibitory action at 10 µg/kg i.v.[58]

WEB 2086 at 0.1 mg/kg i.v. has been shown to prevent totally the PAF (0.125 µg/kg i.v.) -induced tracheobronchial microvascular leakage as assessed histologically using de-tection of a carbon tracer.[59] Specificity for PAF-induced microvascular leakage was evident since the leak to leukotriene D_4 and histamine was not inhibited by WEB 2086.[59] In com-parison with the other structurally unrelated PAF antagonists tested, WEB 2086 was the most potent one *in vivo*.[59]

Also in the rat lung, the hetrazepines brotizolam (1 to 10 mg/kg i.v.),[60] WEB 2086 and

TABLE 4
Inhibition of PAF (100 ng/kg i.v.)-Induced Bronchoconstriction (Changes of Resp. Flow, Tidal Volume, Dynamic Compliance, Resistance) by Oral (p.o.), Intravenous (i.v.), or Inhaled (inh.) WEB 2086 or WEB 2170

	WEB 2170			WEB 2086		
	p.o.[a]	i.v.[a]	inh.[b]	p.o.[a]	i.v.[a]	inh.[b]
Resp. flow	0.01 (0.004—0.057)	0.012 (0.009—0.016)	0.084 (0.025—0.154)	0.04 (0.002—0.17)	0.014 (. . .—0.044)	0.012 (0.022—0.38)
Tidal volume	0.007 (0.0001—. . .)	0.012 (0.009—0.017)	0.105 (0.044—0.19)	0.044 (0.015—0.113)	0.009 (. . .—0.03)	0.112 (0.035—0.25)
Dyn. Compl.	0.004 (0.002—0.009)	0.014 (0.010—0.021)	0.16 (0.10—0.25)	0.058 (0.029—0.125)	0.018 (0.003—0.044)	0.14 (0.086—0.232)
Resistance	0.003 (. . .—. . .)	0.016 (0.005—0.041)	0.19 (. . .—. . .)	0.049 (. . .—. . .)	n.d.	0.095 (. . .—. . .)

Note: n.d. = not determined.

[a] ED_{50} [mg/kg].
[b] EC_{50} [%; mg/100 mL].

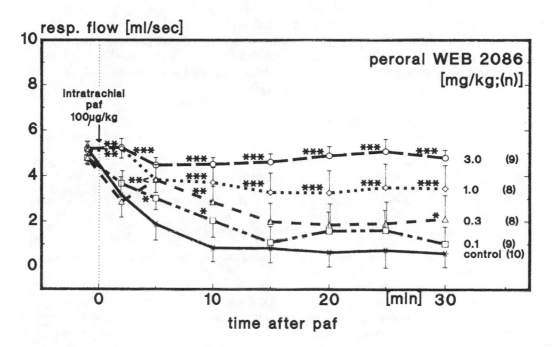

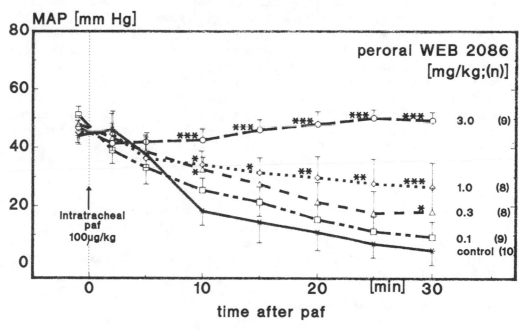

FIGURE 6. Effect of oral WEB 2086 on decrease of respiratory flow and MAP induced by intratracheal PAF (100 μg/kg) in guinea pigs. n in brackets; mean ± SEM; significant differences from controls: * p <0.05, ** P <0.01, *** p <0.001.

WEB 2170 (0.1 to 3 mg/kg i.v.)[61] inhibited the extravasation of the blue dye copper phthalocyanine induced by a bolus of PAF at 100 ng/kg i.v.

Concerning the *extravascular recruitment of platelets and eosinophils*[62] and *chemotaxis of inflammatory cells* into the lung induced by PAF,[62] the action of the hetrazepines brotizolam, WEB 2086, WEB 2170, STY 2108 (orally and i.v.) against the PAF-induced intrathoracic accumulation of [111]Indium-labeled platelets has been previously reported.[15,21,54]

TABLE 5
**ED$_{50}$ Values (mg/kg) of Oral (p.o.), Intravenous (i.v.), and Intratracheal WEB
2086 and WEB 2170 Necessary to Inhibit the Decrease of Respiratory Flow and
MAP and the Lethal Effect in Guinea Pigs Induced by Intratracheal PAF at
100 µg/kg**

	WEB 2170			WEB 2086	
	p.o.	i.v.	tracheal	p.o.	tracheal
Resp. flow	0.044	0.014	0.022	0.69	0.073
	(0.023—0.077)	(0.006—0.019)	(0.016—0.03)	(0.32—1.85)	(0.027—0.14)
MAP	0.034	0.014	0.019	0.66	0.062
	(0.015—0.058)	(0.01—0.018)	(0.013—0.025)	(0.36—1.32)	(0.03—0.100)
Lethality	0.011	0.010	0.012	0.51	n.d.
	(0.000—0.030)	(. . . —0.016)	(0.005—0.017)	(0.013—1.32)	

Note: 95% confidence limits are shown in brackets. Evaluation at 30 min after instillation of PAF. n.d. =
not determined.

Eosinophils are regarded as one of the most prominent inflammatory cells in asthma
and PAF is a very potent chemotactic stimulus for eosinophils. Apart from the *in vitro*
effects on eosinophils particular attention should be paid to PAF-induced extravascular
recruitment and chemotaxis of eosinophils into lung tissue *in vivo*. WEB 2086 inhibited the
eosinophil infiltration into the bronchial walls of guinea pigs induced by PAF.[62] Concerning
the role of PAF in *mucus secretion and mucociliary dysfunction,* an aerosol of PAF decreased
the tracheal mucus velocity in the sheep significantly and WEB 2086 (1 mg/kg i.v.) reversed
this mucociliary dysfunction completely.[63] WEB 2086 at 3 mg/kg i.v. was reported to
counteract the PAF-induced formation of mucus plugs in the lung of guinea pigs.[62]

Late phase responses induced by PAF in the lung have been reported repeatedly. In the
sheep, the PAF-antagonist WEB 2086 (1 mg/kg i.v.) blocked not only the acute bronchoconstriction by aerosolized PAF but also the late phase response.[64] However, this late phase
response by aerosolized PAF was not consistent in all allergic sheep.[64]

Bronchial hyperresponsiveness to PAF has been shown in different models although
increase in bronchial responsiveness to unspecific bronchoconstrictors after PAF-adminis-
tration is not so pronounced (two- to threefold). In an extension of the protocol described
in Reference 65, WEB 2086 prevented the PAF-induced hyperreactivity to sequentially
increasing doses of acetylcholine in guinea pigs, when PAF was infused at 10 ng $\times$ kg^{-1}
$\times$ min^{-1}. Similar blockade of PAF-induced hyperresponsiveness to acetylcholine by 1 mg/kg
i.v. WEB 2086 was reported in another study when hyperreactivity was produced by 600
ng PAF/kg for 1 h.[66]

Cardiovascular Effects and Hypotension *In Vivo*

Systemic hypotension occurring after systemic administration of PAF is assumed to be
platelet independent.[53] Depending on the species and target organ, PAF can induce direct
or indirect vasoconstriction in the pulmonary, coronary, renal, and hepatic circulations upon
systemic administration.[67]

During studies of the antagonism of PAF-induced bronchoconstriction in the guinea pig,
hypotension was also measured and shown to be reversed by oral, intravenous, or intratracheal
PAF-antagonists of the hetrazepine type (WEB 2086, WEB 2170, STY 2108 etc.).[15,21,54]
Although the hypotension caused by intravenous PAF is a platelet-independent phenomenon,
quite similar doses of hetrazepinoic PAF-antagonists could be used to antagonize the hypotension compared with the doses required to antagonize the bronchoconstriction.[15,21,54]

PAF-induced hypotension in the rat is believed not to involve platelets as platelets from

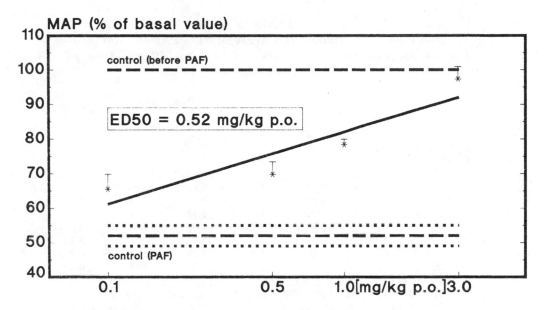

FIGURE 7.   Prevention of PAF-induced hypotension by oral STY 2108 in the rat; mean ± SEM) (n = 6).

the rat are extremely resistant to PAF[68] and this may explain why no relevant bronchoconstriction is observed in the rat after infusion of PAF. In spite of this, rats are still very sensitive to the vasodilating effect of PAF. Infusion of PAF at 30 ng $\times$ kg^{-1} $\times$ min^{-1} in anesthetized rats produced a profound hypotension which remained constant as long as the infusion of PAF continued.[15] Cumulative increasing intravenous doses of the hetrazepines WEB 2086, WEB 2170, WEB 2347, and STY 2108[15,21,22] reversed the PAF-induced hypotension in the rat in a dose-related manner. Compared to structurally unrelated PAF-antagonists, hetrazepines again turned out to be some of the most potent antagonists able to counteract PAF-induced hypotension in the rat.[7]

In contrast, hetrazepines have only a relative weak peroral activity in the rat and the ratio between oral and intravenous effective doses is rather high (Figure 7 exemplifies the antagonistic effect for oral STY 2108); this does not apply to other non-rodent species and to humans. Comparative ED$_{50}$-values for orally to intravenously administered hetrazepinoic PAF-antagonists in the rat are reviewed elsewhere.[9,69] WEB 2170 and WEB 2347 are relative exceptions in this respect; although the ratio between orally and i.v. effective doses is still high, the absolute orally effective doses in the rat are lower.[9,69]

In anesthetized guinea pigs a bolus of PAF at 10 μg/kg i.v. decreased the cardiac output by 70%, increased the end diastolic left ventricular pressure significantly, induced myocardial ischemia (derived from ECG), arrhythmias and blood pressure drop.[70] Pretreatment with WEB 2086 i.v. prevented the cardiac failure and signs of myocardial ischemia completely.[70]

Miscellaneous Effects of PAF In Vivo

Beside the effects on the lung and cardiovascular system PAF induces a number of various other alterations *in vivo*. Inhibition of PAF-induced increase of *vascular permeability* and edema formation may have important implications for the pathophysiology of different diseases. Inhibition of PAF-induced permeability changes and edema formation in the lung have already been reviewed before. PAF-induced increased vascular permeability is also inhibited at other target organs. WEB 2086 was found to inhibit PAF (100 ng/kg i.v.) induced leakage of Evans blue dye in the bladder, nasal mucosa, larynx, and esophagus.[58] Extravasation of Evans blue provoked by intracutaneous PAF (25 ng/site i.c.) in a *skin*

TABLE 6
Inhibition of the Binding and Aggregation to PAF *In Vitro* in Comparison with PAF-Antagonism *In Vivo* Using Different Types of PAF-Antagonists

Substance	Kl (nM) Bind. (a)	IC$_{50}$ (μM) Aggr. (b)	BC/CP (c)	BP/GP (d)	GP/Buxco (e)	BP/Rat (f)
	Platelets			ED$_{50}$mg/kg i.v.		
CV 3988	180	46.2	1.9	1.8	1.0—2.0	0.21
Ro 19.3704	3	0.83	0.09	0.04	0.1	0.2
Ginkgolide B	470	0.82	1.2	1.13	0.7	6.4
L 652.731	130	1.3	2.95	2.05	1.4	0.6
48.740 RP	20,000	48.9	21	15.0	5.2	3.2
52770 RP	22	7.6	1.32	1.39	1.1	6.7
WEB 2086	15	0.17	0.016	0.015	0.01	0.05

Note: Methods models: (a) bindng of ^{3}H-PAF to washed human platelets; (b) PAF (5×10^{-8} *M*)-induced human platelet aggregation — PRP; (c) bronchoconstriction and (d) hypotension in guinea pigs produced by an infusion of PAF at 30 ng/(kg $\times$ min); (e) bronchoconstriction by PAF (100 ng/kg i.v. bolus) measured by the Buxco pulmonary mechanics analyzer. In the table only dynamic compliance is shown; ED$_{50}$ values for the other measured parameters were similar; (f) hypotension in the rat produced by PAF (30 ng/kg $\times$ min).

vascular permeability model in the rat was abrogated by intradermal WEB 2086 in a dose-dependent manner.[15] The ratio between agonist (PAF) and antagonist (WEB 2086) was close to 1. This is in accordance with the effect of two hetrazepine-related PAF antagonists, triazolam and alprazolam, which inhibited the PAF-induced extravasation of a dye when coinjected with PAF in the skin of guinea pigs.[71] In the rabbit skin, local administration of WEB 2086 (10^{-7} moles/site) almost completely blocked the vascular leakage to PAF (10^{-9} moles) + PGE$_2$ (3×10^{-10} moles; PGE$_2$ was used for enhancement of the PAF-response).[72] WEB 2086 was selective in this respect because edema responses to bradykinin, histamine, FMLP, C5a, LTB$_4$, and zymosan were not affected.[72] Contrary to other PAF antagonists, WEB 2086 exhibited no partial agonistic activity.[72]

Also in the rat *mesenteric* microvessels, WEB 2086 abrogated the PAF-associated (1, 10, or 100 μM topically) increased latency period to noradrenaline for complete interruption of blood flow.[73] Also, topically administered WEB 2086 blocked this.[73] In both cases, WEB 2086 failed to block histamine at 100 and 600 μM suggesting a specific inhibition of PAF.[73] In the same study, topically administered PAF enlarged the mesenteric microvessel diameter, an effect which was consistently inhibited by WEB 2086 given i.v. or topically at the same doses as above.[73] Direct effects of WEB 2086 were excluded.[73]

In a rat model of *paw edema,* WEB 2086 (4 to 16 mg/kg i.p. or 2 to 8 mg/kg i.p.) antagonized the intraplantar PAF- (2 μg/paw) or 2-methoxy PAF (0.25 μg/paw) -induced paw edema in a dose-related fashion (Cordeiro, personal communication). WEB 2170 was superior to WEB 2086 in this model (Cordeiro, personal communication). In addition, WEB 2170 very effectively inhibited PAF-induced paw edema in mice.[74]

Synopsis of Data, Antagonism of Exogenous PAF: Potency *In Vitro* and *In Vivo*, Route of Administration, Kinetic Aspects

In comparison to hetrazepine-unrelated PAF-antagonists (PAF-analogs, natural products or their derivatives, other synthetic compounds) WEB 2086 and follow-up compounds turned out to be some of the most potent antagonists of PAF known so far.[7] Table 6 summarizes

TABLE 7

Inhibition of Bronchoconstriction (Decrease of Respiratory Flow) and Hypotension Induced by Infusion of PAF at 30 ng $\times$ kg^{-1} $\times$ min^{-1} in the Guinea Pig

	WEB 2170		WEB 2086	
	Resp. flow	MAP	Resp. flow	MAP
p.o.	0.016	0.011	0.070	0.066
	(0.006—0.03)	(0.001—0.03)	(0.05—0.088)	(0.041—0.087)
i.v.	0.008	0.006	0.018	0.016
	(0.005—0.011)	(0.002—0.010)	(0.011—0.028)	(0.01—0.02)
Tracheal	0.013	0.008	n.d.[a]	n.d.
	(0.005—0.027)	(0.003—0.014)		

Note: ED$_{50}$ values for oral, i.v., and intratracheal WEB 2170 in comparison with ED$_{50}$ values for WEB 2086 (95% confidence limits in parentheses). ED$_{50}$ values (mg/kg) calculated at 30 min after start of infusion on PAF.

[a] n.d. = not determined.

the inhibition of the binding and aggregation to PAF *in vitro* in comparison with PAF-antagonism *in vivo* for representatives of the above mentioned PAF-antagonists.[7]

Comparative data of ED$_{50}$ values of oral, intravenous, or intratracheal WEB 2086 and WEB 2170 for antagonism of intratracheal PAF have already been summarized in Table 5. For comparison of ED$_{50}$ or EC$_{50}$ values for oral, intravenous, or inhaled WEB 2086 and WEB 2170 to antagonize bronchoconstriction induced by an intravenoous bolus of PAF at 100 ng/kg i.v. Table 4 can be referred to. Table 7 summarizes the ED$_{50}$ values of oral and intravenous WEB 2086 in comparison to WEB 2170 when bronchoconstriction is induced by infusion of PAF at 30 ng/kg/min as described in Casals-Stenzel et al.[15] The ED$_{50}$ values (i.v., p.o.) of hetrazepinoic PAF-antagonists to antagonize PAF-induced hypotension in the rat have been reviewed in References 9 and 69. Overall it can be stated that in the guinea pig WEB 2170 is about 10 times more potent than WEB 2086 after oral administration (depending on the model) and about two to five times more potent after intravenous or tracheal administration. In contrast to the guinea pig and man the ratio between intravenously and orally effective doses in the rat is rather high, although the absolute doses of oral WEB 2170 or WEB 2347 are low due to their high *in vivo* potency.[22,23] Also after oral administration to the rabbit, higher doses of WEB 2086 (0.3 to 30 mg/kg) were required in comparison to WEB 2170 (0.01 to 0.5 mg/kg) to antagonize *ex vivo* the PAF-induced platelet aggregation (measured 2 h after oral administration[23]).

Table 8 summarizes the *duration of action* of WEB 2086 and WEB 2170 in guinea pigs and the rat after oral, intravenous, or inhalative/tracheal administration.[23,75] After oral administration the half-time of duration in the guinea pig for both compounds is about twice that estimated in the rat.[23,75] In addition, the half-time of duration of action of WEB 2170 is about twice that of WEB 2086 both in the rat and in the guinea pig (after oral administration[23,75]). In the case of WEB 2347 the half-time of duration of action after oral administration was estimated to be about 1.40 h in the guinea pig and about 10 h in the rat.[22] Thus this again confirms the longer duration of action of hetrazepines in the guinea pig in comparison to the rat. WEB 2347 is a particularly long-acting hetrazepinoic PAF-antagonist.[22] As expected, both WEB 2086 and WEB 2170 exhibited a shorter half-time of duration in the rat after intravenous administration than after oral administration.[23,75]

Since also in humans the ratio between orally and intravenously effective doses of WEB 2086 was about 2:1[76,77] (see below) and on the other hand the duration of action of oral WEB 2086 in man is almost identical with the duration in the guinea pig, the results may

TABLE 8

Estimation of Duration of Action of WEB 2086 and WEB 2170
After Oral Intravenous, or Tracheal/Inhalative Administration
to Guinea Pigs or Rats

		$t_{1/2}$(h)	
Model/parameter/species	Route	WEB 2086	WEB 2170
Guinea pig, bronchoconstriction	p.o.	5.5	12.1
Guinea pig, bronchoconstriction	Tracheal/inhaled	(1.6)[a]	14.8
Rat, PAF-induced hypotension	p.o.	3.1	5.4
	i.v.	0.9—1.2	1.1—2.3

Note: Doses of the PAF-antagonists have been used which provide initially about
100% protection against PAF-induced bronchoconstriction or hypotension.
95% confidence limits in brackets.

[a]   Different protocol used, results not obtained under identical conditions as with
WEB 2170 (WEB 2086 has been aerosolized to guinea pigs).

suggest that the kinetic parameters of hetrazepines estimated in the guinea pig (ratio between orally effective to intravenously effective doses; half-time of duration) may better predict the situation in man than to the results derived from rats.

To study the role of endogenous PAF in disease-related subchronic and chronic models in the rat, oral WEB 2170 or oral WEB 2347 may be better suited due to their longer duration of action and the absolute lower doses required due to their higher oral potency in the rat.[21,23]

ANTAGONISM OF ENDOGENOUS PAF IN DISEASE RELATED MODELS
IN VITRO
Antigen-Induced Changes in Cells or the Lung

At the cellular level, WEB 2086 failed to inhibit the release of histamine from human basophilic leukocytes of atopic patients when these leukocytes were incubated with allergen.[78] The authors conclude that PAF released under these conditions probably does not contribute to a direct positive feedback on the antigen-induced histamine release from the same cell although the action on other target cells is not excluded.[78]

The contractile response of isolated lung parenchymal strips from actively sensitized guinea pigs to immunological challenge is antagonized by the hetrazepine-related PAF-antagonist alprazolam in the presence of an antihistamine and the dual lipoxygenase and cyclooxygenase inhibitor BW 755 C or the leukotriene receptor-antagonist FPL 55712.[79,80] In this study it was already evident that PAF is not the only mediator involved since the PAF-antagonist alprazolam failed to block the anaphylactic response when given alone.[79,80]

The PAF-antagonist WEB 2086 at a concentration of 20 to 50 μM inhibited the antigen-induced contraction of lung parenchymal strips from actively sensitized guinea pigs by 30 to 40%, when contracted by 0.1 to 10 μg ovalbumin in the presence of NDGA, mepyramine, methysergide, indomethacin, and atropine.[45]

In addition, the hetrazepine WEB 2086 blocked the antigen-induced contraction of rabbit peripheral lung strips. Rabbit peripheral lung strips were obtained from animals sensitized from birth so that they synthesized IgE.[81] WEB 2086 failed to counteract the antigen-induced contraction during the first 5 min, but started to relax at 10 min and reached the background level by 40 min.[81] In contrast, the antihistamine chlorpheniramine at 3 μM delayed the beginning of the contraction by 5 min but did not influence the maximal response.[81] A combination of the antihistamine with WEB 2086 eliminated the contractile response to antigen.[81] The results are in agreement with histamine being responsible for the very early contraction and PAF being the major mediator of the maximal response.[81]

When isolated perfused lungs from actively or passively sensitized guinea pigs were provoked by ovalbumin, WEB 2086 significantly reduced the TXB_2 and histamine release from the perfused lungs.[45] Since inhibition of thromboxane synthesis[42] (F. Birke, Boehringer Ingelheim, unpublished) or direct antagonism of histamine has been excluded, the results support the notion that PAF may be a central mediator in the sequence of events in the release of these mediators as well as synergizing with other inflammatory mediators during anaphylaxis.

In a model of rat pulmonary anaphylaxis, perfusion with WEB 2086 prevented the increase of lung weight, increase of pulmonary perfusion pressure, and release of leukotriene D_4 material evoked by an antibody to rat whole serum followed by anti-rat IgG in rat isolated lungs.[44] These data indicate that PAF may be involved in the vasoconstrictor responses and promotion of edema, and releases leukotrienes in a model of allergen-induced rat pulmonary anaphylaxis.[44]

In Vitro Antigen-Induced Changes in the Cardiovascular System

In antigen-perfused guinea pig hearts from actively sensitized guinea pigs WEB 2086 at 0.03 to 1 μM antagonized the antigen-induced increase of coronary perfusion pressure and decrease in cardiac developed tension.[49] In addition, WEB 2086 antagonized the antigen triggered release of LTC_4 but did not significantly inhibit the antigen-induced release of TXB_2.[49]

ANTAGONISM OF ENDOGENOUS PAF IN DISEASE-RELATED MODELS *IN VIVO*

Anaphylaxis and Models of Bronchial Asthma

There is no perfect animal model of bronchial asthma. We are dealing with different models which focus on more or less one aspect of the complex and not fully understood pathophysiology of bronchial asthma.

The results obtained with structurally and even the same antagonists of PAF in models of *in vivo anaphylaxis* are divergent, although most authors do report at least some protective action during passive anaphylaxis in the guinea pig. The divergent results may be due to differing protocols (e.g., testing in the absence of a small dose of an antihistamine) and the different potency and bioavailability of PAF antagonists *in vivo*.

With respect to *anaphylaxis in vivo* and *antigen-induced bronchoconstriction* the hetrazepine related PAF-antagonist alprazolam when tested in the presence of an antihistamine and the lipoxygenase inhibitor BW 755 C increased not only survival from 0 to 64% but also prevented the anaphylactic bronchoconstriction and circulatory failure in actively sensitized guinea pigs.[80,81] The hetrazepinoic PAF-antagonists WEB 2086 and WEB 2170 protected conscious and actively sensitized mice from anaphylactic death in a dose-dependent fashion.[57,82] When actively sensitized (40 μg OA/kg in 100 mg $Al(OH)_3$/guinea pig i.p.) guinea pigs were challenged by ovalbumin, animals died 1 to 2 min after antigen challenge.[82-84] Also, oral WEB 2086 or WEB 2170 given alone failed to protect.[82-84] This has been confirmed in actively sensitized guinea pigs[45] and in actively sensitized rabbits[85] in which WEB 2086 given alone neither inhibited the anaphylactic bronchoconstriction nor circulatory anaphylaxis nor changes in blood cell counts. In contrast, in the presence of an antihistamine (mepyramine) WEB 2086 and WEB 2170 inhibited the anaphylactic bronchoconstriction and in the case of WEB 2170 also the final hypotension.[82-84,86] Thus pretreatment with the antihistamine prevented the immediate death (early histamine predominated component) thereby disclosing the following (PAF predominated) phase which is characterized by a remaining severe anaphylactic bronchoconstriction which can be inhibited by WEB 2086 or WEB 2170 in a dose-dependent manner. Figure 8 illustrates the protective effect of oral WEB 2170 in a model of active anaphylaxis in the guinea pig.

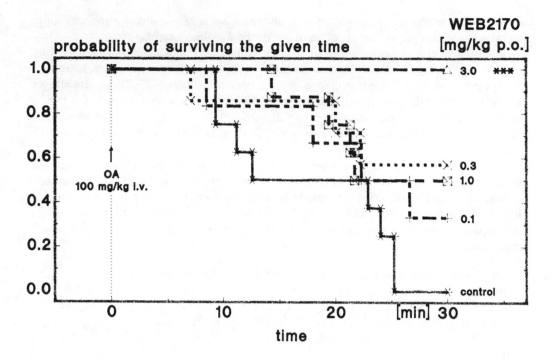

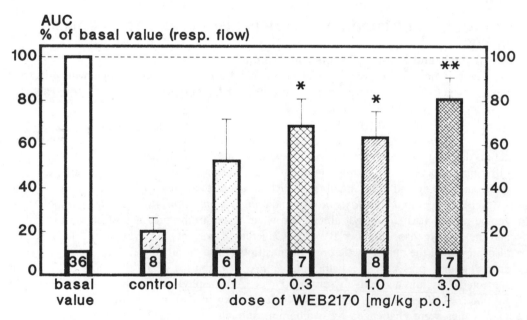

FIGURE 8.   Effect of oral WEB 2170 on mortality (above) and on the anaphylactic decrease of respiratory flow (below; AUC = *A*rea *U*nder *C*urve) during a 30 min observation period. Guinea pigs were sensitized twice with 40 μg ovalbumin/kg in 100 mg Al(OH)$_3$/guinea pig. The actively sensitized guinea pigs were challenged with 100 mg/kg i.v. ovalbumin in the presence of 10 μg/kg i.v. mepyramine. * $p < 0.05$, ** $p < 0.01$, *** $p < 0.001$; n on bottom of the bars; mean ± SEM.

In passively sensitized guinea pigs again neither mepyramine nor WEB 2086 or WEB 2170 alone prevented the antigen-induced death.[57,82] The animals were only protected against intravenous antigen challenge when WEB 2086 or WEB 2170 were administered in the presence of mepyramine.[57,82,86] Also in another series of passive anaphylaxis WEB 2086, again in the presence of mepyramine, markedly suppressed the bronchoconstriction and interestingly, also leukopenia, evoked by 100 µg/kg i.v. ovalbumin.[45]

In contrast, when guinea pigs were exposed to an aerosol of ovalbumin, WEB 2086 given alone protected actively sensitized guinea pigs from anaphylactic bronchoconstriction and the characteristic increase in blood pressure followed by hypotension.[86]

To summarize the action of hetrazepines in different models of antigen-induced anaphylactic bronchoconstriction the results indicate that PAF plays an important role in such models of anaphylaxis. PAF seems to be more important in passive anaphylaxis and during challenge with the antigen by aerosol.[82,86]

The role of PAF in airway *inflammation* and *recruitment of inflammatory cells (particularly eosinophils)* and associated late phase reaction and bronchial hyperreactivity is considered more important than its putative contribution to acute bronchoconstriction. WEB 2086 at the investigated dose of 10 µg/kg i.v. failed to counteract ovalbumin induced airway microvascular leakage in actively sensitized guinea pigs.[58] Although WEB 2086 at similar doses blocked exogenous PAF-induced microvascular leakage in the same model,[58] a final conclusion on the participation of PAF in antigen-induced edema formation cannot be drawn at this point, because WEB 2086 inhibited the antigen-induced edema formation in another model of lung anaphylaxis.[44] With respect to infiltration of eosinophils into lungs, WEB 2086 prevented the eosinophil infiltration in the bronchial walls measured 6 h after antigen challenge in passively sensitized guinea pigs.[62] In addition, also in actively sensitized guinea pigs WEB 2086 inhibited the antigen-induced eosinophil infiltration by about 75% measured by whole lung lavage 4 h after inhaled antigen (Craig Wegner, Boehringer Ingelheim, personal communication). In another study, in actively sensitized guinea pigs WEB 2086 administered 1 h before antigen inhalation inhibited the accumulation of both neutrophils and eosinophils in BAL fluid recovered from the lung at 17 h but not at 72 h after antigen inhalation.[87] In case WEB 2086 was administered 6 h after antigen challenge the numbers of eosinophils and lymphocytes in the BAL at 72 h was significantly reduced, too.[87]

The *late phase response* to antigen and its inhibition by WEB 2086 has been investigated in a new model for investigating the late phase reaction produced by inhalation of ovalbumin to conscious and actively sensitized guinea pigs.[87] Inhalation of antigen produced in the guinea pigs a triphasic reduction of sGaw with maximal reductions at 2, 17, and 72 h after challenge.[87] WEB 2086 administered perorally 1 h before ovalbumin aerosol had little effect on the magnitude but reduced the duration of both the early and late asthmatic response.[87] When WEB 2086 was administered 6 h after antigen challenge, the late asthmatic response at 17 and 72 h, respectively, was inhibited.[87] In another model in the sheep WEB 2086 also blocked antigen-induced late phase response,[64] inflammation (2 h post challenge), and antigen-induced *bronchial hyperreactivity* at the same time.[88]

In *summary*, the results derived from animal models which focus on diverse aspects of the complex pathophysiology of asthma provide increasing support that PAF-antagonists of the hetrazepine type (exemplified by the specific PAF-antagonist WEB 2086) antagonize different symptoms of bronchial asthma.

Diseases of the Heart and Cardiovascular System
Myocardial Ischemia and Reperfusion

In a model of myocardial infarction with reperfusion in the dog WEB 2086 prevented the decrease of coronary vascular resistance and regional blood flow in the stunned myocardium during reperfusion.[89] WEB 2086 reduced the extent of myocardial necrosis for any given flow reduction and selectively improved endocardial flow in the reperfused area.[90] Thus WEB 2086 may be useful for protection of the myocardium after ischemia and reperfusion.

Kidney Diseases

In adriamycin-induced nephropathy in the rat the hetrazepine-related PAF-antagonists triazolam and alprazolam inhibited the proteinuria and the ultrastructural glomerular alterations induced by adriamycin.[91]

Diseases of the Central Nervous System

Concerning *diseases of the CNS* the hetrazepinoic PAF-antagonist brotizolam given curatively (10 mg/kg i.p.), 1 h after declamping, improved the mitochondrial respiration.[92] This was evaluated by the respiratory control ratio in a model of cerebral post-ischemic recovery in the Mongolian gerbil.[92] The possible antiischemic activity of brotizolam is in agreement with the known activity of WEB 2086 to increase survival rate under normobaric hypoxia in mice, both after s.c. or intraventricular pretreatment (G. Schingnitz; Boehringer Ingelheim, personal communication). Preischemic administration of WEB 2086 caused a marked reduction in cortical infarct volume and of total infarct in a model of middle cerebral artery occlusion (MCAO) in the rat.[93] The hetrazepine WEB 2170 also reduced the total infarct volume by 40%.[93]

Models of Shock

PAF may be one of the prominent mediators of shock states like endotoxin-, hemorrhage-, trauma-, or anaphylaxis-associated shock. PAF can mimic most of the pathophysiologic derangements seen in endotoxin shock, like pulmonary hypertension and edema, cardiac failure, derangement of microcirculation with increase of vascular permeability and tissue damage, activation of immune cells with mediator release, and systemic hypotension. Increased levels of PAF-like activity have been reported in blood from endotoxin-treated animals and in septic patients.[94,95]

With respect to the *lethal effect of endotoxin* in animals the role of PAF (as evidenced by a protective effect of selective PAF-antagonists including hetrazepines) remains somewhat controversial. This may be due to different animal species, route of administration of endotoxin, differing kinetic and potency of PAF-antagonists, and different protocols. The lethal effect of endotoxin from *E. coli* in rats was prevented by peroral and intravenous pretreatment with WEB 2086 in a dose-dependent fashion.[96] Also, post-treatment with WEB 2086, starting at 2 h after endotoxin from *Salmonella enteritidis,* significantly improved survival compared to vehicle treatment.[97] When in Balb/C mice the lethality to endotoxin was enhanced by i.v. treatment with propranolol at 8 h after endotoxin, oral WEB 2170 at (1 + 3) to (10 + 30) mg/kg/day protected Balb/C mice from a propranolol induced increase of lethality to endotoxin (observation period 7 days[57,98]). Since tumor necrosis factor (TNF) mimics most of the pathophysiologic aspects of endotoxin, it is of interest that oral WEB 2170 protected Balb/C mice from mortality induced by a combination of endotoxin with TNF.[57,98] Although a first treatment with human recombinant TNF failed to have a lethal effect to Balb/C mice, this primed the mice for an enhanced sensitivity (measured in terms of lethality) to a second challenge 1 week later (Sanarelli-Shwartzman-like phenomenon[98]). The selective and very potent hetrazepinoic PAF-antagonist WEB 2347 at (0.03 + 0.1) to (0.3 + 1.0) mg/kg/day p.o. protected the Balb/C-mice from the lethal effect of TNF in a dose-related manner.[98]

The *hypotensive action of endotoxin* (from *E. coli* 0111:B_4) in the rat was prohibited by oral or intravenous pretreatment WEB 2086, WEB 2170, or STY 2108.[21,96,99] This effect is exemplified by WEB 2086 in Figure 9. In addition, therapeutic intervention at the nadir of endotoxin-induced hypotension at 6 min after endotoxin reversed the endotoxin induced

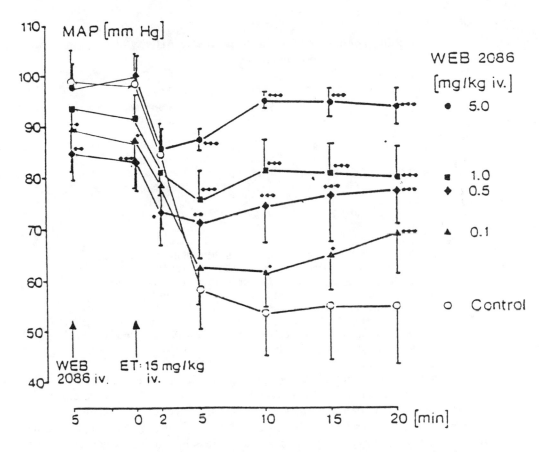

FIGURE 9. Inhibition of the hypotensive activity of *E. coli* endotoxin in rats by i.v. doses of WEB 2086. Mean ± SD; n = 6; * p <0.05, ** p <0.01, *** p <0.001 = significant differences from the control.

hypotension in a dose-dependent fashion.[21,96,99] In opposition to other pharmacological agents, PAF-antagonists only increase blood pressure when lowered by PAF or endotoxin; they do not increase blood pressure per se. Table 9 summarizes the ED_{50}s of preventively (p.o., i.v.) administered WEB 2086, WEB 2170, or STY 2108 in comparison to curatively administered (after administration of endotoxin) PAF-antagonists with respect to their ability to antagonize the endotoxin induced hypotension in the rat.[21,96,99]

In contrast, in endotoxin-induced shock of the pig, WEB 2086 at the tested dose did not attenuate the systemic hypotension occurring after infusion of endotoxin.[100]

The pulmonary hypertension occurring after infusion of endotoxin to the pig was significantly inhibited by treatment with WEB 2086.[100]

When perfusion of the hindlimb and systemic blood pressure was reduced by 30 mg/kg i.v. endotoxin from *E. coli* 0111:B4 in the rat, WEB 2086 (at 10 μM, added to the perfusion medium, plus 1 mg/kg i.v.) reversed the fall in hindlimb perfusion and the fall of systemic blood pressure.[47]

Activation of blood cells (including platelets and leukocytes) with mediator release may particularly contribute to the development of lung injury (ARDS). When conscious guinea pigs were exposed to an aerosol of endotoxin, pretreatment with the hetrazepine brotizolam inhibited the endotoxin-induced pulmonary platelet recruitment in a dose-related manner.[101] Also in the pig WEB 2086 retarded the sharp decline in peripheral white blood cell counts occurring after start of an infusion of endotoxin.[100] In addition the endotoxin associated deterioration in gas exchange and inspiratory pressure were also partially prevented by WEB 2086.[100]

TABLE 9
Inhibition or Reversal of the Hypotensive Activity of
Endotoxin (ET)

	Prophylactic[a] ED_{50} (mg/kg)		Curative[b]
	i.v.	p.o.	ED_{50} (mg/kg i.v.)
WEB 2170	0.099	0.32	0.026
	(. . . — . . .)[c]	(0.001—0.6)	(0.0001—0.084)
STY 2108	0.004	3.51	0.085
	(. . . — . . .)[c]	(1.9—8.77)	(0.055—0.19)
WEB 2086	0.41	6.25	0.34
	(0.052—1.17)	(2.42— . . .)[c]	(0.063—1.62)

Note: The ED_{50} values were calculated on the basis of the BP levels at
the last measurement time point (20 min; in the case of a prophylactic effect) or 6 min after the "curative" administration of the
PAF-antagonist. ED_{50} values in comparison with WEB 2086; 95%
confidence limits in parenthesis.

[a] ED_{50} calculated 20 min after ET.
[b] ED_{50} calculated 6 min after curative administration of PAF-antagonist.
[c]   . . . means confidence limit(s) could not be determined.

Endotoxin-induced *microvascular leakage with edema formation* is judged as one of the
earliest and prominent symptoms in the development of ARDS. With respect to endotoxin-
induced lung injury, WEB 2086 infused at 20 mg/kg/h inhibited the late increase of lymph
flow and lymph protein clearance in the conscious sheep.[102] In contrast, WEB 2086 had
little effect on early pulmonary hypertension and alterations in lung mechanics.[102] In a very
recent study Chang and co-workers[97] reported that WEB 2086 inhibited the lung vascular
leakage not only when given before, but also, more importantly, when given 30 min after
endotoxin.[97] In the same study, post-treatment with WEB 2086 starting at 90 min after
endotoxin attenuated markedly the vascular lung leakage when measured 6 h after endotoxin.[97]

In *hypoxic pulmonary vasoconstriction* in the rat, perfusion with WEB 2086 attenuated
the pulmonary vasoconstrictor response in the isolated, blood perfused, *in situ* ventilated
lung in a concentration-dependent manner.[103] The inhibition of the hypoxic pulmonary
response was complete at the highest concentration.[103]

In a model of *traumatic shock* in anesthetized rats WEB 2086 maintained a higher mean
arterial blood pressure in traumatized rats than those receiving only physiologic saline.[104]
In addition, WEB 2086 increased the overall survival time of traumatized rats.[104] Other
indicators of traumatic shock like accumulation of lysosomal hydrolase, cathepsin D, and
free amino-nitrogen compounds and increase of myocardial depressant factor were also
inhibited by WEB 2086.[104]

Concerning *hemorrhagic shock,* the hetrazepine-related benzodiazepine receptor antagonist and weak PAF-antagonist Ro 15-1788 had a beneficial effect in a rat model of hemorrhagic shock.[105] This is in accordance with an effect of the specific PAF-antagonist WEB
2086 which attenuated hemorrhagic shock (survival and blood pressure drop) in another
model in the rat (R. Reichl, Boehringer Ingelheim KG, personal communication).

Diseases of the Gastrointestinal System

PAF is a potent ulcerogenic agent in the gastrointestinal system. This effect can be
blocked by specific PAF-antagonists.[106] Furthermore, endotoxin-induced gastrointestinal ul-

ceration is assumed to be at least partially mediated via PAF, since this is blocked by PAF-antagonists and PAF is released from the jejunum of endotoxin treated rats.

In mice, treatment with endotoxin (*S. typhosa*) primed mice for an enhanced sensitivity towards PAF resulting not only in decreased gastrointestinal transit velocity, but also in increased mortality.[107] The same priming has been shown between tumor necrosis factor (TNF) and PAF[108-110] which is in line with TNF mimicking most of the pathophysiologic features of endotoxin. This priming effect between endotoxin or TNF towards PAF occurred at doses at which PAF, endotoxin, or TNF given alone did not significantly change these parameters.[109,110] Furthermore, this priming effect of endotoxin/TNF towards PAF with respect to decreased gastrointestinal transit velocity and increased lethality was maximal when the time interval between administration of endotoxin/TNF and subsequently PAF was about 1 to 2 h. WEB 2086 at 0.01 to 1 mg/kg i.p. prevented this enhanced sensitivity to PAF induced by endotoxin/TNF in a dose-dependent fashion.[109,110]

Stress-induced gastric ulceration in the female rat has been reported to be inhibited by the hetrazepine-related PAF antagonist triazolam,[111] although atropine turned out to be more efficient.

In a model of *chronic colitis* in the rat induced by intracolonic administration of trinitrobenzene sulfonic acid (TNB), daily treatment with WEB 2086 or WEB 2170 resulted in significant reduction of the colonic damage.[112]

Miscellaneous Disease-Related Models

In a model of *inflammation* induced by carrageenan, WEB 2086 inhibited the first phase of edema evoked by 300 µg/paw carrageenan in the mice paw but it did not modify the later phase of edema (R. Cordeiro, personal communication).

In another inflammatory model in the rat, WEB 2086 attenuated the inflammatory edema induced by intraplanar injection of an extract from meduse ceventerate.[113] Furthermore, the reversed passive arthus reaction in rats was suppressed by oral pretreatment with WEB 2086 or WEB 2170. WEB 2170 exhibiting higher potency in this model (G. Possanza, Boehringer Ingelheim, personal communication).

CLINICAL PHARMACOLOGY AND SAFETY OF THE PAF-ANTAGONIST WEB 2086

Phase I trials testing the pharmacological activity, safety, and tolerance of WEB 2086 in healthy volunteers have been carried out, and form a basis for performing clinical trials in human diseases. As part of these phase I studies the pharmacological action of WEB 2086 was monitored by measuring *ex vivo* PAF-induced platelet aggregation in platelet rich plasma (PRP).

Three single increasing dose tolerance studies were performed, administering WEB 2086 by oral, intravenous, or inhaled route.[76,114,115]

Six oral dose levels were studied in a first trial: 1.25 mg, 5.0 mg, 20 mg, 100 mg, 200 mg, and 400 mg WEB 2086. The study was performed in a double-blind and placebo-controlled manner.[114] At each dose level eight different volunteers participated. According to randomization, two volunteers were assigned to placebo treatment and six volunteers received WEB 2086.[114] One and three quarter hours after oral dosage, from the dose 20 mg upwards, PAF-induced aggregation was totally inhibited. Even at a dose of only 1.25 mg aggregation was inhibited by 62%.[116]

Intravenously administered drug (infusion over 30 min) was studied in a single, rising dose study.[76,115] Eight different healthy male volunteers took part at each dose level, and according to randomization, two volunteers were allocated to placebo treatment and six volunteers received WEB 2086. Infusions of 0.5 mg, 2.0 mg, 10 mg, 20 mg, or 50 mg

WEB 2086 produced significant inhibition of platelet aggregation *ex vivo* at all dose levels tested.[76,115] In the lowest dose group (0.5 mg), PAF (5×10^{-8} M)-induced platelet aggregation *ex vivo* was attenuated by 68%,[76,115] doses of 10, 20, or 50 mg providing complete inhibition. A placebo-controlled rising dose study design was also used to investigate the effects of inhalatively administered drug. Inhalative administration of 0.5 mg or 1 mg WEB 2086 inhibited PAF (1×10^{-8} M) induced platelet aggregation *ex vivo* by 46 and 64%, whereas 0.05 mg or 0.25 mg WEB 2086 by inhalative route had no significant effect.[76,115]

The time course and dose-dependency of the PAF-antagonistic action of oral WEB 2086 in man was studied in a randomized double-blind, placebo-controlled fourfold cross-over study.[77,114] Twelve healthy male volunteers received either 5, 30, or 90 mg of WEB 2086 via the oral route. PAF-antagonism was monitored over a time period of 24 h using inhibition of 5×10^{-8} M PAF-induced platelet aggregation *ex vivo* as an indicator of pharmacological action. WEB 2086 inhibited PAF-induced aggregation at all doses tested. Maximal inhibition occurred between 1 and 2 h after oral administration.[77,114] Magnitude and duration of inhibition was dose dependent, a significant inhibition was still evident at 10 h after administration at all three dose levels, and at 12 h after administration at the two highest doses (30 and 90 mg;[77,114]). In contrast, platelet aggregation induced by 1×10^{-6} M ADP or 10 $\times 10^{-6}$ M adrenalin were not significantly inhibited by WEB 2086. This confirmed *ex vivo* the specificity of PAF-antagonism in man. Maximal blockade obtained by 5 mg/kg oral WEB 2086 is decreased to 50% at about 4 to 6 h after intake.

In the two subsequent multiple oral dose tolerance studies (randomized, within-subject comparism, twofold cross-over, 12 subjects per dose) 3×100 mg/day or 3×40 mg/day, dose interval 8 h, produced almost complete inhibition throughout the 7-day study period.[114,116] Even if the PAF-concentration was raised to 1×10^{-6} M[114,116] inhibition could not be overcome (Figure 10).

No clinically significant drug-related effects on blood-pressure, pulse-rate, ECG, etc. were observed in all studies. Laboratory parameters (hematology, urinalysis, and serum chemistry) did not show any drug-related changes.[116] All subjects completed the studies. With regard to the structural relationship of WEB 2086 to diazepines it has to be stressed that, up to the highest tested dose (400 mg), no diazepine-characteristic central nervous adverse effects were observed.[116] This confirmed that the reported dissociation of PAF-antagonistic and BDZ-like effects previously reported in animals[5] can be extended to man.

Different clinical trials using WEB 2086 in asthmatics and other human diseases are underway or planned. In a patient with idiopathic thrombocytopenia (ITP) WEB 2086 induced a marked increase of platelet count.[117] After withdrawal of WEB 2086 platelet count dropped again, and rose again when WEB 2086 was reintroduced.[117]

Overall the results from the phase I studies of WEB 2086 in human volunteers suggest that WEB 2086 is a well-tolerated and potent PAF-antagonist in man, independent of the route of administration.

SUMMARY

Hetrazepines are either oxazepines, thiazepines, or diazepines with two annelated 5-membered heterocycles. During the search for leads with PAF-antagonistic activity, the hypnotic brotizolam attracted attention by inhibiting selectively the PAF-induced platelet aggregation. Systematic structure variation in a series of hetrazepines led to a number of potent hetrazepinoic PAF-antagonists which lacked sedative or hypnogenic action. The hetrazepines WEB 2086, WEB 2170, WEB 2347, STY 2108, and other compounds belong to the most potent antagonists of PAF known so far.

WEB 2086, WEB 2170, and others inhibit most exogenous PAF-induced alterations *in*

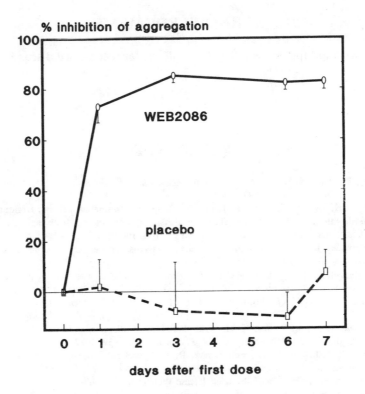

FIGURE 10.   Inhibition of PAF-induced platelet aggregation in human volunteers receiving 3×40 mg WEB 2086/day or placebo for 7 days. Final concentration of PAF $= 1 \times 10^{-6} M$. Each point is the mean $\pm$ SEM of estimations from 12 human volunteers.

vitro and *in vivo* very effectively and irrespective of the route of administration. *In vivo* all PAF-induced alterations on blood cells, in the lung, cardiovascular system, skin, and microcirculation are inhibited.

Results from the effect of hetrazepinoic PAF-antagonists in different disease-related models of asthma suggest a causative role of PAF in (1) allergen-induced bronchoconstriction, (2) infiltrations of eosinophils, (3) edema formation, (4) late phase response, and (5) bronchial hyperreactivity. Based on different disease-related models of shock, the action of specific PAF-antagonists of the hetrazepine type (exemplified by WEB 2086) provide evidence for a role for PAF in (1) endotoxin- or trauma-induced mortality; (2) endotoxin-, trauma-, or hemorrhage-induced systemic blood pressure fall; (3) activation of blood cells with release of enzymes and mediators; (4) edema formation and vascular leakage in target organs of shock; and (5) development of shock organs (like ARDS) and organ failure.

In addition there is support from effects of hetrazepinoic PAF-antagonists in disease-related models that PAF may be involved in myocardial ischemia, cerebral ischemia, kidney disorders, colitis, and other inflammatory diseases.

In the first clinical studies WEB 2086 was shown to be a strong and well-tolerated PAF-antagonist in man independent of whether administered by the oral, intravenous, or inhaled route.

WEB 2086 and related PAF-antagonists may help to investigate the pathophysiological significance of PAF in a broad spectrum of different human diseases and provide an opening in the therapy of these diseases.

ACKNOWLEDGMENT

The author would like to thank Dr. C. J. Meade for reading and discussing the English manuscript.

REFERENCES

1. **Braquet, P., Touqui, L., Shen, T. Y., and Vargaftig, B. B.,** Perspectives in platelet-activating factor research, *Pharmacol. Rev.,* 39, 97, 1987.
2. **Weber, K. H., Kuhn, F. J., Boeke-Kuhn, K., Lehr, E., Danneberg, P. B., Hommer, D., Paul, S. M., and Skolnick, P.,** Pharmacological and neurochemical properties of 1,4-diazepines with two annelated heterocycles ("Hetrazepines"), *Eur. J. Pharmacol.,* 109, 19, 1985.
3. **Casals-Stenzel, J.,** Triazolodiazepines are potent antagonists of platelet activating factor (PAF) in vitro and in vivo, *Arch. Pharmacol.,* 335, 351, 1987.
4. **Casals-Stenzel, J.,** The inhibitory activity of brotizolam and related compounds on platelet activating factor induced effects in vitro and in vivo, in *Proc. 1st Sandoz Research Symposium, New Horizons in Platelet-Activating Factor Research,* Winslow, C. M. and Lee, M. L., Eds., John Wiley & Sons, London, 1987, 277.
5. **Casals-Stenzel, J. and Weber, K. H.,** Triazolodiazepines: dissociation of their PAF (Platelet activating factor) antagonistic and CNS activity, *Br. J. Pharmacol.,* 90, 139, 1987.
6. **Kornecki, E., Ehrlich, Y. H., and Lenox, R. H.,** Platelet-Activating Factor-induced aggregation of human platelets specifically inhibited by triazolodiazepines, *Science,* 226, 1454, 1984.
7. **Heuer, H., Birke, F. W., Casals-Stenzel, J., and Weber, K. H.,** Inhibition of the binding and aggregation to paf in vitro in comparison with paf-antagonsim in vivo: an investigation using different types of paf-antagonists, *Prostaglandins,* 35, 838, 1988.
8. **Weber, K. H. and Heuer, H.,** Structure-activity relationships and effects of PAF-antagonists in the hetrazepine series, *Int. Arch. Allergy Appl. Immunol.,* 88, 82, 1989.
9. **Weber, K. H. and Heuer, H. O.,** Hetrazepines as antagonists of platelet activating factor, *Med. Res. Rev.,* 9, 181, 1989.
10. **Birke, F. W. and Weber, K. H.,** Specific and high affinity binding of WEB 2086 to human platelet PAF receptors, *Clin. Exp. Pharmacol. Physiol. Suppl.,* 13, 2, 1988.
11. **Ukena, D., Dent, G., Birke, F. W., Robaut, C., Sybrecht, G. W., and Barnes, P. J.,** Radioligand binding of antagonists of platelet-activating factor to intact human platelets, *FEBS Lett.,* 228, 285, 1988.
12. **Tahraoui, L., Floch A., Mondot, S., and Cavero, I.,** High affinity specific binding sites for tritiated platelet-activating factor in canine platelet membranes: counterparts of platelet-activating factor receptors mediating patelet aggregation, *Mol. Pharmacol.,* 34, 145, 1988.
13. **Saunders, R. N., Kowal De Lillo, A., Winslow, C. M., Glinka, K. G., Melden, M. K., and Van Valen, R. G.,** Is the human platelet PAF receptor a good screening model for identifying PAF antagonists?, *Clin. Exp. Pharmacol. Physiol. Suppl.,* 13, 10, 1988.
14. **Chesney, C. M., Pifer, D. D., and Cagen, L. M.,** Triazolobenzodiazepines competitively inhibit the binding of platelet activating factor (PAF) to human platelets, *Biochem. Biophys. Res. Commun.,* 144, 359, 1987.
15. **Casals-Stenzel, J., Muacevic, G., and Weber, K. H.,** Pharmacological actions of WEB 2086, a new specific antagonist of platelet activating factor, *J. Pharmacol. Exp. Ther.,* 241, 974, 1987.
16. **Thompson, P. J., Misso, N., Adcock, J., and Gillon, R. L.,** The human platelet aggregatory model used to assess the relative potency of PAF antagonists, *Clin. Exp. Pharmacol. Physiol. Suppl.,* 13, 9, 1987.
17. **O'Donnell, S. R. and Barnett, C. J. K.,** PA$_2$ values for antagonists of platelet activating factor on aggregation of rabbit platelets, *Br. J. Pharmacol.,* 94, 437, 1988.
18. **Stewart, A. G. and Dusting, G. J.,** Characterization of receptors for platelet-activating factor on platelets, polymorphonuclear leukocytes and macrophages, *Br. J. Pharmacol.,* 94, 1225, 1988.
19. **Levy, J. V. and Ezzet, K.,** Schild plot analysis of six putative antagonists of platelet activating factor (PAF) on human platelets, *Pharmacologist,* 29, 219, 1987.
20. **Heuer, H., Birke, F., Brandt, K., Muacevic, G., and Weber, K. H.,** Biological characterisation of the enantiomeric hetrazepines of the paf-antagonist WEB 2170, *Prostaglandins,* 35, 847, 1988.
21. **Heuer, H., Casals-Stenzel, J., Muacevic, G., Stransky, W., and Weber, K. H.,** Effect of WEB 2170 and STY 2108, two hetrazepines with antagonistic activity on platelet activating factor-induced changes in vitro and in vivo, *Clin. Exp. Pharmacol. Physiol. Suppl.,* 13, 7, 1988.

22. **Heuer, H. O. and Weber, K. H.,** Pharmacology of WEB 2347, a new very potent and long acting hetrazepinoic paf-antagonist, *3rd. Int. Conf. on Platelet-Activating Factor and Structurally Related Alkyl Ether Lipids,* Tokyo, May 8—12, 1989, Abstr. book p. 12.

23. **Heuer, H. O., Casals-Stenzel, J., Muacevic, G., Streller, I., and Weber, K. H.,** WEB 2170 — A new and in vivo, more potent PAF-antagonist of the hetrazepine series, *3rd Int. Conf. on Platelet-Activating Factor and Structurally Related Alkyl Ether Lipids,* Tokyo, May 8—12, 1989, Abstr. book p. 96.

24. **Mikashima, H., Takehara, S., Muramoto, Y., Khomaru, T., Terasawa, M., Tahara, T., and Maruyama, Y.,** An antagonistic activity of etizolam on platelet-activating factor (PAF) — In vitro effects on platelet aggregation and PAF receptor binding, *Jpn. J. Pharmacol.,* 44, 387, 1987.

25. **Rubino, A., Tarli, S., Vanni, L., Giotti, A., Montesi, L., and Fantozzi, R.,** Drug modulation of human neutrophil activation evoked by platelet activating factor, *Pharmacol. Res. Commun.,* 20, 7, 1988.

26. **Fukuda, T., Numao, T., Akutsu, I., and Makino, S.,** Possible existence of PAF receptor subtypes on human eosinophils and neutrophils, *J. Allergy Clin. Immunol.,* 83, 193, 1989.

27. **Dent, G., Ukena, D., Chanez, P., Sybrecht, G. W., and Barnes, P. J.,** Characterisation of platelet activating factor (PAF) receptors in human neutrophils and eosinophils using a new competitive PAF antagonist WEB 2086, *FASEB J.,* 2, 1575, 1988.

28. **Kroegel, C., Yukawa, T., Westwick, J., and Barnes, P. J.,** Activation of eosinophils by platelet activating factor (PAF): degranulation and intracellular calcium mobilization, *Biochem. Biophys. Res. Commun.,* 162, 511, 1989.

29. **Yukawa, T., Kroegel, C., Evans, P., Fukuda, T., Chung, K. F., and Barnes, P. J.,** Density heterogeneity of eosinophil leucocytes: induction of hypodense eosinophils by platelet-activating factor, *Immunology,* 68, 140, 1989.

30. **Read, R C., Yukawa, P. J., Kroegel, C., Chung, K. F., Rutman, A., Wilson, R., Cole, P. J., and Barnes, P. J.,** PAF-activated eosinophils damage guinea-pig airway epithelium in vitro, *Am. Rev. Respir. Dis.,* in press.

31. **Ward, S. G. and Westwick, J.,** Antagonism of the platelet activating factor-induced rise of the intracellular calcium ion concentration of U937 cells, *Br. J. Pharmacol.,* 93, 769, 1988.

32. **Ward, S. G., Lewis, G. P., and Westwick, J.,** Differential effect of platelet-activating factor receptor antagonists on human T-lymphocyte proliferation, *Prostaglandins,* 34, 149, 1987.

33. **Rola-Pleszczynski, M., Pouliot, C., Turcotte, S., Pignol, B., Braquet, P., and Bouvrette, L.,** Immune regulation by platelet-activating factor. I. Induction of suppressor cell activity in human monocytes and CD8$^+$ T cells, *J. Immunol.,* 140, 3547, 1988.

34. **Korth, R., Hirafuji, M., Lalau Keraly, C., Delautier, D., Bidault, J., and Benveniste, J.,** Interaction of the PAF-acether antagonist WEB 2086 and its analogues with human platelets and endothelial cells, *Br J. Pharmacol.,* in press.

35. **Hirafuji, M.,** Relative potency of several platelet-activating factor antagonists against activation of human vascular endothelial cells, *3rd Int. Conf. on Platelet-Activating Factor and Structurally Related Alkyl Ether Lipids,* Tokyo, May 8—12, 1989, Abstr. book p. 98.

36. **Schwertschlag, U. S., Tabrizi, K., and Whorton, A. R.,** Platelet activating factor (paf) causes a transient increase in cytosolic Ca^{2+} in vascular smooth muscle cells (VSMC): evidence for homologous and heterologus desensitization, IUPHAR-Satellite, (Brisbane), abstr. book, 1987, 36.

37. **Gomez, J., Bloom, J. W., Yamamura, H. I., and Halonen, M.,** Characterization of specific binding sites for platelet activating factor (PAF) in guinea pig lung membranes, *FASEB J.,* 2, 1577, 1988.

38. **Dent, G., Ukena, D., Mak, J. C. W., Sybrecht, G. W., and Barnes, P. J.,** Platelet-activating factor receptors in human and guinea pig lung: demonstration using the novel antagonist ligand (^{3}H)WEB 2086, *Am. Rev. Respir. Dis.,* 39(Suppl.), A94, 1989.

39. **Anderson, G. and Fennessy, M.,** Effects of REV 5901, a 5-Lipoxygenase inhibitor and leukotriene antagonist, on pulmonary responses to platelet activating factor in the guinea-pig, *Br. J. Pharmacol.,* 34, 1115, 1988.

40. **Del Monte, M. and Subissi, A.,** Platelet activating factor-induced contraction of guinea-pig lung parenchymal strips: involvement of arachidonate metabolites, *Arch. Pharmacol.,* 338, 417, 1988.

41. **Johnson, P. R. A., Armour, C. L., and Black, J. L.,** The action of platelet activating factor and its antagonism by WEB 2086 on human isolated airway smooth muscle, *Eur. Resp. J.,* 3, 55, 1990.

42. **Lawson, A. and Cavero, I.,** Characterization of PAF-induced, hyperresponsiveness of the guinea-pig trachea to potassium, *Br. J. Pharmacol.,* 93, 76P, 1988.

43. **Casals-Stenzel, J., Franke, J., Friedrich T., and Lichey, J.,** Bronchial and vascular effects of Paf in the isolated rat lung are completely blocked by WEB 2086, a novel specific Paf antagonist, *Br. J. Pharmacol.,* 91, 799, 1987.

44. **Christy, L. J., Stewart, A. G., and Dusting, G. J.,** Platelet-activating factor and leukotrienes in rat pulmonary anaphylaxis, *Proc. Austr. Physiol. Pharmacol. Soc.,* 19, 94, 1988.

45. **Pretolani, M., Lefort, J., Malanchere, E., and Vargaftig, B. B.,** Interference by the novel PAF-acether antagonist WEB 2086 with the bronchopulmonary responses to PAF-acether and to active and passive anaphylactic shock in guinea-pigs, *Eur. J. Pharmacol.,* 140, 311, 1987.

46. **Pretolani, M., Lefort, J., and Vargaftig, B. B.,** Limited interference of specific PAF-acether antagonists with hyperresponsiveness to PAF-acether itself of lungs from actively sensitized guinea-pigs, *Br. J. Pharmacol.*, 97, 433, 1989.

47. **Meinig, H. W., Stewart, A. G., and Dusting, G. J.,** Platelet-activating factor contributes to hindlimb vasodilatation in endotoxin shock, *Clin. Exp. Pharmacol. Physiol. Suppl.*, 12, 22, 1988 (*abstr.*).

48. **Stewart, A. G. and Dusting, G. J.,** Direct and indirect actions of platelet-activating factor in guinea-pig isolated hearts, *Clin. Exp. Pharmacol. Physiol. Suppl.*, 13, 32, 1988.

49. **Yaacob, H. B. and Piper, P. J.,** The effects of PAF-antagonist WEB 2086 on paf-induced responses in guinea-pig isolated hearts and in cardiac anaphylaxis, *Br. J. Pharmacol.*, Suppl. 521P, 1988.

50. **Pritze, S. and Simmet, Th.,** Platelet-activating factor (PAF)-induced responses of porcine pulmonary blood vessels in vitro, *Atch. Pharmacol.*, 339, Suppl. R39, 1989.

51. **Buckley, T. L. and Hoult, J. R. S.,** Platelet activating factor is a potent colonic secretagogue with actions independent of specific PAF receptors, in press.

52. **Martins, M. A., Martins, P. M. R. S., Catro Faria Neto, H. C., Bozza, P. T. L., Dias, P. M. F. L., Cordeiro, R. S. B., and Vargaftig, B. B.,** Intravenous injections of PAF-acether induce platelet aggregation in rats, *Eur. J. Pharmacol.*, 149, 89, 1988.

53. **Vargaftig, B. B., Lefort, J., Chignard, M., and Benveniste, J.,** Platelet-activating factor induces a platelet-dependent bronchoconstriction unrelated to the formation of prostaglandin derivates, *Eur. J. Pharmacol.*, 65, 185, 1980.

54. **Heuer, H., Casals-Stenzel, J., Muacevic, G., Stransky, W., and Weber, K. H.,** Activity of the new and specific PAF-antagonists WEB 2170 and STY 2108 on PAF-induced bronchoconstriction and intrathoracic accumulation of platelets in the guinea pig, *Prostaglandins*, 35, 798, 1988.

55. **Terasawa, M., Mikashima, H., Tahara, T., and Maruyama, Y.,** Antagonistic activity of etizolam on platelet-activating factor — in vivo experiments, *Jpn. J. Pharmacol.*, 44, 381, 1987.

56. **Vargaftig, B. B.,** Bronchopulmonary pharmacology of PAF-acether, in *Platelet-Activating Factor and Related Lipid Mediators*, Snyder, F., Ed., Plenum Press, New York, 1987, 341.

57. **Heuer, H. O.,** Action of the new hetrazepinoic paf-antagonist WEB 2170 on shock states induced by paf, antigen or endotoxin/TNF, *Arch. Pharmacol.*, 339, Suppl. R78, 1989.

58. **Evans, T. W., Dent, G., Rogers, D. F., Aursudkij, B., Chung, K. F., and Barnes, P. J.,** Effect of a PAF antagonist, WEB 2086, on microvascular leakage in the guinea-pig and platelet aggregation in man, *Br. J. Pharmacol.*, 94, 164, 1988.

59. **O'Donnell, S. R., Barnett, C. J. K.,** Specificity of PAF antagonist drugs, *Clin. Exp. Pharmacol. Physiol. Suppl.*, 13, 11, 1988.

60. **Muacevic, G. and Casals-Stenzel, J.,** Increase of vascular permeability by platelet activating factor (paf) in the rat lung: inhibition by brotizolam, *6th Int. Conf. on Prostaglandins and Related Compounds*, (Florence, June), abstr. book, 1986, 296.

61. **Muacevic, G.,** Inhibition of PAF-induced vascular permeability in rats, by the PAF-antagonist WEB 2086 and WEB 2170, *Prostaglandins*, 35, 839, 1988.

62. **Lellouch-Tubiana, A., Lefort, J., Simon, M. T., Pfister, A., and Vargaftig, B. B.,** Eosinophil recruitment into guinea-pig lungs after PAF-acether and allergen administration: modulation by prostacyclin, platelet depletion and selective antagonists, *Am. Rev. Respir. Dis.*, 137, 948, 1988.

63. **Homolka, J., Abraham, W. M., Rubin, E., Nieves, L., and Wanner, A.,** Effect of platelet activating factor on tracheal mucus velocity in conscious sheep, *Am. Rev. Respir. Dis.*, 135, part II, (Suppl.) 160A, 1987.

64. **Stevenson, J. S., Tallent, M., Blinder, L., and Abraham, W. M.,** Modification of antigen-induced late responses with an antagonist of platelet activating factor (WEB 2086), *Fed. Proc.*, 46, 1461, 1987.

65. **Heuer, H. O.,** Wechselwirkung der hetrazepinartigen Paf-antagonisten WEB 2086 und WEB 2170 mit etablierten Antiasthmatika — Untersuchungen zur Hyperreaktivität, in *Bochumer Treff Juni 1988*, Ulmer, W. T. Ed., Verlag Gedon & Reuss, München, in press.

66. **Dixon, E. J. A., Wilsoncroft, P., Robertson, D. N., and Page, C. P.,** Paf does not contribute to bronchial hyperreactivity induced by indomethacin or propranolol, *Br. J. Pharmacol.*, 93, Proc. Suppl., 218P, 1988.

67. **Feuerstein, G. and Goldstein, R. E.,** Effect of PAF on the cardiovascular system, in *Platelet-Activating Factor and Related Lipid Mediators*, Snyder, F., Ed., Plenum Press, New York, 1987, 403.

68. **Sanchez-Crespo, M., Alonso, F., Inarrea, P., Alvarez, V., and Egido, J.,** Vascular actions of synthetic PAF-acether (a synthetic platelet activating factor) in the rat: evidence for a platelet independent mechanism, *Immunopharmacology*, 4, 173, 1982.

69. **Heuer, H. O.,** Hetrazepinoic antagonists of platelet activating factor, *Drug Design and Delivery*, 5, 31, 1989.

70. **Felix, S. B., Baumann, G., Berdel, W., and Raschke, P.,** Platelet activating factor-induced shock state development — separation of cardiac from respiratory events, *1st Int. Symp. on Heart Failure — Mechanism and Management, Jerusalem*, May 15—21, 1989.

71. **Torley, L., Kohler, C., and Wrenn, S.,** Characterisation of paf induced skin lesions, *Fed. Proc.*, 46, 739, 1987.

72. **Hellewell, P. G. and Williams, T. J.,** Antagonism of PAF-induced inflammation in rabbit skin, *Clin. Exp. Pharmacol. Physiol. Suppl.,* 13, 37, 1987.

73. **Lagente, V., Fortes, Z. B., Garcia-Leme, J., and Vargaftig, B. B.,** Effect of PAF-acether on rat mesenteric microvessels: interference by antagonists and lyso-PAF, *Clin. Exp. Pharmacol. Physiol. Suppl.,* 13, 32, 1987.

74. **Henriques, M. G. M. O., Cordeiro, R. S. B., Weg, V. B., Fernandes, P. O., Martins, M. A., Martins, P. R. S., and Vargaftig, B. B.,** Paf-acether in the carrageenan-induced inflammatory reaction in mice, *Prostaglandins,* 35, 840, 1988.

75. **Casals-Stenzel, J. and Heuer, H. O.,** Use of WEB 2086 and its analogue WEB 2170, two platelet activating factor (PAF) antagonists, in *Methods in Enzymology,* 187, 455, 1990.

76. **Adamus, W. S., Heuer, H., and Meade, C. J.,** Paf-induced platelet aggregation ex vivo as a method for monitoring pharmacological activity in healthy volunteers, *Meth. Find. Exp. Clin. Pharmacol.,* 11, 415, 1989.

77. **Adamus, W. S., Heuer, H., Meade, C. J., Frey, G., and Brecht, H. M.,** Inhibitory effect of oral WEB 2086, a novel selective PAF-acether antagonist, on ex vivo platelet aggregation, *Eur. J. Clin. Pharmacol.,* 35, 237, 1988.

78. **Kleine-Tebbe, J., Schaefer, I., and Kunkel, G.,** Der Einfluss eines spezifischen Paf-antagonisten WEB 2086 auf die Antigen-induzierte Histaminfreisetzung aus menschlichen Basophilen, *Allergology,* 10, 426, 1987.

79. **Darius, H., Smith, J. B., and Lefer, A. M.,** Inhibition of the platelet activating factor mediated component of guinea pig anaphylaxis by receptor antagonists, *Int. Arch. Allergy Appl. Immunol.,* 80, 369, 1986.

80. **Darius, H., Lefer, D. J., Bryan-Smith, J., and Lefer, A. M.,** Role of platelet-activating factor-acether in mediating guinea pig anaphylaxis, *Science,* 232, 58, 1986.

81. **Dunn, A. M., Palmer, J. D., and Halonen, M.,** Platelet activating factor (PAF) and histamine mediate antigen-induced contraction of rabbit peripheral lung strips, *FASEB J.,* 2, 1577, 1988.

82. **Casals-Stenzel, J.,** Effects of WEB 2086, a novel antagonist of platelet activating factor, in active and passive anaphylaxis, *Immunopharmacology,* 13, 117, 1987.

83. **Heuer, H.,** Inhibition of active anaphylaxis in the guinea pig by the selective hetrazepinoic paf-antagonist WEB 2170, *Arch. Pharmacol.,* 338, Suppl. R 58, 1988.

84. **Heuer, H. O.,** Inhibition of active anaphylaxis in mice and guinea pigs by the new hetrazepinoc PAF-antagonist WEB 2170, *Eur. J. Pharmacol.,* in press.

85. **Lohman, I. C. and Halonen, M.,** Effects of a PAF antagonist on IgE anaphylaxis in rabbits, *FASEB J.,* 2, 1577, 1988.

86. **Heuer, H. and Casals-Stenzel, J.,** Effect of the PAF-antagonist WEB 2086 on anaphylactic lung reaction: comparison of inhalative and intravenous challenge, *Agents Actions Suppl.,* 23, 207, 1988.

87. **Hutson, P. A., Holgate, S. T., and Church, M. K.,** Effect of WEB 2086 on early and late airway responses to ovalbumin challenge in conscious guinea-pigs, *Br. J. Pharmacol.,* 95 (Proc. Suppl.), 770P, 1988.

88. **Soler, M., Sielczak, M. W., and Abraham, W. M.,** Platelet-activating factor (PAF) contributes to antigen-induced airway hyperresponsiveness and inflammation in allergic sheep: modulation by a selective PAF-antagonist, *J. Appl. Physiol.,* 67, 406, 1989.

89. **Schroeder, E., Van Mechelen, H. Maldague, P., Vuylsteke, A., Keyeux, A., Rousseau, M. F., and Pouleur, H.,** Increased coronary vascular resistance in the stunned myocardium: role of the platelet activating factor, *Circulation,* 78 (4), part II (Suppl.), 77, 1988.

90. **Pouleur, H., Schroeder, E., and Van Mechelan, H.,** Effects of dipyridamole and of the platelet-activating factor antagonist WEB-2086 on post-reperfusion myocardial damage in a low flow, high demand model of ischemia, submitted.

91. **Egido, J., Robles, A., Ortiz, A., Ramirez, F., Gonzalez, E., Mampaso, F., Sanchez Crespo, M., and Braquet, P.,** Role of platelet activating factor in adriamycin-induced nephropathy in rats, *Eur. J. Pharmacol.,* 138, 119, 1987.

92. **Spinnewyn, B., Blavet, N., Clostre, F., Bazan, N., and Braquet, P.,** Involvement of platelet-activating factor (PAF) in cerebral post-ischemic phase in mongolian gerbils, *Prostaglandins,* 34, 337, 1987.

93. **Bielenberg, G. W. and Wagener, G.,** Paf antagonists reduce infarct size in a rat stroke model, *Arch. Pharmacol.,* 339, Suppl. R107, 1989.

94. **Bussolino, F., Porcellini, M. G., Varese, L., and Bosia, A.,** Intravascular release of platelet activating factor in children with sepsis, *Thromb. Res.,* 48, 619, 1987.

95. **Schierenberg, M., Darius, H., Lohmann, H. F., Meyer, J., Treese, N., and Heuer, H. O.,** Paf-like activity in the plasma from patients with septicemia and other diseases, *3rd. Int. Conf. on Platelet Activating Factor and Structurally Related Alkyl Ether Lipids,* Tokyo, May 8—12, 1989, Abstr. book p. 220.

96. **Casals-Stenzel, J.,** Protective effect of WEB 2086, a novel antagonist of platelet activating factor in endotoxin shock, *Eur. J. Pharmacol.,* 135, 117, 1987.

97. **Chang, S.-W., Fernyak, S., and Voelkel, N. F.,** Post-treatment with WEB 2086, a platelet-activating factor antagonist, decreases lung injury in endotoxin-treated rats, *Am. Rev. Respir. Dis.,* in press.

98. **Heuer, H. O.,** Effect of hetrazeponoic PAF-antagonists (WEB 2170 and WEB 2347) on shock states induced by endotoxin and/or tumour necrosis factor, *3rd Int. Conf. on Platelet Activating Factor and Structurally Related Alkyl Ether Lipids,* Tokyo, May 8—12, 1989, Abstr. book p. 216.

99. **Heuer, H.,** Activity of the hetrazepines WEB 2170 and STY 2108, two new and potent paf-antagonists on paf-induced changes in vitro and endotoxin- or paf-induced hypotension in the rat, *Arch. Pharmacol.,* 337, Suppl. R70, 1988.

100. **Siebeck, M., Weipert, J., Jochum, M., Mryka, J., Keser, C., Kempe, E. R., and Schweiberer, L.,** A new triazolodiazepine platelet activating factor receptor antagonist reduces pulmonary dysfunction in endotoxin shock of the pig, *Am. Rev. Respir. Dis.,* in press.

101. **Beijer, L., Botting, J., Crook, P. Oyekan, O. A., Page, C. P., and Rylander, R.,** The involvement of platelet activating factor in endotoxin-induced pulmonary platelet recruitment in the guinea-pig, *Br. J. Pharmacol.,* 92, 803, 1987.

102. **Purvis, A. W., Christman, B. W., McPherson, C. D., Miller, R. F., Lefferts, P. L., and Snapper, J. R.,** WEB 2086, a platelet activating factor antagonist, attenuates the response to endotoxin in awake sheep, *Am. Rev. Respir. Dis.,* 137, part II (Suppl.), 99, 1988.

103. **McCormack, D. M., Barnes, P. J., and Evans, T. W.,** Evidence for platelet-activating factor as a mediator of hypoxic pulmonary vasoconstriction, *Clin. Sci.,* 75 (Suppl. 19), 21P, 1988.

104. **Stahl, G. L., Bitterman, H., and Lefer, A. M.,** Protective effects of a specific platelet activating factor (PAF) antagonist, WEB 2086, in traumatic shock, *Thromb. Res.,* 53, 327, 1989.

105. **Bitterman, H., Lefer, D. J., and Lefer, A. M.,** Beneficial actions of Ro 15-1788, a benzodiazepine receptor antagonist, in hemorrhagic shock, *Meth. Find. Exp. Clin. Pharmacol.,* 9, 341, 1987.

106. **Brambilla., A., Ghiorzi, A., and Giachetti, A.,** WEB 2086 a potent PAF antagonist exerts protective effect toward PAF-induced gastric damage, *Pharmacol. Res. Commun.,* 19, 147, 1987.

107. **Heuer, H., Casals-Stenzel, J., and Weber, K. H.,** Activity of a new and specific PAF antagonist, WEB 2086, against PAF- and endotoxin-induced changes in mortality and intestinal transit velocity, *Clin. Exp. Pharmacol. Physiol. Suppl.* 13, 50, 1988.

108. **Heuer, H. and Weber, K. H.,** Effect of a new and specific PAF-antagoniist, WEB 2086, on PAF and tumor necrosis factor induced changes in mortality and intestinal transit velocity, *Prostaglandins,* 35, 814, 1988.

109. **Heuer, H. O., Letts, G., and Meade, C. J.,** Tumour necrosis factor (TNF) and endotoxin prime effects of paf in vivo, *J. Lipid Mediators,* 2, 5101, 1990.

110. **Heuer, H.,** Effect of a new and specific paf-antagonist, WEB 2086, on paf and endotoxin/tumour necrosis factor induced changes in mortality and intestinal transit velocity, in *Progress in Clinical and Biological Research,* Subseries Vienna Shock Forum, Alan R. Liss, New York, 1989, 919.

111. **Braquet, P., Etienne, A., Mencia-Huerta, J.-M., and Clostre, F.,** Effects of the specific platelet-activating factor antagonists, BN 52021 and BN 52063, on various experimental gastrointestinal ulcerations, *Eur. J. Pharmacol.,* 150, 269, 1988.

112. **Wallace, J. L., Ibbotson, G. C., and Keenan, C. M.,** Mediatory role of platelet-activating factor in intestinal inflammation and ulceration, in *Ginkgolides — Chemistry, Biology, Pharmacology and Clinical Perspectives,* Vol. 2, Braquet, P., Ed., J. R. Prous, Barcelona, 1990.

113. **Cordeiro, R. S. B., Fierro, I. M., Martins, P. M. R. S., Henriques, M. G. M. O., and Martins, M. A.,** Inflammatory activity of a crude extract of coelenterate tentacles (dactilometra) and the possible paf-acether involvement, *Prostaglandins,* 35, 836, 1988.

114. **Adamus, W. S., Heuer, H., Meade, C. J., and Brecht, H. M.,** Effect of peroral WEB 2086 on ex vivo platelet activating factor induced platelet aggregation in man, *Prostaglandins,* 35, 836, 1988.

115. **Adamus, W. S., Heuer, H., Meade, C. J., Kempe, E. R., and Brecht, H. M.,** Effect of intravenous or inhalative WEB 2086 on ex vivo platelet activating factor induced platelet aggregation in man, *Prostaglandins,* 35, 797, 1988.

116. **Adamus, W. S., Heuer, H., Meade, C. J., and Brecht, H. M.,** Safety, tolerability and pharmacologic activity in man of multiple doses of the new PAF-acether antagonist, WEB 2086, *Clin. Pharmacol. Ther.,* 45, 270, 1989.

117. **Lohmann, H. F., Adamus, W. S., and Meade, C. J.,** Idiopathic thrombocytopenia treated with paf-acether antagonist WEB 2086, *Lancet,* II, 1147, 1988.

Chapter 9

STRUCTURE-ACTIVITY RELATIONSHIPS IN PYRROLO[1,2-c]THIAZOLES PAF RECEPTOR ANTAGONISTS

Daniel Lavé

INTRODUCTION

Involvement of PAF in various pathological conditions[1] prompted many research teams, soon after its identification in 1979,[2-4] to look for products blocking the effects of this potent biological mediator.

The principal chemical approach was the synthesis of PAF-related derivatives such as CV 3988,[5] which was the first published PAF antagonist. However, PAF antagonist activity was also soon reported for natural products such as kadsurenone.[6]

STRUCTURE-ACTIVITY RELATIONSHIPS IN THE PYRROLO[1,2-c]THIAZOLE FAMILY

Nonlipid synthetic compounds with PAF receptor antagonist properties were unknown until the synthesis of RP 48740[7-9] (Figure 1) which was the first member of the potent pyrrolo[1,2-c]thiazole family of PAF receptor antagonists. This product, synthesized according to the reactional scheme shown in Figure 2, displayed interesting pharmacological properties and a very low toxicity, and was therefore selected for clinical trials.

Optimization of the PAF receptor antagonist activity of the pyrrolo[1,2-c]thiazole family was performed by preparing compounds of general formula (I) according to the reactional scheme outlined in Figure 3.

OPTIMIZATION OF THE SUBSTITUENTS OF THE PYRROLO[1,2-c]THIAZOLE NUCLEUS

Introduction of additional substituents R_1, R_2, R_3, and R_4 on the pyrrolo[1,2-c]thiazole nucleus of RP 48740 (Figure 3, Z = $CONH_2$) was shown to lead to less active or inactive products. Moreover, PAF receptor antagonist activity is lost by replacement of pyridine of RP 48740 by a benzene or a quinoline ring or by introduction of extra substituents on the pyridine nucleus.

Compounds (II), resulting from the substitution of other functions for the primary carboxamide function of RP 48740 are less interesting (Table 1). Two products, the methyl ketone and the carboxamide oxime, are more active than RP 48740 in inhibiting PAF-evoked platelet aggregation in rabbit platelet rich plasma (PRP) but are less selective since these compounds also show a slight activity in inhibition of collagen-induced platelet aggregation. It is noteworthy that the acid compound is completely inactive. Therefore, 3-(3-pyridyl)-1H,3H-pyrrolo[1,2-c]thiazole-7-carboxamides (III) were thoroughly studied.

OPTIMIZATION OF THE NATURE OF THE CARBOXAMIDE FUNCTION OF 3-(3-PYRIDYL)-1H,3H-PYRROLO[1,2-c]THIAZOLE-7-CARBOXAMIDES

These compounds could be very easily synthesized according to the reactional scheme shown in Figure 4.

The N-methyl and the N-butyl compounds were shown to be more potent than RP 48740 in inhibition of PAF-induced platelet aggregation in rabbit PRP but the N-benzyl derivative

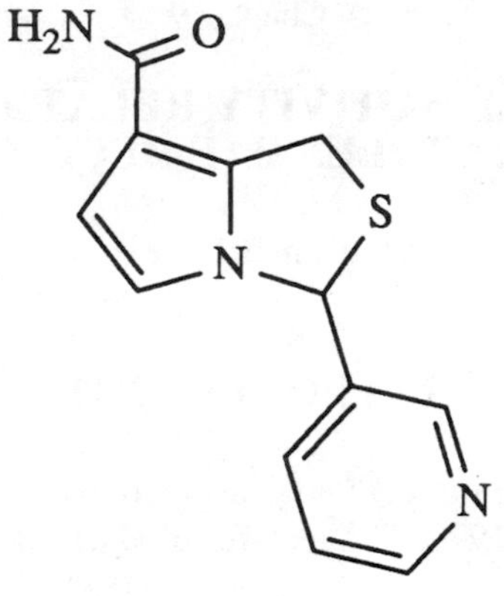

FIGURE 1.   Chemical structure of RP 48740.

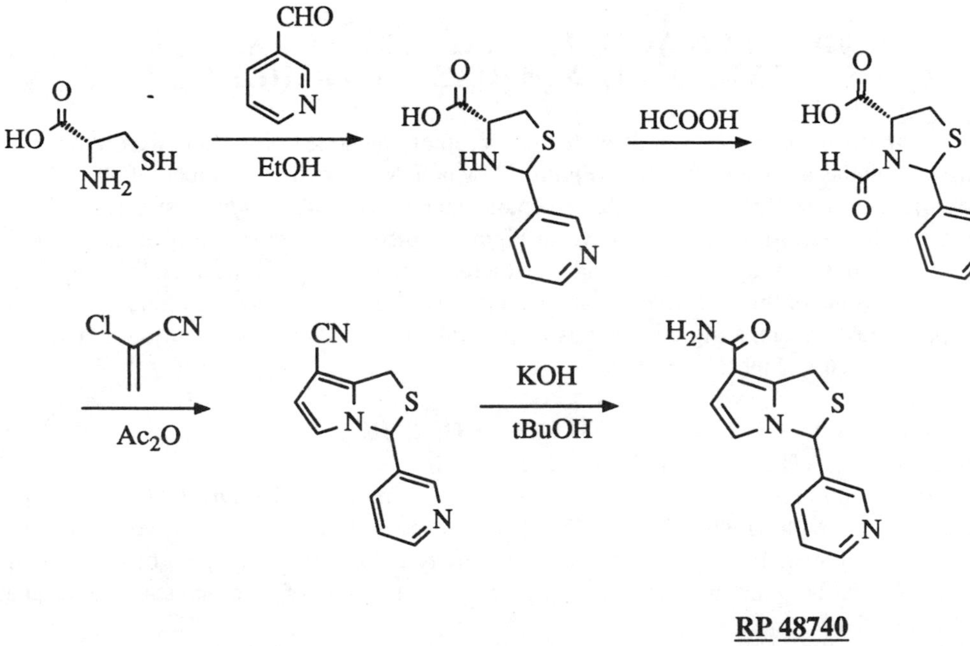

FIGURE 2.   Synthesis of RP 48740.

is nearly inactive (Table 2). Substitution of the carboxamide function by an aromatic or a pyridinic ring increases significantly the PAF receptor antagonist activity: as a matter of fact, the *N*-phenyl amide RP 51944 and the *N*-(2-pyridyl) compound RP 52758 are about 13-fold, respectively, 80-fold more potent as selective inhibitors of PAF-evoked platelet aggregation in rabbit PRP than RP 48740. On the other hand, the *N,N*-dimethyl tertiary amide was found less selective than RP 48740, since it is slightly active in inhibition of collagen-induced platelet aggregation. Furthermore, it was shown that secondary alkyl amides carrying a basic or acidic substituent on the alkyl chain and that tertiary cyclic amides are less interesting than RP 51944 and RP 52758, either because of a lower activity or a lower selectivity.

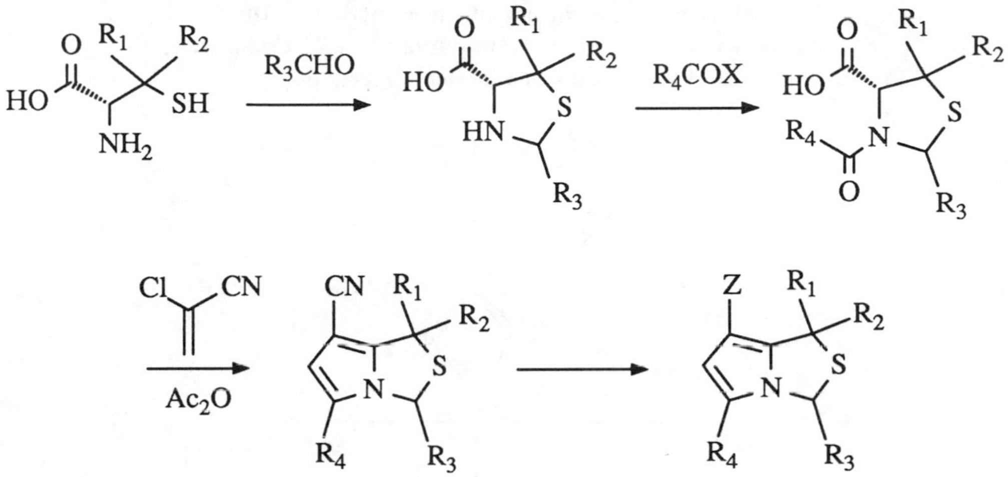

(I)

FIGURE 3. General synthetic scheme of compounds (I).

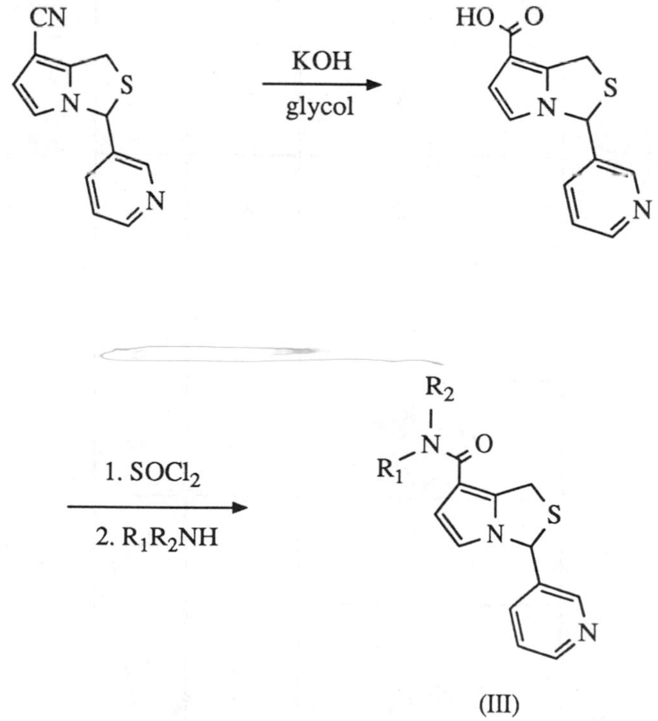

(III)

FIGURE 4. General synthetic scheme of pyrrolo[1,2-c]thiazole-7-carboxamides (III).

TABLE 1
Influence of the Nature of the Function on the
Potencies of Compounds (II) as Inhibitors of Collagen-
and PAF-Induced Platelet Aggregation

(II)

Z	Platelet Aggreg. IC_{50} (μM)	
	collagen	PAF
$CONH_2$	>407	24.5
$CSNH_2$	>383	65
COOH	>407	>407
$CONHNH_2$	38.5	77
$COCH_3$	53	9
$C{\underset{NH_2}{\overset{NOH}{\diagup}}}$	126	23
CN	326	22
$C{\underset{NH_2}{\overset{NN(CH_3)_2}{\diagup}}}$	244	9.8

TABLE 2
Influence of the Nature of the Substituent(s) on the Carboxamide Function of Pyrrolo[1,2-c]thiazoles on the Potencies of Compounds (III) as Inhibitors of Collagen- and PAF-Induced Platelet Aggregation in Rabbit PRP

(III)

R_1	R_2	Platelet Aggreg. IC_{50} (µM)	
		collagen	PAF
H	CH_3	> 138	6.9
H	C_4H_9	> 331	2.3
H	$CH_2C_6H_5$	> 300	113
H	C_6H_5	> 312	1.9
H		40.5	1.2
H		> 300	0.3
CH_3	CH_3	64	16.5
H	H	> 407	24.5

TABLE 3

Influence of the Position of the Chloro or Methoxy Substituent on the Aromatic Ring of *N*-Phenyl pyrrolo[1,2-c]thiazole-7-carboxamides on the Potency of Compounds (IV) as Inhibitors of collagen- and PAF-Induced Platelet Aggregation in Rabbit PRP and as Displacers of [³H]-PAF Binding in Washed Rabbit Platelets

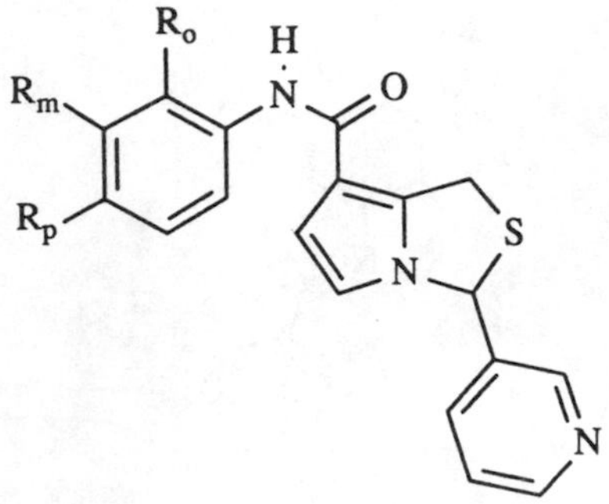

(IV)

R_o	R_m	R_p	Platelet Aggr. IC$_{50}$ (μM) collagen	PAF	[³H]-PAF Binding K_i (nM)
OCH$_3$	H	H	> 280	0.39	28
H	OCH$_3$	H	> 280	0.3	13.3
H	H	OCH$_3$	> 285	3.4	167
Cl	H	H	> 280	1.4	26.7
H	Cl	H	> 280	0.3	7
H	H	Cl	52	7.9	66.7
H	H	H	> 310	0.84	22.7

OPTIMIZATION OF THE *N*-ARYL- AND *N*-(2-PYRIDYL)-3-(3-PYRIDYL)-1H,3H-PYRROLO[1,2-c]THIAZOLE-7-CARBOXAMIDE FAMILY

On account of the great potency of RP 51944 and RP 52758, the influence of the nature and position of substituents on the phenyl ring of RP 51944 and on the 2-pyridyl ring of RP 52758 on the PAF receptor antagonist activity was investigated. It was clearly shown in the family of RP 51944 that the activity is increased generally by addition of a substituent in the meta position of the aromatic ring. Moreover, for a given substituent, the potency is maximum for the meta compound and minimum for the para derivative. Table 3 presents

TABLE 4

Influence of the Position of the Chloro Substituent on the Pyridinic Ring of *N*-(2-pyridyl) pyrrolo[1,2-c] thiazole-7-carboxamides (V) on the Potency of these Compounds as Displacers of [^{3}H]-PAF Binding in Washed Rabbit Platelets

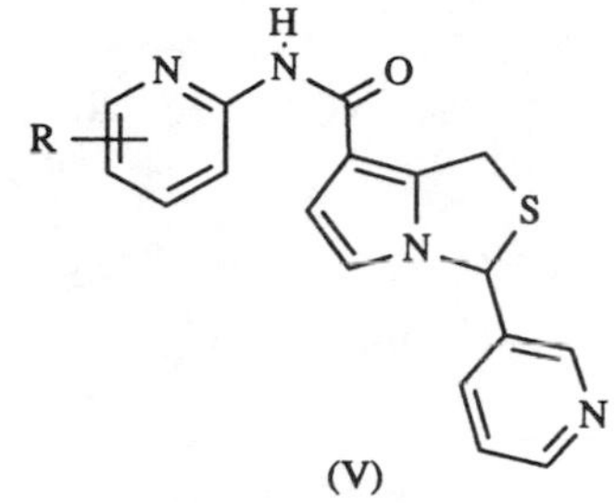

(V)

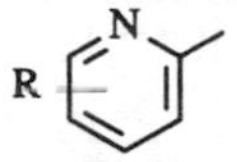 R	[^{3}H]-PAF Binding K_i (nM)
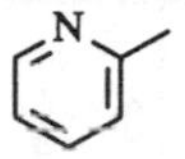	73
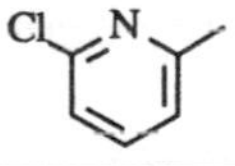	5
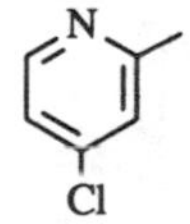	6
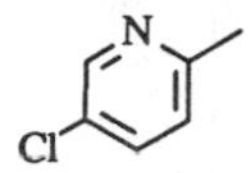	73

the results obtained with the *N*-phenyl-3-(3-pyridyl)-1H,3H-pyrrolo[1,2-c]thiazole-7-carboxamides (IV), substituted either with a chlorine atom or a methoxy group on the aromatic ring. In this family, two products exhibit a high PAF receptor antagonist activity and were selected for further biological investigations: RP 52629 (R_o = R_p = H; R_m = OCH$_3$) and RP 52770 (R_o = R_p = H; R_m = Cl) with a K_i of 13.3 n*M* and 7 n*M*, respectively, in antagonism of [^{3}H]-PAF binding in washed rabbit platelets.

Table 4 shows that similar structure-activity relationships are observed in the family of RP 52758: the introduction of a chlorine atom in the 4 or 6 position of the pyridinic ring of RP 52758 increases the PAF receptor antagonist potency whereas no improvement of the activity is obtained with the compound resulting from the substitution of a chlorine atom in the 5 position of the pyridinic ring. Several other pyridinic compounds of general formula (VI) were prepared. Their biological results are reported in Table 5.

Observation that the introduction of an aromatic or a pyridinic ring on the carboxamide function of pyrrolo[1,2-c]thiazole-7-carboxamides increases the PAF antagonist activity led to the synthesis of compounds (VII) (Table 6), where the amide group is substituted by various aromatic or heterocyclic rings. Unfortunately, none of these products showed an interesting activity.

TABLE 5
Biological Activity of Compounds (VI) as Antagonists
of [³H]-PAF Binding in Washed Rabbit Platelets

(VI)

R₁	R₂	[³H]-PAF Binding K_i (nM)
F	H	11.8
CH₃O	H	18.7
H	OCH₃	5.5
CH₃	H	15.7
H	CH₃	6.9
CH₃	CH₃	6.1

PHARMACOLOGICAL PROFILE OF RP 52770

Further biological experiments on RP 52770 confirmed the high potency of this compound which was shown to be 26 times more potent than L-652,731 in inhibiting PAF-induced platelet aggregation in washed rabbit platelets.[10] Moreover, RP 52770 is approximately twice as potent when administered intravenously as L-652731 in antagonizing PAF-evoked hypotension in rat.[10] In addition, [³H]-RP 52770 (Figure 5) was shown to be a potent radioligand of PAF binding sites, not only in intact rabbit platelets and crude membrane preparations,[10] but also in human polymorphonuclear leukocytes.[11] Besides, the two enantiomers of RP 52770 were synthesized from racemic 3-(3-pyridyl) 1H,3H-pyrrolo[1,2-c]thiazole-7-carboxylic acid. The dextrorotatory isomer, RP 56972, was found to be the active isomer, being about 700 times, respectively, 300 times more potent than the levorotatory enantiomer, RP 56973, in displacing [³H]-PAF and [³H]-RP 52770 from its binding sites in intact rabbit platelets. It is beyond doubt that the commercial availability (NEN Products) of [³H]-RP

TABLE 6
Biological Activities of Compounds (VII) as Displacers
of [³H]-PAF Binding in Washed Rabbit Platelets

(VII)

Ar	[³H]-PAF Binding K_i (nM)
	18.7
	15.3
	107
	213
	327
	40
	207
	52

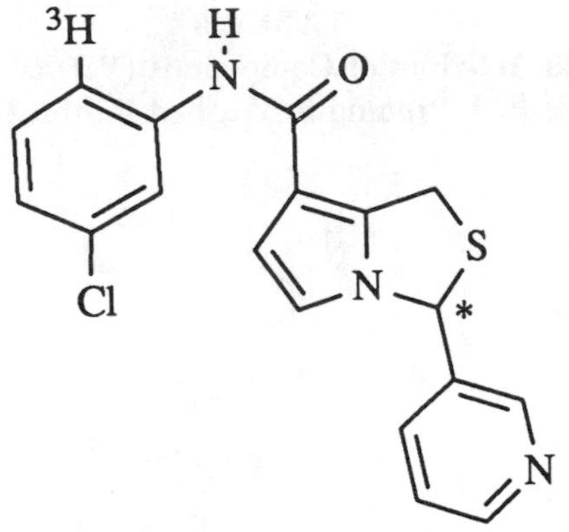

FIGURE 5. Chemical structure of [³H]-RP 52770 (racemic compound) and of [³H]-RP 56972 (dextrorotatory isomer). The asterisk indicates the position of the asymmetric carbon.

56972 [[³H]-(+)RP 52770] may be helpful in understanding the role of PAF binding sites in pathophysiological processes.

OPTIMIZATION OF THE NATURE OF THE SUBSTITUENT ON THE PHENYL RING OF N-ARYL-3-(3-PYRIDYL)-1H,3H-PYRROLO[1,2-c]THIAZOLE-7-CARBOXAMIDE FAMILY

Introduction of additional substituents on the aromatic ring of RP 52629 or of RP 52770 does not improve the PAF receptor antagonist activity (Table 7). However, analogs (IX) of RP 52629 where the methoxy group is replaced by aromatic ether substituents are more potent than RP 52629 and RP 52770 (Table 8). On account of the interesting results obtained, both *in vitro* and *in vivo*, with the compound RP 56626 carrying a 3-phenoxy substituent, synthesis of analogs (X) of this derivative where the oxygen of the phenoxy group is replaced by an other heteroatom or by a carbon atom was performed (Table 9). Two products, the 3-benzyl derivative and the 3-benzoyl compound RP 58467, were found more potent than RP 56626 in displacing [³H]-PAF from its binding sites in washed rabbit platelets. On the contrary, the thio analog of RP 56626 is more potent than RP 52770 and RP 52629, but is less active than RP 56626. As replacement of the terminal phenyl ring of RP 58467 by a heteroaromatic ring or introduction of additional substituents on the aromatic rings of RP 58467 does not yield more potent compounds than this product (Tables 10 and 11), RP 58467 was selected for further biological and chemical investigations.

As this compound was found to display a very high potency in antagonizing *in vivo* and *in vitro* the effects of PAF, its two enantiomers were synthesized. The first batches of these derivatives were obtained according to the same reactional scheme as for RP 52770, which involves a resolution of the racemic acid derivative. The results obtained (Table 12) showed that the dextrorotatory isomer, RP 59227, is about 200 and 450 times more potent than the levorotatory enantiomer in inhibition of PAF-induced platelet aggregation in rabbit PRP and in displacement of [³H]-PAF binding in washed rabbit platelets, respectively.[12] This high stereoselectivity suggested that RP 59227 should be developed in clinical studies. Accordingly, an efficient stereospecific synthesis of this compound was developed in six steps from L-cysteine as outlined in Figure 6.[13-14]

TABLE 7
Biological Activity of Phenyl Polysubstituted Compounds (VIII) as
Displacers of [³H]-PAF

(VIII)

-R$_2$	-R$_3$	-R$_4$	-R$_5$	-R$_6$	[³H]-PAF Binding K$_i$ (nM)
-H	-OCH$_3$	-H	-H	-H	13.3
-H	-OCH$_3$	-OCH$_3$	-OCH$_3$	-H	67
-H	-OCH$_3$	-H	-OCH$_3$	-H	20
-H	-OCH$_3$	-OCH$_3$	-H	-H	420
-H	-Cl	-H	-H	-H	7
-H	-Cl	-H	-Cl	-H	233
-CH$_3$	-Cl	-H	-H	-H	27
-Cl	-Cl	-H	-H	-H	320
-H	-Cl	-H	-H	-Cl	17

TABLE 8
Influence of the Nature of the Ether Substituent on the Potencies of Compounds (IX) as Inhibitors of PAF-Induced Platelet Aggregation in Rabbit PRP and as Antagonists of [³H]-PAF Binding in Washed Rabbit Platelets

(IX)

R—	PAF Platelet Aggr. IC$_{50}$ (μM)	[³H]-PAF Binding K$_i$ (nM)
CH$_3$—	0.3	13.3
⟨phenyl⟩	0.44	2.5
⟨pyridyl⟩	0.41	7.3

PHARMACOLOGICAL PROFILE OF RP 59227

RP 59227 exhibits a very high activity and selectivity, both *in vitro* and *in vivo*. RP 59227 was found to behave as a competitive antagonist of [³H]-PAF binding in dog and human platelets with respective K$_i$ values of 7.9 ± 1.5 and 1.9 ± 0.7 nM.[12,15-16] Moreover, in the same species, RP 59227 inhibits the PAF-induced platelet aggregation in PRP with IC$_{50}$ of 0.29 ± 0.01 and 0.26 ± 0.05 μM, respectively, but does not interfere with the platelet aggregation evoked by classical proaggregant agents.[12]

The same high activity and selectivity is also observed *in vivo*, in inhibition of PAF- and endotoxin-induced hypotension and hemoconcentration,[17,18] and in antagonism of PAF-evoked bronchoconstriction.[12]

Accordingly, the high activity of RP 59227 in antagonizing the PAF-evoked effects suggests that this compound may be of great interest in treating the pathological manifestations where PAF may be involved.

TABLE 9

**Potencies of Compounds of Formula (X) as Inhibitors
of PAF-Induced Platelet Aggregation in Rabbit PRP
and as Antagonists of [³H]-PAF Binding in Washed
Rabbit Platelets**

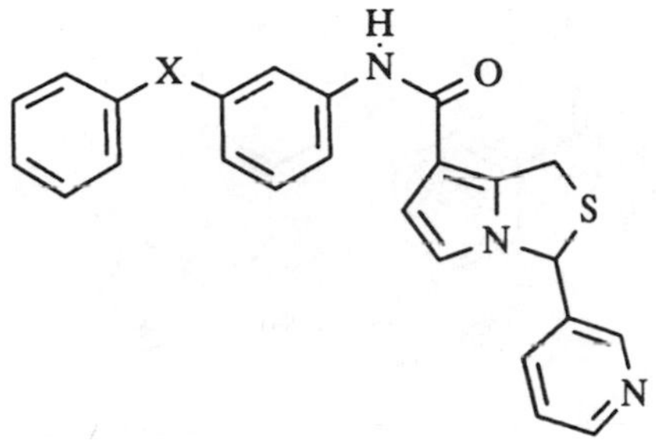

(X)

- X -	PAF Platelet Aggr. IC$_{50}$ (µM)	[³H]-PAF Binding K$_i$ (nM)
-O-	0.44	2.5
-S-	21	3.8
-CH$_2$-	0.95	1.8
-CO-	0.2	1.5
-CH(OH)-	2.34	64

CONCLUSION

All these results show the great interest of this potent new chemical entity: the results of clinical trials performed with RP 48740 and its dextrorotatory isomer, RP 55778, as well as those expected with RP 59227 may be helpful for ascertaining the potential therapeutic usefulness of PAF receptor antagonists. On the other hand, [³H]-RP 56972 may be a very valuable tool to elucidate the role of PAF binding sites in pathophysiological processes.

TABLE 10
Influence of the Nature of the Terminal Ring on the
Potencies of Compounds (XI) as Inhibitors of PAF-
Induced Platelet Aggregation in Rabbit PRP and as
Antagonists of [^{3}H]-PAF Binding in Washed Rabbit
Platelets

(XI)

Ar -	PAF Platelet Aggreg. IC$_{50}$ (μM)	[^{3}H]-PAF Binding K$_i$ (nM)
	0.2	1.5
	0.39	4.4
	0.15	6.7
	0.2	4.6
	0.52	3.5

TABLE 11

Influence of Substituents on the Aromatic Rings on the Potencies of Compounds (XII) as Inhibitors of PAF-Induced Platelet Aggregation in Rabbit PRP and as Antagonists of [³H]-PAF Binding in Washed Rabbit Platelets

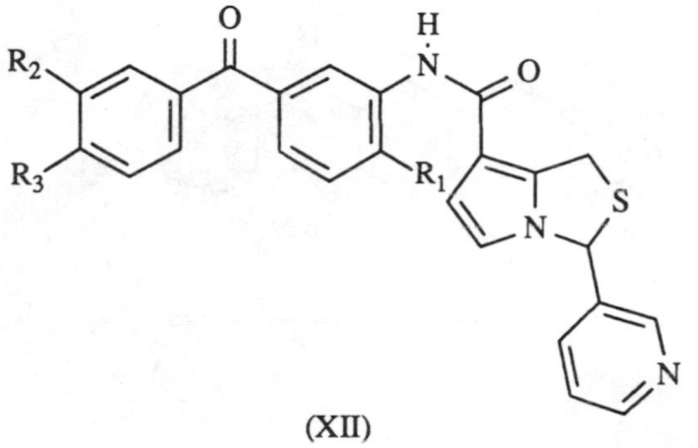

(XII)

R_1	R_2	R_3	PAF Platelet Aggr. IC_{50} (μM)	[³H]-PAF Binding K_i (nM)
H	H	H	0.2	1.5
H	H	OCH_3	0.13	9.3
H	H	Cl	0.13	6.7
H	H	CH_3	0.14	2.3
H	CH_3	H	0.25	2.3
NMe_2	H	H	0.18	6.3

TABLE 12
Potencies of Racemic RP 58467 and of its Two
Enantiomers RP 59227 and RP 59228 in Inhibiting
PAF-Induced Platelet Aggregation in Rabbit PRP and
in Antagonizing [³H]-PAF Binding in Washed Rabbit
Platelets

Product	PAF Platelet Aggr. IC_{50} (μM)	[³H]-PAF Binding K_i (nM)
Racemic RP 58467	0.20	1.5
(+) (R) RP 59227	0.16	1.18
(-) (S) RP 59228	74.5	330

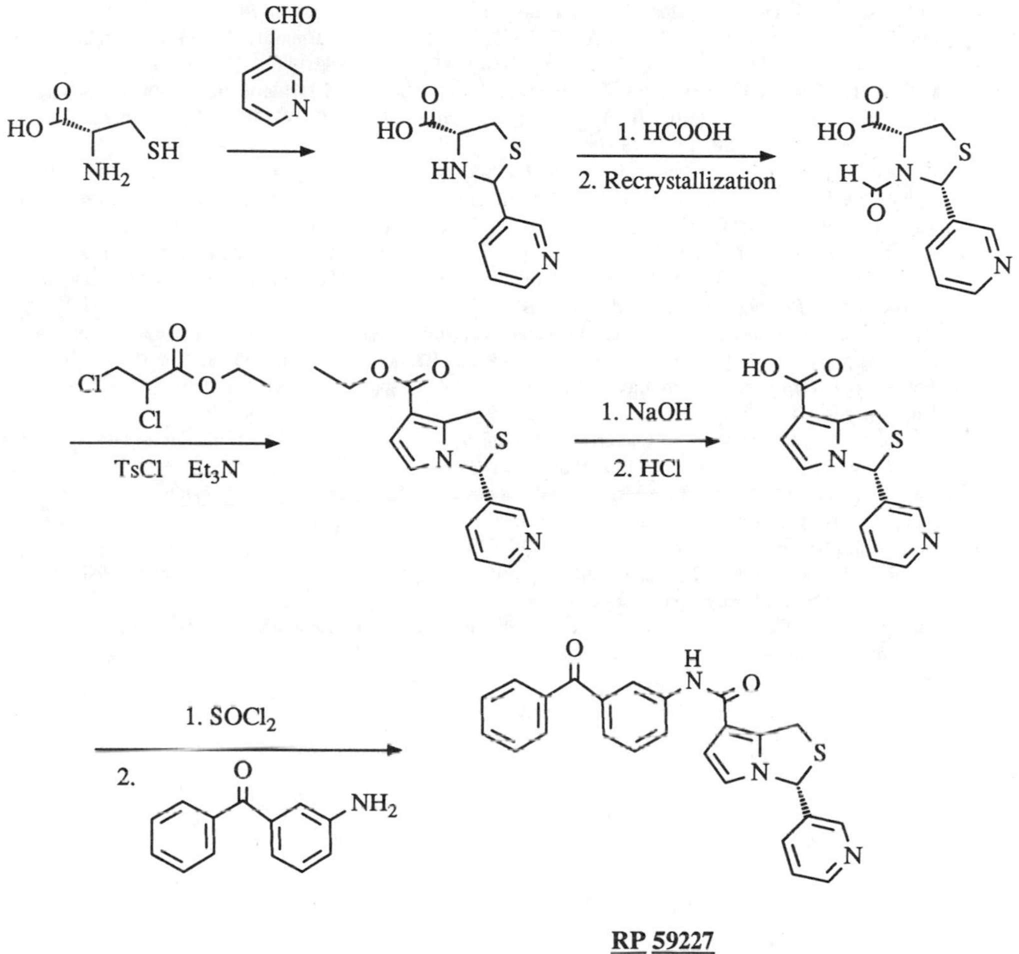

FIGURE 6.   Stereospecific synthesis of RP 59227.

REFERENCES

1. **Braquet, P., Touqui, L., Shen, T. Y., and Vargaftig, B. B.,** Perspectives in platelet-activating factor research, *Pharmacol. Rev.,* 39, 97, 1987.
2. **Benveniste, J., Tence, M., Varenne, P., Bidault, J., Boullet, C., and Polonski, J.,** Semisynthèse et structure proposée du facteur activant les plaquettes: PAF-Acéther, un alkyl éther analogue de la lyso-phosphatidylcholine, *C. R. Acad. Sci. (Paris) Ser. D.,* 289, 1037, 1979.
3. **Demopoulos, C. A., Pinckard, R. N., and Hanahan, D. J.,** Platelet activating factor. Evidence for 1-O-alkyl-2-acetyl-sn-glyceryl-3-phosphorylcholine as the active component (a new class of lipid chemical mediators), *J. Biol. Chem.,* 254, 9355, 1979.
4. **Blanck, M. L., Snyder, F., Byers, L. W., Brooks, B., and Muirhead, E. E.,** Antihypertensive activity of an alkyl ether analog of phosphatidylcholine, *Biochem. Biophys. Res. Commun.,* 90, 1194, 1979.
5. **Terashita, Z., Tsushima, S., Yoshioka, Y., Nomura, H., Inada, Y., and Nishikawa, K.,** CV-3988 — a specific antagonist of platelet activating factor (PAF), *Life Sci.,* 32, 1975, 1983.
6. **Shen, T. Y., Hwang, S. B., Chang, M. N., Doebber, T. W., Lam, M.-H., Wu, M. S., Wang, X., Han, G. Q. and Li, R. Z.,** Characterization of a platelet-activating factor receptor antagonist isolated from haifenteng *(Piper futokadsura)*: specific inhibition of in vitro and in vivo-platelet-activating factor-induced effects, *Proc. Natl. Acad. Sci. U.S.A.,* 82, 672, 1985.

7. **Fabre, J. L., Farge, D., James, C., and Lavé, D.,** European Patent 115979, 1983.

8. **Sédivy, P., Caillard, C. G., Floch, A., Folliard, F., Mondot, S., Robaut, C. and Terlain, B.,** 48740 RP: a specific PAF-acether antagonist, *Prostaglandins,* 30, 688, 1985.

9. **Lefort, J., Sédivy, P., Desquand, S., Randon, J., Coëffier, E., Maridonneau-Parini, I., Floch, A., Benveniste, J., and Vargaftig, B. B.,** Pharmacological profile of 48740 R.P., a PAF-acether antagonist, *Eur. J. Pharmacol.,* 150, 257, 1988.

10. **Robaut, C., Durand, G., James, C., Lavé, D., Sédivy, P., Floch, A., Mondot, S., Pacot, D., Cavero, I., and Le Fur, G.,** PAF binding sites: characterization by [^{3}H]-52770 RP, a pyrrolo[1,2-c]thiazole derivative, in rabbit platelets, *Biochem. Pharmacol.,* 36, 3221, 1987.

11. **Marquis, O., Robaut, C., and Cavero, I.,** [^{3}H]-52770 RP, a platelet-activating factor receptor antagonist, and tritiated platelet-activating factor label a common specific binding site in human polymorphonuclear leukocytes, *J. Pharmacol. Exp. Ther.,* 244, 709, 1988.

12. **Robaut, C., Mondot, S., Floch, A., Tahraoui, L., and Cavero, I.,** Pharmacological profile of a novel potent and specific PAF receptor antagonist, the 59227 RP, *Prostaglandins,* 35, 838, 1988.

13. **Fabre, J. L., James, C., and Lavé, D.,** European Patent Application 253711, 1986.

14. **Rajoharison, H.,** European Patent Application 297987, 1987.

15. **Tahraoui, L., Floch, A., and Cavero, I.,** Optimisation for a viable [^{3}H]-PAF binding to human platelet membranes, *Prostaglandins,* 35, 794, 1988.

16. **Tahraoui, L., Floch, A., Mondot, S., and Cavero, I.,** High affinity specific binding sites for tritiated platelet-activating factor in canine platelet membranes: counterparts of platelet-activating factor receptors mediating platelet aggregation, *Mol. Pharmacol.,* 34, 145, 1988.

17. **Mondot, S. and Cavero, I.,** Cardiovascular profile of 59227 RP, a novel potent and specific PAF receptor antagonist, *Prostaglandins,* 35, 827, 1988.

18. **Floch, A. and Cavero, I.,** Studies on the mechanisms of the hemoconcentration produced by PAF and endotoxin in rats, *Prostaglandins,* 35, 808, 1988.

Chapter 10

STRUCTURE ACTIVITY RELATIONSHIPS IN 5-ARYL-2,3-DIHYDROIMIDAZO[2,1a]ISOQUINOLINE PAF ANTAGONISTS

William J. Houlihan

INTRODUCTION

The search for substances that can antagonize PAF (Figure 1) by a receptor-mediated mechanism has resulted in the discovery of a variety of compounds that can be classified as charged and non-charged PAF receptor antagonists.[1-9] The charged antagonists contain a formal positive charge as a zwitterion, quaternary alkyl ammonium, or heterocyclic group and were designed using the PAF molecule as a template. Some examples of charged PAF antagonists are CV-3988, CV-6209, and SRI 63-441 (Figure 2). Non-charged PAF antagonists, of which ginkgolide B and brotizolam (Figure 3) are representative examples, lack a formal charge and were discovered by screening of natural products, known pharmacological agents, and synthetic compounds. The imidazo[2,1-a]isoquinolines[10,11] represent the first class of non-charged PAF receptor antagonists that were designed using the PAF molecule as a template.[12,13]

IMIDAZO[2,1-a]ISOQUINOLINES

PHARMACOLOGICAL ASSAYS

The primary *in vitro* screen used for detecting PAF antagonism activity was the inhibition of PAF-induced platelet aggregation in human platelet-rich plasma.[14] The ability to displace or compete with [³H]PAF for the high affinity binding sites on isolated human platelets was then used to classify a compound as a specific PAF receptor antagonist.[15]

In vivo assays involved i.v. PAF-induced hypotension in the rat[16] and hemoconcentration and bronchoconstriction changes in the guinea pig.[17]

DESIGN

It was recognized that the PAF-16 molecule could be divided into a lipophilic (atoms 1—16), polarizable (atoms 17—21), and charged zones (atoms 22—27) for purposes of structure modification (Figure 4A). Replacement of the charged group by a polar group was postulated to enhance oral absorption and compounds of the general formulae (B) and (C) in Figure 4 were suggested as models to develop potential PAF antagonists. The postulate was tested by preparing the thioimidazolinyl and imidazolinyl compounds **1** and **2** which showed weak inhibition of PAF-induced aggregation, or receptor activity on human platelets (Table 1). Further modification of **2** to structures **3** and then **4** where the alkyl chain in **3** is bound to the ortho position of the phenyl group gave a compound with good receptor and anti-aggregation activity. Replacement of the octyl side-chain in **4** by a phenyl group gave 5-phenyl-2,3dihydroimidazo[2,1-a]isoquinoline (**5**), a compound that served as a lead for further development.

QSAR STUDIES

The initial phase of the QSAR study on structure **5** focused on substituents at positions 8 and 9 of ring C and a variety of mono-, di-, and tri-substituents at the 2′- to 5′- positions of ring D (Figure 5). The most active compounds against PAF-induced aggregation and

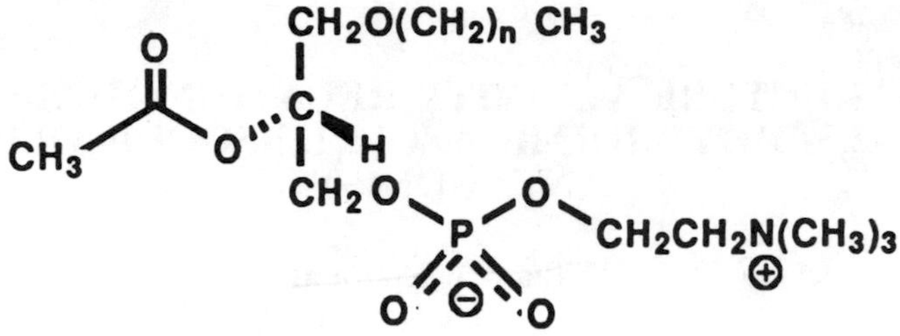

R - Enantiomer   n = 15, 17

FIGURE 1.   Absolute configuration of natural PAF.

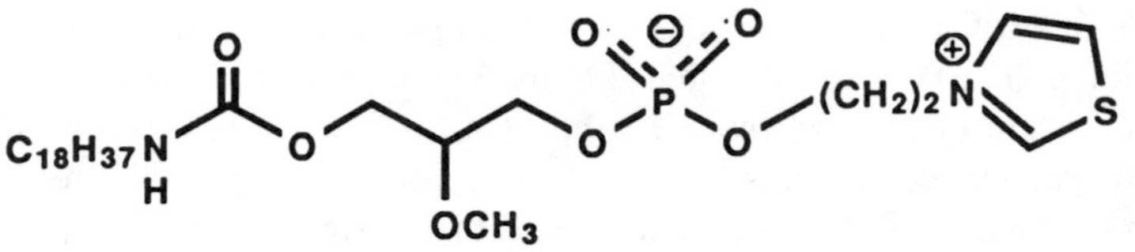

CV-3988

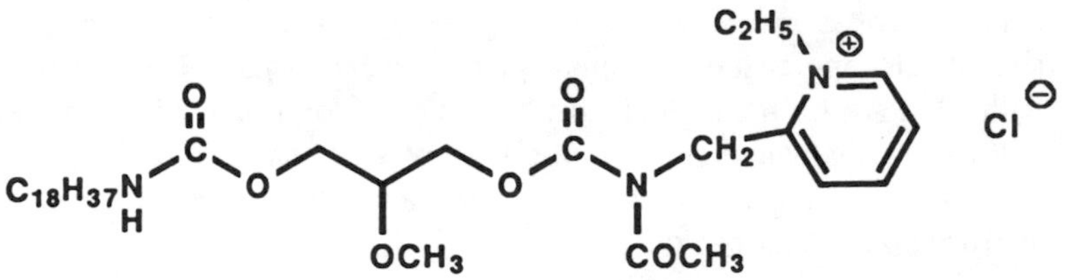

CV-6209

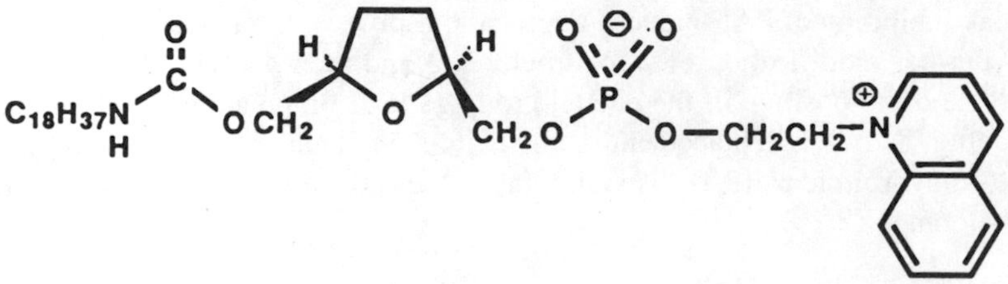

SRI   63-441

FIGURE 2.   Charged PAF receptor antagonists.

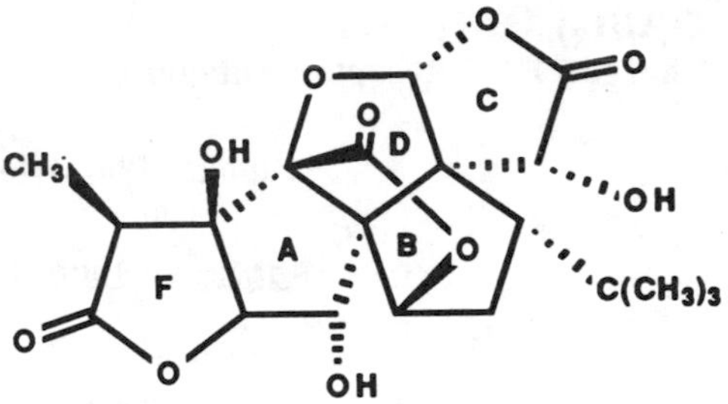

Ginkgolide B

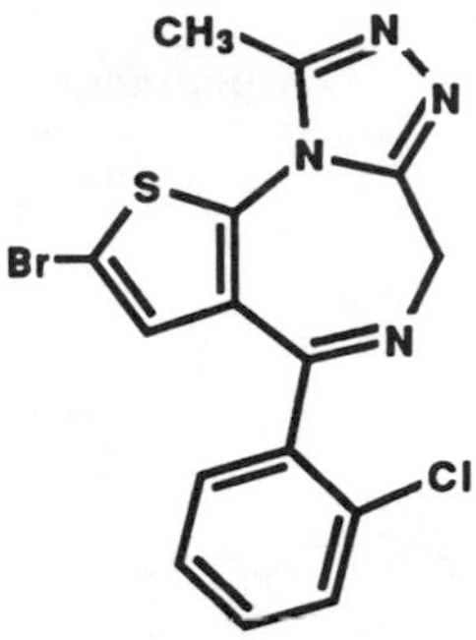

Brotizolam

FIGURE 3. Non-charged PAF receptor antagonists.

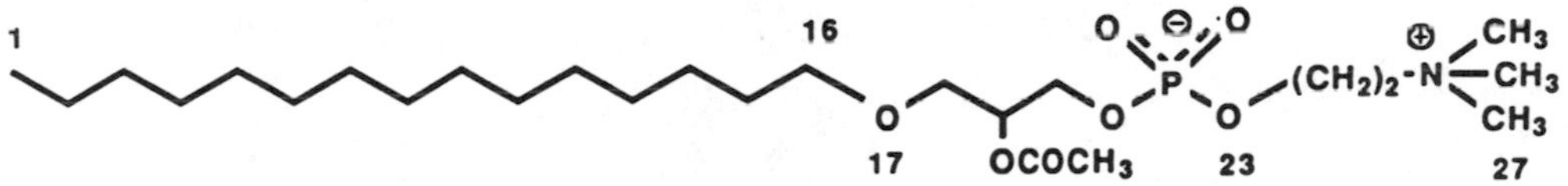

(A) LIPOPHILIC ZONE (1–16) — POLARIZABLE ZONE (17–21) — CHARGED ZONE (22–27)

(B) LIPID CHAIN — POLARIZABLE ZONE — POLAR GROUP

(C) LIPID CHAIN — POLAR GROUP

FIGURE 4. PAF zones and derived structures.

competition of [^{3}H]PAF binding were the lipophilic alkyl, aryl, or an O- or N-linked benzyl group at position 4′- of ring D (Table 2).

The next phase of the QSAR study (Table 3) involved adding one or more halogen, alkyl, and alkoxy groups at the 2″- to 6″-positions of the phenyl ring in 5-[4′-benzyloxy-phenyl]-2,3-dihydroimidazo[2,1-a]isoquinoline (**9**). The compounds (**9, 11—20**) possessed a good level of PAF receptor antagonism (IC_{50} = 0.14 to 0.85 μM) with the most active in both assays being the 2″-Cl, 4″-F (**13**); 2″-Cl, 6″-F (**14**); 4″-OCH_3 (**16**); 2″, 3″, 4″-(OCH_3) (**19**); and 3″, 4″, 5″-$(OCH_3)_3$ (**20**) derivatives. Evaluation of these compounds in the guinea pig at 100 mg/kg orally revealed that the two halogen compounds **13** and **14** possessed strong to moderate CNS stimulant-like activity, the methoxy analogue **16** had a weak stimulant activity and the two trimethoxy derivatives **19** and **20** were free of CNS activity up to doses of 200 mg/kg.

Further work with compound **20** showed that when the 3″,4″,5″-trimethoxybenzyloxy group was moved from position 4′- of ring D to the 3′-position a fivefold drop in receptor activity (IC_{50} = 0.74 μM) occurred while a 250-fold drop in activity (IC_{50} = 35.5 μM) occurred when moved to the 2′-position.

The final QSAR study involved varying the length and atom composition of the OCH_2 linking group in compound **20** (Table 4). Very good receptor activity, IC_{50} values of 0.06 to 0.30 μM, was maintained with a linking chain of one to five atoms composed of all CH_2

TABLE 1
Development of a Non-Charged PAF Receptor Antagonist

| | Cmpd. No. | Human Platelets IC$_{50}$, μM | |
		Aggr.	Receptor
(structure 1)	1	>100	34.8
(structure 2)	2	48.0	>100
(structure 3)	3	68.0	50.0
(structure 4)	4	31.2	2.0
(structure 5)	5	4.8	11.2

groups (**23**, **24**, and **27**) or a mix of O and CH$_2$ groups (**20, 25, 26,** and **28**). A similar trend, except for the CH$_2$OCH$_2$ linked **26** was observed for the PAF-induced platelet aggregation. The most active member of this series, compound **24** (SDZ 64-412), was selected for further studies as its hydrochloride salt.

SDZ 64-412
Structural Comparison with PAF
In a structural comparison of PAF-16 and SDZ 64-412 hydrochloride (Figure 6), it was postulated that the $^+$N(CH$_3$)$_3$ and PO$_4^-$ groups in PAF are mimicked by the C=NH$^+$ and the benzene ring, respectively, in the isoquinoline portion of SDZ 64-412. The ether oxygen at position 10 in PAF, which has been demonstrated[18] to be very important in anchoring to the PAF receptor was mimicked by the double bond at position 9 and 10 in SDZ 64-412. No attempt was made to incorporate the OCOCH$_3$ group at position 8 in PAF since its presence is usually associated with PAF agonist activity.[18] The C-16 alkyl group in PAF was replaced by the trimethoxyphenylethylphenyl group.

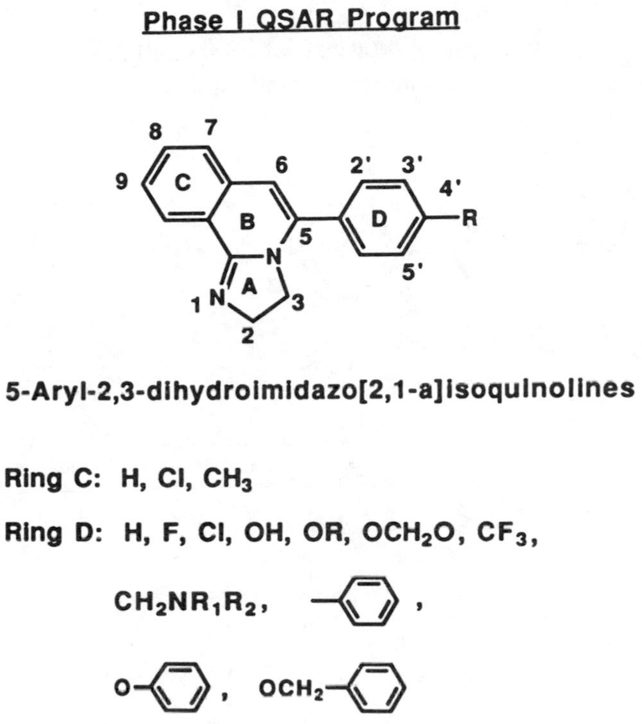

Phase I QSAR Program

5-Aryl-2,3-dihydroimidazo[2,1-a]isoquinolines

Ring C: H, Cl, CH$_3$

Ring D: H, F, Cl, OH, OR, OCH$_2$O, CF$_3$,

CH$_2$NR$_1$R$_2$,

O—, OCH$_2$—

FIGURE 5. Phase 1 QSAR study.

TABLE 2
Most Interesting Compounds from
Phase I QSAR Study

No.	R in Figure 5	Human platelets (IC$_{50}$, μM)	
		Aggr.	Receptor
6	t-C$_4$H$_9$	1.6	0.9
7	C$_6$H$_5$	4.8	3.4
8	OC$_6$H$_5$	2.2	2.8
9	OCH$_2$C$_6$H$_5$	1.2	0.9
10	CH$_2$N(CH$_2$C$_6$H$_5$)$_2$	0.2	1.3

Pharmacology

SDZ 64-412 inhibited PAF-induced human platelet aggregation (IC$_{50}$ 60 $\pm$ 18 nM) and competed in a dose response manner with [³H]PAF in receptor binding (IC$_{50}$ 60 $\pm$ 23 nM) on human platelets. At 100 μM, SDZ 64-412 did not inhibit epinephrine-induced aggregation, and had a weak effect on collagen (21%) or ADP-induced (22%) aggregation of human platelets.[19-21]

SDZ 64-412 given orally 2 h before PAF administration to anesthetized guinea pigs was effective in inhibiting bronchoconstriction (ED$_{50}$ = 5.2 mg/kg p.o.) and hemoconcentration (ED$_{50}$ = 4.2 mg/kg p.o.). At 20 mg/kg p.o. in the guinea pig maximal inhibition of the PAF-induced responses occurred 2 h after dosing with 50% inhibition being retained up to 10 h post-dosing.[21]

When SDZ 64-412 was given at 20 mg/kg as a single oral treatment 2 h before an i.v. acetylcholine or histamine challenge to ovalbumin-sensitized guinea pigs, it significantly

TABLE 3
Substituted 5-[4'-benzyloxyphenyl]-2,3-dihydroimidazo[2,1-a]isoquinolines

No.	R	Human platelets (IC$_{50}$ μM) Aggr.	Receptor	CNS[a] activity Guinea pig (100 mg/kg, p.o.)
9	H	1.20	0.85	+
11	4"-F	0.25	0.66	+ + +
12	2"-Cl	1.80	0.35	+ + +
13	2"-Cl, 4"-F	0.12	0.23	+ + +
14	2"-Cl, 6"-F	0.16	0.22	+ +
15	2", 6"-Cl$_2$	0.60	0.50	+ +
16	4"-OCH$_3$	0.30	0.47	+
17	3", 4"-(OCH$_3$)$_2$	1.37	0.40	+
18	3", 4"-(CH$_3$)$_2$	0.80	0.20	+
19	2", 3", 4"-(OCH$_3$)$_3$	0.19	0.23	None
20	3", 4", 5"-(OCH$_3$)$_3$	0.23	0.14	None

[a]   + = Weak; + + = moderate; + + + = strong

TABLE 4
Effect of Varying Linking Chain X-Y in Compound *20*

No.	X-Y	Human platelets (IC$_{50}$, μM) Aggr.	Receptor
23	CH$_2$	0.11	0.10
20	OCH$_2$	0.23	0.14
24	CH$_2$CH$_2$	0.06	0.06
25	OCH$_2$CH$_2$	0.20	0.13
26	CH$_2$OCH$_2$	4.23	0.11
27	CH$_2$CH$_2$CH$_2$	0.50	0.30
28	OCH$_2$CH$_2$CH$_2$CH$_2$	1.00	0.22

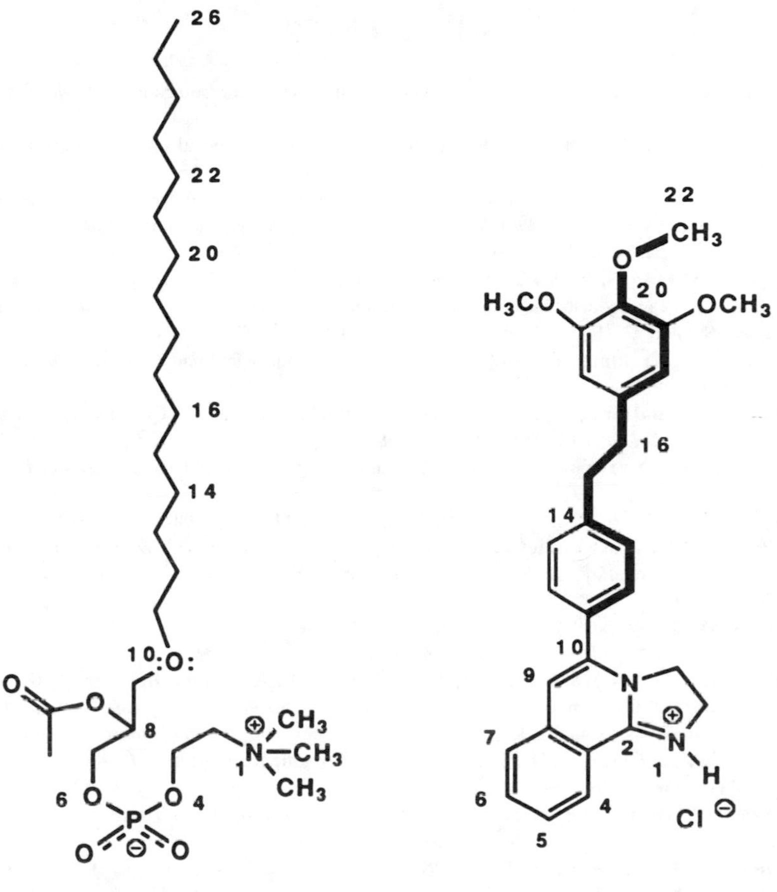

FIGURE 6.   Structural comparison of PAF-16 and SDZ 64-412.

inhibited the development of airway hyperreactivity. The compound had no effect on bron-choalveolar eosionphil recruitment.[22] In contrast, SDZ 64-412 at 20 mg/kg oral was effective in blocking eosinophil accumulation in the pulmonary airways of guinea pigs exposed to aerosols of PAF.[23]

PAF-induced hypotension in the anesthetized rat was inhibited in a dose-dependent manner both parenterally (ED_{50} = 0.23 µg/kg i.v.) and orally (ED_{50} = 13.0 mg/kg p.o.).[21]

Anesthetized primates given SDZ 64-412 orally 3 h before PAF challenge showed a dose-response inhibition of the mean hemoconcentration changes with ED_{50} values of 13 mg/kg and 10 mg/kg p.o. at 3 and 6 h post-drug administration.[21]

Both PAF and endotoxin (*Escherichia coli* 011-B$_4$LPS) induced lethality in mice was blocked by SDZ 64-412 in a dose-dependent manner. At 20 mg/kg p.o. SDZ 64-412 improved PAF-induced lethality (LD_{75} = 75 µg/kg i.v.) survival from 25 ± 4% to 77 ± 8%. Complete protection against endotoxin-induced lethality (LD_{90} = 7.5 mg/kg i.v.) was given by SDZ 64-412 where the ED_{50} was 45 mg/kg twice predose.[21,24]

ACKNOWLEDGMENTS

The assistance of Mrs. Ellen Brennan in typing and Dr. Charles Jewell in preparing the artwork for this chapter is greatly appreciated.

REFERENCES

1. **Saunders, R. N. and Handley, D. A.,** Platelet-activating factor antagonists, *Annu. Rev. Pharmacol. Toxicol.,* 27, 237, 1987.
2. **Hanahan, D. J. and Kumar, R.,** Platelet activating factor; chemical and biochemical characteristics, *Prog. Lipid Res.,* 26, 1, 1987.
3. **Braquet, P. and Godfroid, J. J.,** Conformational properties of the PAF-acether receptor on platelets based on structure-activity studies, in *Platelet-Activating Factor and Related Lipid Mediators,* Snyder, F., Ed., Plenum Press, New York, 1987, 191.
4. **Shen, T. Y., Hwang, S.-B., Doebber, T. W., and Robbins, J. C.,** The chemical and biological properties of PAF agonists, antagonists and biosynthetic inhibitors, in *Platelet-Activating Factor and Related Lipid Mediators,* Snyder, F., Ed., Plenum Press, New York, 1987, 153.
5. **Piwinski, J. J., Kreutner, W., and Green, M. J.,** Pulmonary and antiallergy agents, *Annu. Rep. Med. Chem.,* 22, 73, 1987.
6. **Godfroid, J. J. and Braquet, P.,** PAF-acether specific binding sites. 1. Quantitative SAR study of PAF-acether isosteres, *Trends Pharmacol. Sci.,* 7, 368, 1986.
7. **Handley, D. A.,** Development and therapeutic indications for PAF antagonists, *Drugs Future,* 13, 137, 1988.
8. **Chang, M. N.,** PAF and PAF antagonists, *Drugs Future,* 11, 867, 1986.
9. **Houlihan, W. J.,** Platelet activating factor antagonists, in *Platelet Activating Factor in Endotoxin and Immune Disease,* Handley, D., Saunders, R., Houlihan, W. J., and Tomesch, J., Eds., Marcel Dekker, New York, 1990, 31.
10. **Houlihan, W. J.,** World Pat. 88/00587, January 28, 1988.
11. **Houlihan, W. J.,** World Pat. 88/06157, August 25, 1988.
12. **Houlihan, W. J., Cheon, S. H., Larson, D. A., Parrino, V. A., Reitter, B., Schmitt, G., and Winslow, C. M.,** 5-Aryl-2,3-dihydroimidazo[2,1-a]isoquinolines. A novel class of platelet-activating factor (PAF) receptor antagonists structurally derived from the PAF molecule, *Prostaglandins,* 35, 848 (1988).
13. **Houlihan, W. J., Cheon, S. H., Handley, D. A., Larson, D., Parrino, V. A., Reitter, B., Schmitt, G., and Winslow, C. M.,** 5-Aryl-2,3-dihydroimidazo[2,1-a]isoquinolines. A novel class of platelet activating factor (PAF) receptor antagonists structurally derived from the PAF molecules, *10th Int. Symp. on Medicinal Chemistry,* Budapest, August 15—19, 1988, 93.
14. **Winslow, C. M., Anderson, R. C., D'Aries, F. J., Frisch, G. E., DeLillo, A. K., Lee, M. L., and Saunders, R. N.,** Toward understanding the mechanism of action of PAF receptor antagonists, in *New Horizons in Platelet Activating Factor Research,* Winslow, C. M. and Lee, M. L., Eds., John Wiley & Sons, New York, 1987, 153.
15. **Valone, F. H., Coles, E., Reinhold, V. R., and Goetzl, E. J.,** Specific binding of phospholipid platelet activating factor by human platelets, *J. Immunol.,* 129, 1637, 1982.
16. **Handley, D. A., VanValen, R. G., Melden, M. K., Flury, S., Lee, M. L., and Saunders, R. N.,** Inhibition and reversal of endotoxin-, aggregated IgG- and PAF-induced hypotension in the rat by SRI 63-072, a PAF receptor antagonist, *Immunopharmacology,* 12, 11, 1986.
17. **Handley, D. A., Tomesch, J. C., and Saunders, R. N.,** Inhibition of PAF-induced responses in the rat, guinea pig, dog, and primate by the receptor antagonists SRI 63-441, *Thromb. Haemostasis,* 56, 40, 1986.
18. **Braquet, P., Touqui, L., Shen, T. Y., and Vargaftig, B. B.,** Perspectives in platelet-activating factor research, *Pharmacol. Rev.,* 39, 97, 1987.
19. **Handley, D. A., Van Valen, R. G., Melden, M. K., Houlihan, W. J., Parrino, V. A., Cheon, S. H., and Saunders, R. N.,** SDZ 64-412: an orally-active and potent antagonist to platelet activating factor, *Taipei Conference on Prostaglandin and Leukotriene Research,* Taipei, Taiwan, R.O.C., abstr. 1988.
20. **Saunders, R. N., Van Valen, R. G., Melden, M. K., Houlihan, W. J., and Handley, D. A.,** Pharmacology of the PAF antagonist SDZ 64-412, *FASEB J.,* 2, 1988.
21. **Handley, D. A., Van Valen, R. G., Melden, M. K., Houlihan, W. J., and Saunders, R. N.,** Biological effects of the orally active platelet activating factor receptor antagonist SDZ 64-412, *J. Pharmacol. Exp. Ther.,* 247, 617, 1988.
22. **Havill, A. M., Van Valen, R. G., and Handley, D. A.,** Prevention of non-specific airway hyperreactivity after allergen challenge in guinea-pigs by the PAF receptor antagonist SDZ 64-412, *Br. J. Pharmacol.,* 99, 396, 1990.
23. **Sanjar, S., Aoki, S., Boubekeur, K., Chapman, I. D., Smith, D., Kings, M. A., and Morley, J.,** Eosinophil accumulation in pulmonary airways of guinea-pigs induced by exposure to an aerosol of platelet-activating factor: effect of anti-asthma drugs, *Br. J. Pharmacol.,* 99, 267, 1990.
24. **Van Valen, R. G., Handley, D. A., Houlihan, W. J., Cheon, S. H., and Saunders, R. N.,** Protection against PAF or endotoxin-induced BALB/C mice; SDZ 64-412, *FASEB J.,* 2, 1988.

Chapter 11

N-[ω-(HETEROARYL)ALKYL]CARBOXAMIDE DERIVATIVES AS PLATELET ACTIVATING FACTOR ANTAGONISTS: STRUCTURE-ACTIVITY RELATIONSHIPS AND BIOLOGICAL DATA

Jefferson W. Tilley and Margaret O'Donnell

INTRODUCTION

Platelet-activating factor (1-O-alkyl-2-sn-glycerophosphoryl choline, PAF) is a phospholipid mediator generated in a variety of inflammatory and allergic reactions.[1-5] It exerts a vast array of biological activities including induction of platelet and neutrophil aggregation, bronchoconstriction, increased vascular permeability, and hypotension.[5,6] As our understanding of the range of PAF's biological properties has increased, there has also been a corresponding increase in the evidence implicating PAF's involvement in a variety of human disease states including asthma.[7-10] An intensive effort to find drugs which attenuate the effects of PAF has resulted in the discovery of a number of specific PAF antagonists,[11,12] some of which are currently undergoing clinical trials.

As part of an effort to identify novel PAF antagonists, a binding assay employing whole, washed dog platelets as the receptor source and [^{3}H]PAF as the ligand was established in our laboratories several years ago.[13,14] Using this system, we have found that two pyrido [2,1-b]quinazoline derivatives, **3** and **5** (Table 1), were relatively potent inhibitors of PAF binding.[15] In this report, we describe the structure-activity relationships among compounds of the pyridoquinazoline and related classes of PAF antagonists and the steps which led from our initial observations to the design and characterization of the more potent and long acting pentadieneamide class of PAF antagonists. We also present a detailed summary of the pharmacology of one member of the latter series, **126** (Ro 24-0238), which was selected for further development based on its *in vivo* profile.

PYRIDOQUINAZOLINE CARBOXAMIDE DERIVATIVES

Since members of the pyridoquinazoline series were under active consideration as spasmolytic agents at the time of their discovery as PAF antagonists,[16-18] a large number of these compounds were on hand and we were able to quickly establish certain elements of their structure-activity relationship in the binding assay. From comparison of the isopropyl substituted pyridoquinazoline derivatives **1-6** in Table 1, it was apparent that the compounds with four (4) and six (6) carbon chains between the carboxamide nitrogen atom and the pyridine ring were the most interesting. Holding the connecting chain length and heterocyclic ring constant, compounds **7—15** (Table 2) were examined to compare the effect of substitution in the pyridoquinazoline 2- and 3-positions on potency. These limited results suggest that dialkyl substitution is preferable, but that a variety of substitutions are reasonably well tolerated and are not positionally specific.

In order to determine the contribution of the heterocyclic moiety to binding, a variety of analogs with four carbon connecting chains and differing heteroaromatic species were investigated (Table 3). Among the positionally isomeric pyridine derivatives, the order of potency with respect to the position of connecting chain attachment is 3 > 4 > 2. The 5-substituted pyrimidines **18** and **20** in which the heteroaromatic nitrogen atoms and point of chain attachment are in a *meta* relationship was approximately equipotent to the corresponding

TABLE 1
2-Isopropyl-*N*-[(3-Pyridinyl)alkyl]-11-oxo-11H-pyrido[2,1-b]-
quinazoline-8-carboxamides

Compd	n	Inhibition of PAF Binding IC_{50} (nM)[a]
1	2	2,500
2	3	>1,000 (5)
3	4	350
4	5	>1,000 (9)
5	6	400
6	7	>1,000 (19)

[a] For compounds with IC_{50}s of >1000 nM, the number in parentheses is the percent inhibition of specific binding observed at a concentration of 1000 nM.

3-substituted pyridines **3** and **9**, respectively. The more basic imidazole **19**, which also has a heteroaromatic nitrogen atom in a 1,3-relationship with the connecting chain linkage, was approximately an order of magnitude less active in this assay while the phenyl derivative **21** was inactive. In order to test a hypothesis that a protonated heterocyclic ring might mimic the quaternary nitrogen atom of PAF at the receptor site, the quaternized analogs **22—24** were prepared, but all were inactive in the PAF binding assay.[15]

Our previous experience with the pyridoquinazoline carboxamide **19** suggested that related compounds may be subject to the action of amidases *in vivo*,[19] therefore, we were interested in designing modifications to the amide moiety of the lead PAF antagonist **3** which would render it more metabolically stable. Compounds **25—30** in Table 4 represent attempts to find isosteric replacements for the amide, all of which led to a decrease of activity. However, addition of a single methyl group alpha to the carboxamide nitrogen atom (compound **31**) did not attenuate potency in the PAF binding assay whereas the corresponding alpha, alpha-dimethyl derivative **34** had only about one third the potency of **3**. Comparison of the (R)- and (S)-enantiomers of **31**, compounds **32** and **33**, respectively, revealed that PAF binding inhibition is enantioselective with the (R)-enantiomer being the more potent by a factor of about 2.5.

In order to determine whether inclusion of an alpha-methyl group would have an effect on hydrolysis rates, studies were carried out in liver homogenates derived from guinea pig, squirrel monkey, and dog in which the initial rates of formation of the pyridoquinazoline carboxylic acid **35** from the amides **3** and **31—34** were compared. Since preliminary experiments indicated that amidase activity was present in both the particulate and supernatant fractions of rat liver, further work was carried out on whole liver homogenates. Reaction

TABLE 2
N-[4-(3-Pyridinyl)butyl]-11-oxo-11H-pyrido[2,1-b]-quinazoline-8-carboxamides

Compd	R_1	R_2	Inhibition of PAF Binding IC_{50} (nM)
7	H	H	1,800
8	CH_3	H	500
9	CH_3	CH_3	250
10	HO-	H	1,200
11	CH_3O-	H	1,000
12	Br	H	700
13	$(CH_3)_2CHO-$	H	600
14	H	Cl	1,000
15	H	CH_3O-	370

rates were linear over the first 15 min of incubation and tended to fall after longer periods, presumably due to instability of the amidase preparation. Thus, for comparison purposes, incubations were carried out for 10 min at an enzyme saturating concentration of 0.4 mM of substrate and the amount of **35** which had formed was determined by HPLC as previously described.[19]

35

From the results in Table 5, it is apparent that the racemic (**31**) and (S)-alpha methyl (**33**) amides were hydrolyzed at substantially the same *initial* rates by guinea pig and squirrel monkey liver homogenates and somewhat more slowly than the parent compound **3** which lacks the alpha methyl group. In contrast, the (R)-enantiomer **32** was only slowly hydrolyzed by guinea pig and at a nondetectable rate by squirrel moneky and dog liver homogenates. Thus, we concluded that the hydrolysis observed with the racemate **31** was due to the presence of the (S)-enantiomer and that an alpha methyl group in the R configuration confers considerable metabolic stability to the amide linkage.[15]

Having established that inhibition of PAF binding is highly sensitive to the presence of

TABLE 3
N-[(Heteroaryl)butyl]-11-oxo-11H-pyrido[2,1-b]-quinazoline-8-carboxamides

Compd	R_1	R_2	HET	Inhibition of PAF Binding IC_{50} (uM)[a]
16	$(CH_3)_2CH-$	H		5,000
17	$(CH_3)_2CH-$	H		1,300
18	$(CH_3)_2CH-$	H		450
19	$(CH_3)_2CH-$	H		3,500
20	CH_3	CH_3		100
21	CH_3	CH_3		>1,000 (0)
22	CH_3	CH_3		>1,000 (0)
23	CH_3	CH_3		>1,000 (0)
24	CH_3	CH_3		>1,000 (0)

[a]   For compounds with IC_{50} s >1000 nM, the number in parentheses is the percent inhibition of specific binding observed at a concentration of 1000 nM.

a N-[4-(3-pyridinyl)butyl]carboxamide moiety, we were interested in determining whether the pyrido[2,1-b]quinazoline was also an essential feature of this class of PAF antagonists. Table 6 shows binding data for a variety of aromatic *N*-[4-(3-pyridinyl)butyl]carboxamides and indicates that simple mono- and bicyclic derivatives are not active but that more complex structures containing two aromatic rings joined either by an ether or carbonyl bridge and tricyclic analogs such as the xanthone **43** are comparable to the corresponding pyridoquinazolines in potency.

BIPHENYL CARBOXAMIDES

The above findings led to the hypothesis that the presence of the aromatic ring marked "a" in structure **47** was an important element for receptor binding, particularly when conjugated to the carboxamide, and that the acceptor region of the PAF receptor comprises

TABLE 4
2-Isopropyl-8-substituted-11-oxo-11H-pyrido[2,1-b]quinazolines

Compd	X	R_1	R_2	Inhibition of PAF Binding IC_{50} (nM)[a]
25	$(CH_2)_2$	H	H	>1,000 (15)
26	CH_2NH	H	H	>1,000 (15)
27	CO_2	H	H	>1,000 (16)
28	SO_2NH	H	H	>1,000 (7)
29		H	H	>1,000 (16)
30		H	H	900
31[b]	CONH	CH_3	H	400
32	CONH	CH_3	H	250
33	CONH	H	CH_3	600
34	CONH	CH_3	CH_3	1,200

[a] For compounds with IC_{50} s >1000 nM, the number in parentheses is the percent inhibition of specific binding observed at a concentration of 1000 nM.
[b] Racemic.

at minimum, a hydrophibic area which associates with the aromatic ring marked ''a'', a hydrogen bond donor which interacts with the amide of **47** and a π donor which interacts

47

TABLE 5
Relative Rate of Hydrolysis of PAF Antagonists in Whole Liver Homogenates[a]

COMPOUND	SPECIES		
	GUINEA PIG	SQUIRREL MONKEY	DOG
3	1.0 (n = 1)		
3 1	0.35 ± 0.18 (n = 5)	0.49 ± 0.18 (n = 4)	1.9 ± 0.7 (n = 3)
3 2	0.063 ± 0.015 (n = 3)	<0.01 (n = 2)	<0.01 (n =1)
3 3	0.50 ± 0.07 (n = 3)	0.26 (n = 2)	6.8 (n = 1)
3 4	<0.01 (n = 1)		

[a]   nmol of 2-isopropyl-11H-11-oxopyrido[2,1-b]quinazoline-8-carboxylic acid formed/10 min with 21 mg of fresh liver and 0.4 mM substrate.

From Tilley, J.W. et al., *J. Med. Chem.*, 31, 466, 1988. With permission.

TABLE 6
Aryl-*N*-[4-(3-pyridinyl)butyl]carboxamides

Compd	Aryl	Inhibition of PAF Binding IC$_{50}$ (nM)[a]	Compd	Aryl	Inhibition of PAF Binding IC$_{50}$ (nM)[a]
3 6		>1,000 (19)	4 2		350
3 7		>1,000 (31)	4 3		350
3 8		>1,000 (11)	4 4		800
3 9		>1,000 (18)	4 5		1,000
4 0		400	4 6		>1,000 (11)
4 1		700			

[a]   For compounds with IC$_{50}$s >1,000 nM, the number in parentheses equals percent inhibition of specific binding at 1,000 nM.

with the electron deficient pyridine ring. Molecular modeling studies indicated that the [1,1′]biphenyl-4-carboxamide derivatives **48** fulfilled the requirements of this model as they

possess a suitably located aromatic ring connected through a conjugated π system to a substituted carboxamido group and thus might represent a new class of PAF antagonists even though when positioned for the best overall correspondence, the groups R_1 and R_2 were not coincident.[20]

Accordingly, the biphenylcarboxamide derivatives listed in Table 7 were synthesized and evaluated for PAF antagonist activity in the binding assay. Variation of the substituents in the 3′- and 4′-positions had only a modest effect on potency in keeping with our previous observations in the pyridoquinazoline series. Surprisingly, comparison of **52** with **53** and **56** with **57** indicate that incorporation of a methyl group in the connecting chain led to a 10- to 20-fold increase in potency in the binding assay, suggesting that the mode of interaction of these biphenyl carboxamides with the dog platelet receptor was modified from that of the pyridoquinazoline derivatives.

Comparison of the structures of these biphenyl derivatives with that of the 5,5-bis (4-methoxyphenyl)pentadienamide **86**, (*vide infra*), suggested that that hydrophobic region of the binding site would tolerate additional bulk and prompted us to prepare a number of analogs bearing substituents in the 2-position (Table 8). Compounds **58—62** in which a nitro, bromo, or methoxy moiety is present in the biphenyl 2-position were approximately equipotent to the corresponding unsubstituted analog **56**, but were also insensitive to the presence or absence of an alkyl group on their connecting chains. The high affinity binding observed with the analogs **63—68** indicates that saturated and unsaturated aliphatic groups of up to four carbon atoms in the 2-position are well tolerated.

The compounds of Tables 7 and 8 which had binding IC_{50}s of $\leqslant 500$ nM were further evaluated in guinea pigs for their ability to prevent PAF-induced bronchoconstriction. In this model, as described in more detail later in this chapter, guinea pigs were administered 1 mg/kg of the drug substance 1 min prior to intravenous challenge with a maximally constrictory dose of PAF (1 μg/kg) and the ability of the drug to inhibit the ensuing bronchoconstriction relative to control animals was determined. Compounds which caused a $\geqslant 50\%$ inhibition of the response were further evaluated at multiple doses to determine an intravenous ID_{50} and were tested at a trial doe of 50 mg/kg, orally, 2 h prior to PAF challenge. Oral ID_{50} values and the percent inhibition 6 h after a 50 mg/kg oral dose were also determined for compounds which caused a $\geqslant 50\%$ inhibition of bronchoconstriction response in the initial screen.

The amides **53** and **57**, each of which incorporate a side chain methyl group and are potent in the binding assay, and **52** which was less potent in the binding assay, inhibited PAF-induced bronchoconstriction by $>50\%$ after intravenous administration of a 1 mg/kg dose. Compound **57** was also effective 2 h after oral dosing, with an oral ID_{50} of 30 mg/kg, comparable to the more potent compounds of this series. The analogs of **57** bearing substituents in the 2-position (**58—66, 68**) had comparable activity after intravenous (ID_{50} 0.19 to 0.80 mg/kg) and 2 h after oral dosing (ID_{50} 14 to 39 mg/kg) despite relatively wide

TABLE 7
PAF Antagonist Activity of N-[4-(3-pyridiny)butyl]-1,1'-biphenyl-4-carboxamides[a]

No.	R_1	R_2	R	Inhibition of PAF Binding IC_{50}, nM	% Inhibition 1 mg/kg iv[b]	GUINEA PIG BRONCHOCONSTRICTION ASSAY			
						ID_{50} mg/kg iv[b]	% Inhibition, 50 mg/kg, po 2 Hr	6 Hr	ID_{50} mg/kg, po[c]
49	H	H	H	630	42±7				
50	F	H	H	2,100	0±11				
51	CH_3	H	H	500					
52	CH_3O	H	H	280	70±10	0.51	55±17		50
53	CH_3O	H	CH_3	20	74±6	0.45	44±13		
54	OH	H	H	300	7±7				
55	CH_3	CH_3	H	200	0±4				
56	CH_3O	CH_3O	H	400	8±3				
57	CH_3O	CH_3O	CH_3	15	65±9	0.62	88±5	29±11	30

From Tilley, J. W. et al., *J. Med. Chem.*, 32, 1814, 1989. With permission.

[a]

[b] 1 min pretreatment time.

[c] 2 h pretreatment time.

TABLE 8

PAF Antagonist Activity of 2-Substituted 3',4'-Dimethoxy-N-[4-(3-pyridinyl)butyl]-1,1'-biphenyl-4-carboxamides[a]

No.	R_1	R	Inhibition of PAF Binding IC_{50}	% Inhibition, 1 mg/kg iv 1 Min mg/kg iv[b]	GUINEA PIG BRONCHOCONSTRICTION ASSAY			
					ID_{50} mg/kg, iv[b]	% Inhibition, 50 mg/kg, po 2 Hr	6 Hr	ID_{50} mg/kg, po[c]
58	NO_2	H	200	81±15	0.76	62±15	4±4	39
59	NO_2	CH_3	200	97±0.7	0.19	89±8	36±14	22
60	Br	H	220	81±10	0.40	74±12	1±2	19
61	Br	CH_3	180	98±0.7	0.40	97±1	59±21	14
62	CH_3O	H	300	58±10	0.52	64±12	13±9	
63	HC≡C-	CH_3	5	22±10				
64	C_2H_5	CH_3	4	93±1	0.34	89±5	23±7	24
65	⌇	CH_3	80	80±11	0.33	93±3	26±7	24
66	nC_3H_7	CH_3	50	28±12				
67	nC_4H_9	H	18	6±4				
68	nC_4H_9	CH_3	4	55±12	0.80	91±1	55±18	25

[a] From Tilley, J. W. et al., *J. Med. Chem.*, 32, 1814, 1989. With permission.

[b] 1 min pretreatment time.

[c] 2 h pretreatment time.

variations in their potencies in the binding assay. Among the 2-nitro (**58** and **59**) and 2-bromo (**60** and **61**) pairs for which both the unsubstituted and methyl substituted side chains were prepared, it is apparent that the methyl group conferred a slight enhancement of oral activity at the 2 h time point, as reflected in lower ID_{50} values, and a more marked enhancement at the 6 h time point. The influence of the side chain methyl was even more evident in the case of the pair of 2-butyl derivatives **67** and **68** in which the linear chain compound **67** was inactive in contrast to its branched chain homolog.

It is apparent from this work on biphenyl carboxamide derivatives that the PAF binding assay employing dog platelets is useful for the identification of potential PAF antagonists, but not for predicting relative potencies of compounds in the guinea pig bronchoconstriction assay. The *in vitro* and *in vivo* activity of the 2-substituted analogs implies that co-planarity and conjugation of the biphenyl aromatic rings is not essential for PAF antagonist activity in the guinea pig.[20]

PENTADIENEAMIDES

The diphenylethylenylpiperidine **69** was also identified in our screening efforts as a relatively potent inhibitor of PAF binding (IC_{50} 100 nM) although it was devoid of activity *in vivo*. Molecular modeling experiments indicated that low energy conformations of **47**, **48**, and **69** exist in which the aromatic ring of **69** marked ''a'' can be superimposed with the corresponding rings of **47** and **48**, the piperidine nitrogen is superimposed with the carboxamide nitrogen atoms of **47** and **48**, while the pyridine rings with their side chains are free to adopt the same conformation in all three molecules. When fit in this manner, a correspondence between the second aromatic ring of **69**, marked ''b'' and the carbonyl group of the pyridoquinazoline **47** is also seen.

The likelihood that all three molecules interact with the PAF receptor in a similar manner encouraged us to consider ring opened derivatives of **69**, such as **70**.[21]

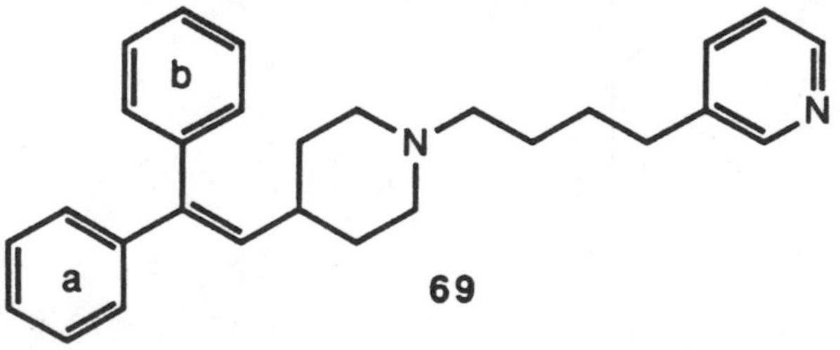

69

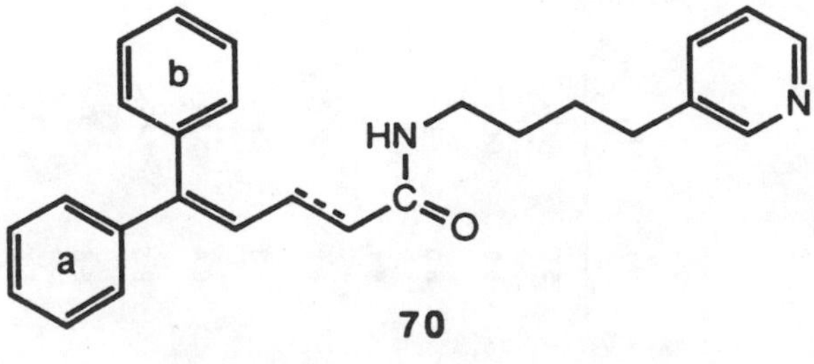

70

In order to determine whether compounds of structure **70** might be useful as PAF antagonists, the derivatives listed in Table 9 were evaluated in the PAF binding assay and compounds which had binding IC_{50} values of $\leqslant$500 n*M* were further evaluated in guinea pigs for their ability to prevent PAF-induced bronchoconstriction. Compounds **71** and **78** met our threshold activity criteria both in the binding assay and after intravenous adminis-

TABLE 9
PAF Antagonist Activity of
N-[4-(3-Pyridiny)butyl]alkenamides[a]

No.	X	Inhibition of PAF Binding IC_{50} nM	Guinea Pig Bronchoconstriction Assay		
			% Inhibition 0.5 mg/kg, iv[b]	ID_{50} mg/kg iv[b]	% Inhibition 50 mg/kg, po[c]
71	bond	450	66±10	0.58	28±4
72	CH$_2$	>1000			
73	(CH2)$_2$	100	21±2		
74	(CH$_2$)$_3$	>1000			
75	(CH$_2$)$_4$	550	15±6		
76	(CH$_2$)$_5$	>1000			
77	/==	400	-1±2		
78	⋏	55	60±8	0.62	35±2

[a] From Guthrie, R. W. et al., *J. Med. Chem.*, 32, 1820, 1989. With permission.
[b] 1 min pretreatment time.
[c] 2 h pretreatment time.

tration. Furthermore, both showed a modest, but significant inhibition of PAF-induced bronchocostriction after oral administration which was sufficient to encourage us to pursue each series. Below, we describe a series of pentadienamide analogs based on the lead provided by **78**.

Compounds **79—90**, direct analogs of **78** bearing various substituents on the aromatic rings are described in Table 10. Consistent with our previous findings, it is apparent that potency in the PAF binding assay and intravenous PAF inhibitory activity are relatively independent of substitution in the 3- and 4-positions. A number of these compounds also demonstrated oral activity with the variations being presumably due to differences in absorption and metabolsim. The 4,4'-dimethoxy analog **86**, is of particular interest as it is not only one of the most potent members of this series, but also retained a high level of inhibition 6 h after oral dosing.

In order to determine whether the introduction of an alkyl substutient on the carbon atom alpha to the carboxamide nitrogen would result in a stereoselective enhancement of oral potency in this series as well, compounds **91—110** (Table 10) were prepared. Comparison, particularly of the *in vivo* data for several pairs of enantiomeric alpha methyl analogs (**91 and 92, 93 and 94, 95 and 96, 97 and 98**) provided convincing evidence that compounds of the R configuration have superior activity as PAF antagonists with the corresponding S enantiomers having significant, but considerably diminished potency. The analog **99** with two alpha methyl groups is less potent orally than either of the corresponding monomethyl enantiomers **97** or **98**. In order to probe the steric limitations of the alpha alkyl substutient, several examples (**104—110**) in the bis-(4-methoxyphenyl) series were prepared which incorporated homologous alkyl substituents.

TABLE 10
PAF Antagonist Activity of (E)-N-[4-(3-Pyridinyl)butyl]-5,5-diphenylpentadienamides[a]

No.	R₁	R₂	R₃	R₄	Inhibition of PAF Binding IC₅₀ nM	Guinea Pig Bronchoconstriction Assay				
						% Inhibition, iv[b] 1.0 mg/kg[b]	ID₅₀ mg/kg iv[b]	% Inhibition, 50 mg/kg, po 2 Hr	6Hr	ID₅₀, po[c]
79	3-F	3-F	H	H	20	71±17[d]	0.34	37±24		50
80	4-F	4-F	H	H	40	91±0	0.38	89±9		28
81	3-Cl	3-Cl	H	H	25	76±14	0.47	23±7		50
82	4-Cl	4-Cl	H	H	60	95±2[d]	0.18	54±11		
83	3-NO₂	3-NO₂	H	H	115	78±6[d]	0.26			
84	2-OCH₃	2-OCH₃	H	H	40	40±2				
85	3-OCH₃	3-OCH₃	H	H	2	69±9[d]	0.36	31±11		80
86	4-OCH₃	4-OCH₃	H	H	25	92±3	0.25	82±12	71±8	12
87	3,4-diOCH₃	3,4-diOCH₃	H	H	55	78±6	0.54	71±12	17±11	27
88	4-CH₃	4-CH₃	H	H	60	95±1	0.26	67±15	11±6	43
89	3-F	3-OCH₃	H	H	40	90±5	0.25	1±8		
90	3-OCH₃	3-F	H	H	25	88±4	0.46	25±14		
91	3-F	3-F	CH₃	H	170	73±6	0.22	91±3	87±9	37
92	3-F	3-F	H	CH₃	250	34±7[d]		46±15		
93	4-F	4-F	CH₃	CH₃	250	70±9[d]	0.31	53±22		

No.									
94	4-F	4-F	H	CH3	275	21±10			
95	3-OCH3	3-OCH3	CH3	H	35	88±3	0.21	86±11	12±7	29
96	3-OCH3	3-OCH3	H	CH3	300	36±4		10±8		4
97	4-OCH3	4-OCH3	CH3	H	65	98±0	0.25	98±1	93±4	29
98	4-OCH3	4-OCH3	H	CH3	200	59±12	0.84	90±2	56±18	55
99	4-OCH3	4-OCH3	CH3	CH3	85	97±0	0.27	54±9		
100	H	4-OCH3	CH3	H	2	89±4	0.16	95±1	53±10	
101	4-OCH3	H	CH3	H	4	74±11	0.50	0±2		
102	3,4-diOCH3	3,4-diOCH3	CH3	H	50	99±1	0.14	67±19	2±8	26
103	4-CH3	4-CH3	CH3	H	250	97±2	0.30	91±7	14±16[f]	18
104	4-OCH3	4-OCH3	C2H5	H	120	99±4	0.16	99±1	85±12[f]	6
105	4-OCH3	4-OCH3	H	C2H5	400	44±8				
106	4-OCH3	4-OCH3	nC3H7[e]	H	>1000	24±13				
107	4-OCH3	4-OCH3	CH(CH3)2[e]	H	800	87±7	0.43	57±19		26
108	4-OCH3	4-OCH3	△[e]	H	60	98±1	0.20	99±0.3	82±12	6
109	4-OCH3	4-OCH3	nC4H9[e]	H	>1000	42±7				
110	4-OCH3	4-OCH3	⬠[e]	H	>1000	19±14				

[a] From Guthrie, R. W. et al., *J. Med. Chem.*, 32, 1820, 1989. With permission.

[b] 1 min pretreatment time.

[c] 2 h pretreatment time.

[d] Screening dose of 0.5 mg/kg, i.v.

[e] Racemic.

[f] 8 h pretreatment time.

It is apparent that ethyl in the R, but not the S configuration and cyclopropyl are tolerated very well, but that activity falls off rapidly as substituents of greater size are introduced. Thus a decrease in activity is seen as the size of the alkyl group is increased from cyclopropyl to isopropyl and the *n*-propyl and *n*-butyl derivatives had only minimal activity.

In order to ascertain effect of restriction of the conformation of the aromatic rings of compounds of this type, the tricyclic analogs **111—113** were synthesized, but were found

111, X = bond
112, X = CH$_2$CH$_2$
113, X = S

to be essentially inactive in the PAF binding assay (IC$_{50}$ > 1000 n*M*).

Compounds **114** and **115** (Table 11) were prepared in order to test a proposal that the pyridinyl carbon-nitrogen double bond of this class of PAF antagonists mimics the acetoxy carbonyl group of PAF at its receptor. According to our speculation, positions 1 and 2 of the pyridine would correspond to the acetoxy carbonyl and the carbon atom in the pyridine 3-position, which is bound to the side chain, would correspond to the acetoxy oxygen atom of PAF. Given the tight steric requirements of the PAF acetyl group, we anticipated that the 2-methylpyridinyl analog **114** would be more active than the 6-methylpyridinyl analog **115** and this proved to be the case, although neither compound was as active as the corresponding unsubstituted derivative **86**.

The other compounds in Table 11 were prepared to further characterize the limitations on the pyridinealkanamide side chain. The poor activity of the ethers **116** and **117** suggest that an all carbon side chain is optimal. The relatively high potency of the 3-pyridinylanalide **118** was a surprise. This finding combined with the observation that the homolog **119** is virtually inactive *in vivo* is useful in defining the distance requirements between the amido moiety and the pyridine nitrogen atom. However, it also suggests that binding site models which attempt to relate the receptor binding of the *N*-[4-(3-pyridinyl)butyl]carboxamides to that of PAF itself, with the carboxamide mimicking the PAF ether oxygen atom and the pyridine ring, the acetyl moiety, are invalid due to impossible distance constraints.

Concerns about the possible toxicological implications of the extended π system of compounds such as **86**, prompted us to consider analogs in which one or both of the anisole rings were replaced with an alkyl moiety. As the data in Table 12 indicate, when the anisole ring which is *syn*-to the amide is replaced with an alkyl group, intravenous activity in the bronchoconstriction assay increases to a maximum as the alkyl chain length is increased from 0 to 5 carbon atoms and remains relatively constant as the chain is further extended to 8 carbon atoms. Oral activity, particularly when measured at the 6-h time point after dosing, is more sensitive to alkyl chain length in this series, maximal activity is seen with the *n*-butyl and *n*-pentyl derivatives **125** and **126**, respectively. This is presumably due to differences in metabolism and absorption among the different homologs. Two compounds (**131** and **132**) were prepared in which the *anti*-aromatic ring was replaced by an alkyl group, both were substantially less potent in the guinea pig bronchoconstriction assay than their geometric isomers **126** and **130**, respectively.

TABLE 11

PAF Antagonist Activity of (E)-N-Substituted-5,5-bis-(4-methoxyphenyl)pentadienamides[a]

Compd.	R	Inhibition of PAF Binding IC_{50} nM	Guinea Pig Bronchoconstriction Assay				
			% Inhibition, iv		% Inhibition, 50 mg/kg, po		ID_{50} mg/kg, po[c]
			% Inhibition, 1.0 mg/kg[b]	ID_{50} mg/kg iv[b]	2 Hr	6 Hr	
114		30	47±10	1.1			
115		700	5±6				
116		250	48±7				
117		300	43±7				
118		10	97±1	0.15	82±12	77±16	29
119		250	3±7				

[a] From Guthrie, R. W. et al., *J. Med. Chem.*, 32, 1820, 1989. With permission.
[b] 1 min pretreatment time.
[c] 2 h pretreatment time.

TABLE 12
PAF Antagonist Activity of (E)-N-[4-(3-Pyridinyl)butyl]-5,5-di-(substituted)pentadienamides[a]

No.	R_1	R_2	Inhibition of PAF Binding IC_{50} nM	% Inhibition, iv 1.0 mg/kg[b]	Guinea Pig Bronchoconstriction Assay ID_{50} mg/kg iv[b]	% Inhibition, 50 mg/kg, po 2 Hr	6 Hr	ID_{50} mg/kg, po[c]
120	H	CH_3O–C$_6$H$_4$	30	-17±13				
121	CH_3	CH_3O–C$_6$H$_4$	25	42±16				
122	C_2H_5	CH_3O–C$_6$H$_4$	30	72±13	0.68	84±2	9±11	35
123	nC_3H_7	CH_3O–C$_6$H$_4$	50	86±7	0.52	9±13		
124	$CH(CH_3)_2$	CH_3O–C$_6$H$_4$	40	89±3	0.41	71±14	20±5	30
125	nC_4H_9	CH_3O–C$_6$H$_4$	14	99±1	0.68	98±1	69±15	12
126	nC_5H_{11}	CH_3O–C$_6$H$_4$	40	99±1	0.06	100±1	71±4	4
127	nC_6H_{13}	CH_3O–C$_6$H$_4$	9	100±1	0.07	96±1	14±10	8
128	nC_8H_{17}	CH_3O–C$_6$H$_4$	5	98±1	0.10	84±8	27±10	13

129	nC5H11		100	78±7	0.64	4±4	
130	nC5H11		20	73±17	0.21	97±1	12±10
131	nC5H11		10	57±1	0.78	13±7	10
132			20	18±12			

From Guthrie, R. W. et al., *J. Med. Chem.*, 32, 1820, 1989. With permission.

[a] From Guthrie, R. W. et al., *J. Med. Chem.*, 32, 1820, 1989. With permission.

[b] 1 min pretreatment time.

[c] 2 h pretreatment time.

ARYLPROPENEAMIDES

Since the pyridoquinazolines **47** in which the key aromatic ring "a" is part of a planar heteroaromatic ring are generally less potent PAF antagonists than the biphenylcarboxamides **48** or the pentadienamides **70** in which rotation of the corresponding aromatic ring out of conjugation with the remainder of the π-system is possible, we were interested to determine the effect of constraining analogs of **70** such that the aromatic ring would be held in conjugation with the olefin and amide portions of the molecule. Thus, we have prepared a number of propenamide derivatives of general formula **133** in which an *o*-position of the

133

aromatic ring has been fused to C_4 of the pentadienamide moiety through a one or two atom linking unit "A".

Since the carboxamides listed in Table 13 by design bear a close structural relationship to the more active members of the pentadienamide series of PAF antagonists, it was not unexpected that most showed high levels of activity in the binding assay. Comparison of *in vivo* efficacy among the naphthalenepropenamides (**134—139**) reveals that oral PAF antagonist activity is highly sensitive to the position of the methoxy group. All of these compounds except **137** effectively attenuated PAF-induced bronchoconstriction after intravenous administration. However, after oral administration, compounds bearing a methoxy group in the 4- or 6-positions were highly efficacious while those substituted in the 5- or 7-positions, including the 4,7-dimethoxy analog **138**, were devoid of activity. The profound sensitivity of oral bioavailability to the position of methoxy substitution was not seen in th more flexible pentadienamide series and may be related to changes in metabolic pathways. The dihydronaphthalene derivatives **140** and **141** were approximately equipotent to the corresponding naphthalenes **134** and **135** after intravenous administration, but were less potent or shorter acting after oral dosing.

Those substances in which the linking unit "A" is included in a 5-membered carbocyclic (**142**) or heteroaromatic ring structure (**143—145**) exhibited levels of inhibition in the binding assay and after intravenous administration that essentially mirrored those found for the lead pentadienamide **126**. However, when these compounds were examined for oral activity, the indene (**142**) and benzofuran (**143**) derivatives were totally inactive while the benzothiophene **144** and indole **145** were among the most potent and long-acting agents of this class yet encountered.

The naphthalenes monosubstituted with methoxy groups in the 4- or 6-positions, the benzothiophene **144** and the indole **145** all show profiles of activity similar to that of the lead compound. These results suggest that while the aromatic ring "a" in structures **47, 48, 70**, and **133** is an important element for PAF antagonist activity, its precise orientation with respect to the extended π system is not critical. We speculate that the relatively inferior levels of potency found in the pyridoquinazolinecarboxamides, wherein the corresponding phenyl ring is part of a rigid planar heteroaromatic ring system may be due to unfavorable electronic effects of the pyridine nitrogen atom and carbonyl groups present in the pyridoquinazoline heteroaromatic system. A second possibility is that the connecting π system may be preferably in or close to a *s*-cis conformation as in partial structure **146** for good PAF antagonist activity rather than the *s-trans* conformation (**147**). If valid, this steric

146   **147**

requirement could be readily accommodated by both the phenylpentadienamides and the biphenylcarboxamides but obviously not by the pyridoquinazolinecarboxamides.

In conclusion, we have described a new class of PAF antagonists which is characterized by a *N*-[4-(3-pyridinyl)butyl]carboxamide attached to an unsaturated, lipophilic moiety. The binding site for these agents comprises a large lipophilic region, possibly at the receptor protein-membrane interface, which is tolerant of steric bulk, but provides recognition for the aromatic ring marked "a" in structures **47, 48,** and **70**. More specific recognition comes from a polar interaction with the carboxamide moiety and either a π-interaction with the pyridine ring or an association of receptor elements with the pyridine nitrogen lone pair. From the above work, compound **126** (Ro 24-0238) was selected for in-depth evaluation based on its long duration of action in the guinea pig bronchoconstriction test and its good safety profile in preliminary toxicological testing. The studies which have been carried out to date are summarized below.

PHARMACOLOGY OF COMPOUND 126 (RO 24-0238)

INTRODUCTION

The strategy used in evaluating **126** as a PAF receptor antagonist involved testing its pharmacological activity in numerous *in vitro* and *in vivo* model systems designed to measure antagonism of PAF-mediated activities. In the sections which follow, the profile of **126** in these models is compared with that of the corresponding S-enantiomer **148** and the literature

126, R-enantiomer
148, S-enantiomer

TABLE 13
PAF Antagonist Activity of (E)-N-[4-(3-Pyridinyl)butyl]-2-propenamides

No	R_1 [a]	R_2	A	R_3	Inhibition of PAF Binding IC_{50} (nM)	Guinea Pig Bronchoconstriction Assay				
						% Inhibition, iv		% Inhibition, 50 mg/kg, po		ID_{50} mg/kg
						1.0 mg/kg	ID_{50} mg/kg	2 Hr	6 Hr	
134	6-CH$_3$O	CH$_3$O–C$_6$H$_4$–	CH=CH	CH$_3$	55	92 ± 3	0.18	79 ± 2	55 ± 19	12
135	6-CH$_3$O	CH$_3$(CH$_2$)$_3$	CH=CH	CH$_3$	7	95 ± 1	0.45	92 ± 2	71 ± 10	4.2
136	5-CH$_3$O	CH$_3$(CH$_2$)$_3$	CH=CH	CH$_3$	6	50 ± 12	1.0	4 ± 2		
137	7-CH$_3$O	CH$_3$(CH$_2$)$_3$	CH=CH	CH$_3$	15	0				
138	7-CH$_3$O	CH$_3$(CH$_2$)$_3$	CH$_3$OC=CH	CH$_3$	3	80 ± 12	0.44	16 ± 8		
139	H	CH$_3$(CH$_2$)$_3$	CH$_3$OC=CH	CH$_3$	1	90 ± 5	0.11	95 ± 2	52 ± 15	2.8
140	6-CH$_3$O	CH$_3$O–C$_6$H$_4$–	CH$_2$CH$_2$	CH$_3$	30	95 ± 2	0.15	75 ± 2	1 ± 10	17
141	6-CH$_3$O	CH$_3$(CH$_2$)$_3$	CH$_2$CH$_2$	CH$_3$	90	94 ± 2	0.46	50 ± 2		50

No.	R_1	R_3	A	R_2						
142	6-CH_3O	$CH_3(CH_2)_4$	CH_2	CH_3	33	96 ± 1	0.05	0		
143	6-CH_3O	$CH_3(CH_2)_4$	O	CH_3	40	89 ± 1	0.06	0		
144	6-CH_3O	$CH_3(CH_2)_4$	S	CH_3	24	98 ± 1	0.11	97 ± 1	97 ± 1	5.4
145	6-CH_3O	$CH_3(CH_2)_4$	NCH_3	CH_3CH_2	26	98 ± 0	0.07	99 ± 1	96 ± 2	3.0

TABLE 14
Inhibition of Canine Platelets

Compound	PAF Binding	PAF Aggregation
	IC_{50}, nM[a]	
126	40±9 (4)[b]	470±120 (3)
148	120±18 (3)	500±100 (3)
149	200±34 (5)	280±70 (4)

[a] IC_{50} values (mean ± SEM) are the concentrations required to inhibit by 50% PAF-induced binding and aggregation.

[b] Values in parentheses are the number of experiments.

PAF antagonist WEB 2086 (**149**), which is one of the most potent and long-acting PAF antagonists described to date.[22]

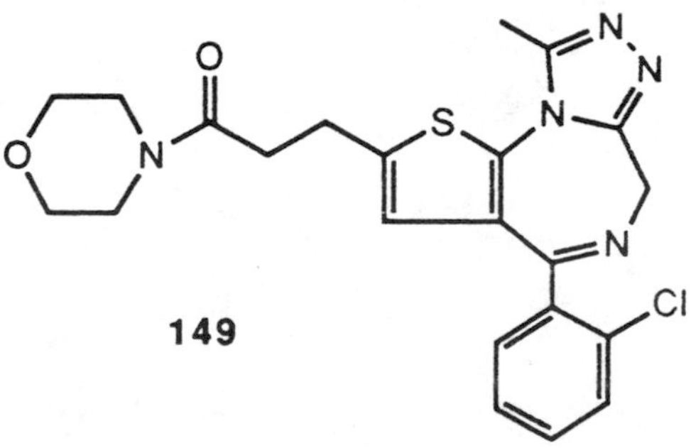

149

IN VITRO STUDIES

PAF Receptor Ligand Binding Assay

Platelets were prepared from dog platelet rich plasma, packed, washed with 1 mM EDTA and resuspended in saline buffer containing 0.1% BSA. The standard assay mixture contains buffer, 1.0 nM [³H]PAF and the platelets (2 × 10⁷) in a final volume of 25 μl. The binding reaction takes place in a 400 μl microfuge tube containing 50 μl of silicone oil, and is carried out at 20°C for 10 min. Separation of bound from free [³H]PAF is performed by rapid centrifugation of platelets through the oil layer. Radioactivity contained in the platelet pellet is measured in 10 ml of Aquasol. Specific binding is defined as that displaced by 1 μM unlabeled PAF and is 70 to 80% of total binding.

Competition studies (Table 14) demonstrated that there was a threefold difference between **126** and the corresponding S-enantiomer, **148**, at displacing [³H]PAF from its binding site (IC_{50}s of 40 vs. 120 nM). Compound **126** was fivefold more potent than the reference PAF antagonist **149** (IC_{50} of 200 nM).

Canine Platelet Aggregation Assay

The aggregation of canine platelets in whole blood was induced by addition of PAF (0.1 μM). The inhibitory effect of the compounds was tested by adding them to a volume of 500 μl whole blood 1 min before addition of the aggregating agent. Each of **126, 148,** and **149** inhibited PAF-induced platelet aggregation in a concentration-dependent manner. Comparison of their IC_{50} values (Table 14), show **126** and **148** were approximately equipotent (IC_{50}s of 470 nM vs. 500 nM) and both were about twofold less potent than **149** (IC_{50} of 280 nM).

TABLE 15
Inhibition of Ionophore-Induced Arachidonic Acid Metabolism in Rat Peritoneal Macrophages

Compound	Inhibition Of Production Formation IC_{50} (µM)		
	TBX_2	PGE_2	LTB_4
126	0.03	0.2	1
148	0.07	0.9	4
149	Inact[a]	Inact[a]	Inact[a]
Dazoxiben	0.3	10	Inact[b]
Indomethacin	0.1	0.1	60
Takeda AA861	2.0	5	0.2

[a] No significant inhibition at a concentration of 50 µM.
[b] No significant inhibition at a concentration of 100 µM.

Effect on Arachidonic Acid Metabolizing Enzymes

The rat peritoneal macrophage assay measures the ability of a test compound to influence the release of arachidonic acid from membrane phospholipd stores and/or its subsequent metabolism through the cyclooxygenase and lipoxygenase pathways to the final products secreted by the cells: LTB_4, PGE_2, and TXB_2 (stable form of TXA_2). The amounts of these products are then measured by radioimmunoassay.

Macrophages were obtained from rats by peritoneal lavage with phosphate buffered saline minus Ca^{2+} and Mg^{2+} (PBS). Cells were washed three times with PBS and resuspended in Delbecco's Modified Eagle medium containing L-glutamine an D-glucose (Gibco Laboratories) and supplemented with 10% fetal calf serum. Cells were counted on a Coulter ZBI cell counter and then resuspended to a concentration of 4×10^6 cells/ml. Three milliliters of the cell suspension was added to plastic culture dishes (3 cm) and the cells were then allowed to adher to the dishes for 90 min at 37°C. Dishes were washed three times with PBS to remove nonadherent cells. Approximately 54 µCi/mmol of [^{14}C]arachidonic acid was added to the cells (1 µCi/dish) and incubated for 90 min. The cell layer was again washed three times with PBS to remove unincorporated [^{14}C]arachidonic acid. Cells were incubated with test compounds or the solution used to dissolve the test compounds (control) for 30 min at 37°C and were then stimulated with the Ca-ionophore A 23187 (0.5 µM) for 20 min. The extracellular fluid was removed and release of [^{14}C] into this fluid from arachidonic acid metabolism was measured. The effect of the test compound was calculated as a percent inhibition of the maximum effect produced in the presence of A 23187 and expressed as an IC_{50}.

Table 15 shows the effects of **126, 148,** and **149** compared to the standard drugs, dazoxiben, indomethacin, and Takeda AA861 on the production of TXA_2, PGE_2, and LTB_4 in this assay. Both **126** and **148** were inhibitors of arachidonic acid metabolism in macrophages, whereas **149** was not. In fact **126** was about tenfold more potent as an inhibitor of thromboxane production (IC_{50} 0.03 µM) than dazoxiben (IC_{50} 0.3 µM). Compound **126** alsc produced a concentration-dependent inhibition of PGE_2 and LTB_4 production, however, at concentrations which were 7-fold and 33-fold higher, respectively. The inhibition of thromboxane formation by **126** did not appear to be stereoselective, since the S-enantiomer, **148,** was only slightly less potent (IC_{50} 0.07 µM).

IN VIVO STUDIES
Antagonism of PAF-Induced Bronchoconstriction in Guinea Pigs

PAF has a number of biological properties relevant to the pathogenesis of asthma. One of the most important is that PAF is a potent bronchoconstrictor in several species including guinea pig,[23] rabbit,[24] baboon,[25] and man.[26,27] PAF induces bronchoconstriction in guinea pigs with intravenous doses as small as 30 ng/kg and is 20-fold more potent than LTD_4, 400-fold more potent than histamine and 3000-fold more potent than arachidonic acid. As noted above, those compounds meeting threshold activity criteria in the binding assay were evaluated by intravenous and oral administration for their potency and duration of action as PAF antagonists in an exogenous, PAF-induced bronchoconstriction test in guinea pigs.

The intravenous technique utilized male guinea pigs (Hartley strain, Charles River) weighing 400 to 600 g. Animals were anesthetized with urethane (2 g/kg) intraperitoneally and a polyethylene cannula was inserted into the jugular vein for intravenous drug administration. Tracheal pressure (cm of H_2O) was recorded from a Statham pressure transducer (P 23AA). Propranolol was administered 5 min prior to challenge with PAF. Two minutes later spontaneous breathing was arrested with succinylcholine chloride (1.2 mg/kg) administered intravenously, and the animals were ventilated with a Harvard (Model 680) small animal respirator set at 40 breaths/min and 4.0 cc stroke volume. Control vehicle or test drug was administered through the cannula into the jugular vein 1 min before the animals were challenged with a maximum constrictory dose of PAF (1.0 μg/kg) given intravenously. For determination of oral activity, animals were dosed with test compound or vehicle 2 h prior to challenge with PAF (1.0 μg/kg, i.v.). Compounds were initially evaluated at a dose of 1.0 mg/kg intravenously or 50 mg/kg orally. The change in tracheal pressure was averaged for four control and four drug-treated animals and percent inhibition was calculated. The median inhibitory dose (ID_{50}) was determined for drugs that inhibited PAF-induced bronchoconstriction by >50%. For determination of the time course of inhibition for various drugs, the time between administration of drug and challenge with PAF was varied. Data on the ability of compounds which meet the threshold criteria for activity in the binding assay to inhibit PAF-induced bronchoconstriction is summarized in earlier sections of this chapter.

When administered intravenously, **126**, its stereosiomer, **148**, and the thienodiazepine, **149**, produced dose-dependent inhibition of PAF-induced bronchoconstriction. Comparison of the ID_{50} values (Table 16) shows that, by the intravenous route, **126** (ID_{50} 0.06 mg/kg) was 18 times more potent than its S-enantiomer, **148** (ID_{50} 1.1 mg/kg) and nearly equipotent to **149** (ID_{50} 0.03 mg/kg).

To assess specificity, all three compounds were evaluated for their ability to inhibit leukotriene D_4 (LTD_4)-, histamine-, and arachidonic acid-induced bronchoconstriction by techniques similar to those described above except that equiactive doses of intravenous LTD_4 (25 μg/kg), histamine (50 μg/kg) and arachidonic acid (500 μg/kg) were employed. At doses of 10 mg/kg i.v., none of the PAF antagonists showed inhibitory activity toward the bronchoconstrictor effects of LTD_4 or histamine.

Arachidonic acid is thought to cause bronchoconstriction through generation of thromboxane A_2.[28] Although **149** showed no inhibitory activity against arachidonic acid, **126** produced dose-related inhibition (ID_{50} 1.4 mg/kg). Its activity in this model is presumably a reflection of its ability to inhibit thromboxane synthase. It should be noted that, by the intravenous route, **126** was 23-times more potent as an antagonist of PAF-induced bronchoconstriction than arachidonic acid-induced bronchoconstriction.

After oral administration, all three PAF antagonists **126, 148,** and **149** produced dose-related inhibition of PAF-induced bronchoconstriction. Comparison of the ID_{50} values in Table 16 show that **126** was 22-fold more potent than its S-enantiomer, **148**, and about 3-fold less potent than **149**. The results of oral duration of action studies with **126** and **149**,

TABLE 16
Intravenous and Oral Potency of 126, 148, and 149 at Antagonizing the Effects of Bronchoconstrictor Agents in Guinea Pigs

Bronchoconstrictive Agent	126	148	149
Intravenous ID_{50}, mg/kg			
PAF	0.06	1.1	0.03
LTD_4	Inact[a]	Inact[a]	Inact[a]
Histamine	Inact[a]	Inact[a]	Inact[a]
Arachidonic Acid	1.4	15	Inact[a]
Oral ID_{50}, mg/kg			
PAF	4.1	88	1.2

[a] No significant inhibition at an intravenous dose of 10 mg/kg

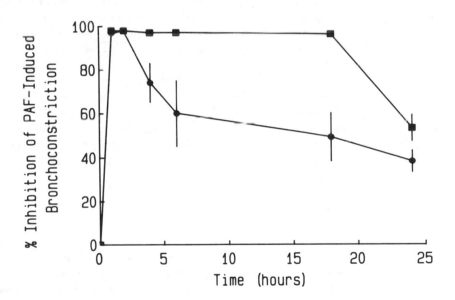

FIGURE 1. Time course for oral **126** (●) and **149** (■) inhibition of PAF-induced bronchoconstriction. The compounds were administered orally at a dose of 50 mg/kg. Responses are presented as percent inhibition of control responses. Each point represents the mean ± SEM for determinations made on four animals.

administered at a dose of 50 mg/kg in the PAF-induced bronchoconstriction test indicate that both exhibit long durations of action as illustrated in Figure 1.

Antagonism of PAF-Induced Changes in Vascular Permeability

Another activity of PAF which may be relevant to its role in mediating asthma and inflammatory processes in general is its ability to increase capillary permeability, and thereby participate in the edema and inflammatory cell exudation associated with these processes. The ability of **126** to block PAF-mediated increases in capillary permeability was assessed utilizing PAF-induced skin wheal tests in rats and guinea pigs.

TABLE 17
Intravenous and Oral Potency of 126 and 149 at Antagonizing the Effects of PAF in the Rat and Guinea Pig Vascular Permeability Test

	Rat Skin Test ID_{50}, mg/kg		Guinea Pig Skin Test ID_{50}, mg/kg	
Compound	Intravenous	Oral	Intravenous	Oral
126	1.7	70	3.0	65
149	0.64	45	2.5	35

In these tests, anesthetized Sprague-Dawley rats or Charles River guinea pigs were pretreated for 30 min by intraperitoneal injection of an antihistamine (50 mg/kg of pyrilamine maleate) and a serotonin antagonist (4 mg/kg of methysergide maleate). For determination of intravenous activity, PAF (5 ng/site in 0.05 ml of saline) was injected intradermally 1 min after intravenous administration of test compound or vehicle. In each case, 1.0 ml of 0.5% Evans blue dye was injected into the tail vein of the rat or the ear vein of the guinea pig. Thirty minutes later, the animals were sacrificed by cervical dislocation and, in order to quantitate the increase in capillary permeability induced by PAF, the average diameter of each wheal on the dorsal rat or guinea pig skin was measured with a metric vernier caliper. Oral activity was determined by dosing animals with test compound or vehicle 2 h prior to challenge with PAF. For determination of ID_{50} values, five animals were used in the control group (four injection sites per animal) and five animals in each drug treatment group (4 injection sites per animal).

The ability of **126** and **149** to prevent PAF-induced increases in vascular permeability in rats and guinea pigs is summarized in Table 17. These studies indicate that both compounds produced dose-related inhibition in the rat and guinea pig skin and **126** was only slightly less potent than **149** by the intravenous and oral routes.

Antagonism of Endotoxin-Induced, PAF-Mediated Shock in Rats

Septic shock is the body's response to Gram-negative bacteremia and is characterized by systemic hypotension, increased vascular permeability, bronchoconstriction, pulmonary hypertension, and gastrointestinal ulceration. The symptoms are reproduced in various animal models by intravenous administration of endotoxin, hence the name endotoxin shock. Endotoxin induces a dual-phase hypotensive response involving multiple pathophysiological mechanisms which are still unclear. Previous investigations[29-32] suggest a participation of arachidonic acid metabolites such as leukotrienes or thromboxane A_2 in the early hypotensive phase of shock, but this remains controversial.

The second shock hypotensive phase is characterized by an increase in permeability leading to a loss of fluid from the circulatory system and eventual lung failure. PAF has been suggested as a key mediator in the development of the second phase of endotoxin shock because: (a) PAF mimics the symptomatology — a single injection of PAF in animals produces microvascular permeability changes associated with extravasation of fluid in interstitial spaces and prolonged hypotension, (b) PAF has been found in the plasma of endotoxin-treated animals,[33] and (c) a number of chemically dissimilar PAF antagonists [Takeda's CV 3988,[34,35] Ipsen-Beaufour's BN-52021,[36] Sandoz's SRI 63-072,[37] and Boehringer Ingelheim's **149**[38]] have been shown to have a protective effect against endotoxin shock in animals. Thus studies were undertaken to comparatively evaluate the ability of the PAF antagonists, **126** and **149**, to inhibit and reverse this process in rats.

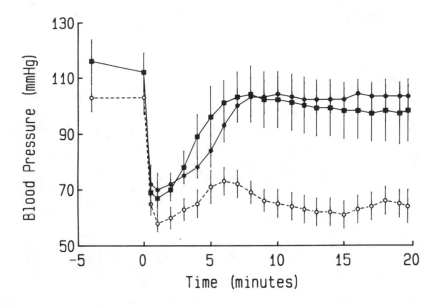

FIGURE 2. Effects of **126** (●), **149** (■), or vehicle (○) pretreatment on endotoxin-induced hypotension in anesthetized rats. The compounds were administered intravenously (10 mg/kg) 5 min prior to challenge with endotoxin (30 mg/kg, i.v.) at time 0. Values are means ± SEM (n = 6).

Male Sprague-Dawley rats (300 to 500 g) were anesthetized with sodium pentobarbital (50 mg/kg, i.p.), and the right common carotid artery was cannulated (PE 50 tubing) and connected to a p50 pressure transducer. Mean arterial pressures were calculated by an on-line Cardiovascular Computer (Buxco Electronics, Sharon CT) and were recorded simultaneously on a Hewlett Packard 7758 physiograph (Hewlett Packard, Paramus, NJ). As the biological activity of endotoxin was variable depending on the lot, the strain, and the age of rats used, the optimal dose of endotoxin was established in preliminary experiments. A dose of 30 mg/kg was selected for use in all experiments because it produced a fall in blood pressure of 45 ± 3 mmHg within 1 min which was sustained for at least 20 min. In the protection series of experiments, **126** or **149** were given intravenously 5 min before the endotoxin (30 mg/kg) was injected intravenously. In the reversal studies, the PAF antagonists were given intravenously when the blood pressure was maximally reduced 10 min after the endotoxin had been injected intravenously. The changes in blood pressure were monitored every minute for 20 min after the endotoxin was injected.

The ability of **126** and **149** to prevent endotoxin-induced decreases in blood pressure is illustrated in Figure 2. Neither compound affected basal blood pressure or inhibited the first phase of hypotension. At an intravenous dose of 10 mgdikg, **126** and **149** were equiactive in inhibiting the second phase of endotoxin-induced hypotension (approximately 70% inhibition).

Figure 3 compares the reversal of endotoxin-induced hypotension by **126** and **149**. Both compounds were capable of producing rapid reversal of endotoxin-induced hypotensin (within 2 min), however **126** was more efficacious. At an intravenous dose of 10 mg/kg, **126** produced a maximal reversal of 100%, whereas **149** produced a maximal reversal of 52%.

These data provide further evidence for the involvement of PAF in the pathophysiology of endotoxin shock in rats. Compound **126** was shown to partially attenuate and completely reverse the hypotension of endotoxemia and thus may be a beneficial drug for septic shock.

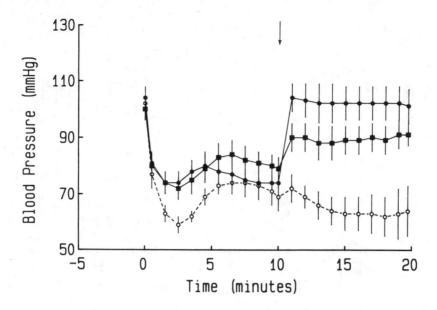

FIGURE 3.   Reversal of endotoxin-induced hypotension by **126** (●), **149** (■) or vehicle (○) in anesthetized rats. Endotoxin (30 mg/kg, i.v.) was given at 0 min, and 10 min later, when the maximum decrease in blood pressure had been achieved, 10 mg/kg of drug or 0.1 ml/kg of vehicle were administered intravenously. Values are means ± SEM (n = 6).

SUMMARY

In conclusion, we have described a new class of PAF antagonists which are characterized by a *N*-[4-(3-pyridinyl)butyl]carboxamide attached to an unsaturated, lipophilic moiety. The results of our structure-activity studies suggest that the binding site for these agents comprises a large lipophilic region, possibly at the receptor protein-membrane interface, which is tolerant of steric bulk, but provides recognition for the aromatic ring marked "a" in structures **48, 49, 69**, and **70**. More specific recognition comes from a polar interaction with the carboxamide moiety and either a π-interaction with the pyridine ring or an association of receptor elements with the pyridine nitrogen lone pair. The inclusion of a lower alkyl group on the carboxamide side chain and in the R-configuration is important for achieving a long duration of action, presumably by inhibiting the action of amidases which would otherwise degrade the molecule by hydrolysis.

In-depth pharmacological evaluation of the lead structure **126** (Ro 24-0238) indicates that this compound is an effective, orally active PAF antagonist with a long duration of action in guinea pigs and rats. This compound inhibits PAF induced bronchocostriction in guinea pigs after intravenous and oral administration with somewhat lower potency than the thienodiazepine **149** (WEB 2086), but is nearly equipotent to **149** in attenuating PAF-induced capillary permeability changes in rats and guinea pigs and more effective in reversing the secondary hypotensive phase of endotoxin-induced shock in rats. We speculate that the activity of **126** in the latter model may be a reflection of a synergy between its ability to block access of PAF to its receptors and its ability to inhibit the formation of thromboxane A_2. Because bronchial asthma and endotoxemia are complex disorders probably not attributable to a single causative factor, an agent such as **126** with the combined properties of PAF antagonism and thromboxane synthase inhibition may prove to be therapeutically beneficial.

ACKNOWLEDGMENT

We gratefully acknowledge B. Burghardt, C. Burghardt, J. W. Clader, H. Crowley, K. E. Fahrenholtz, R. W. Guthrie, D. Janero, G. Kaplan, R. W. Kierstead, R. A. LeMahieu, F.-J. Leinweber, J. Lind, F. Mennona, D. Morgan, J. Mullin, M. Wirkus, A. Welton, and S. Zawoiski, all of whom contributed importantly to the work described herein.

REFERENCES

1. **Braquet, P., Touqui, L., Shen, T. Y., and Vargaftig, B. B.,** Perspectives in platelet activating factor research, *Pharmacol. Rev.,* 39, 97, 1987.
2. **Henson, P. M. and Pinckard, R. N.,** Platelet activating factor (PAF). A possible direct mediator of anaphylaxis in the rabbit and a trigger for the vascular deposition of circulating immune complexes, *Monogr. Allergy,* 12, 13, 1977.
3. **Chang, M. N.,** PAF and PAF antagonists, *Drugs Future,* 11, 869, 1986.
4. **Saunders, R. N. and Handley, D. A.,** Platelet-activating factor antagonists, *Annu. Rev. Pharmacol. Toxicol.,* 27, 237, 1987.
5. **Vargaftig, B. B., Chignard, M., Benveniste, J., Lefort, J., and Wal, F.,** Background and present status of research on platelet-activating factor (PAF-acether), *Ann. N.Y. Acad. Sci.,* 370, 119, 1981.
6. **Pinckard, R. N., McManus, L. M., Halonen, M., and Hanahan, D. J.,** Biological activities of acetyl glyceryl ether phosphorylcholine in experimental animals and man, in *Role of Chemical Mediators in the Pathophysiology of Acute Illness and Injury,* McConn, R., Ed., Raven Press, New York, 1982, 81.
7. **Page, C. P.,** The role of platelet-activating factor in asthma, *J. Allergy Clin. Immunol.,* 81, 144, 1988.
8. **Barnes, P. J.,** Platelet activating factor and asthma, *J. Allergy Clin. Immunol.,* 81, 152, 1988.
9. **Chung, K. F. and Barnes, P. J.,** PAF antagonists. Their potential therapeutic role in asthma, *Drugs,* 35, 93, 1988.
10. **Morley, J.,** Platelet activating factor and asthma, *Agents Actions,* 19, 100, 1986.
11. **Godfroid, J. J. and Braquet, P.,** PAF-acether specific binding sites. I. Quantitative SAR study of paf-acether isosteres, *Trends Pharmacol. Sci.,* 7, 368, 1986.
12. **Braquet, P. and Godfroid, J. J.,** PAF-acether specific binding sites. II. Design of specific antagonists, *Trends Pharmacol. Sci.,* 7, 397, 1986.
13. **Janero, D. R., Burghardt, B., and Burghardt, C.,** Specific binding of 1-O-alkyl-2-acetyl-sn-glycero-3-phosphocholine (platelet-activating factor) to the intact canine platelet, *Thrombosis Res.,* 50, 789, 1988.
14. **Janero, D. R., Burghardt, B., and Burghardt, C.,** Radioligand competitive binding methodology for the evaluation of platelet-activating factor (PAF) and PAF-receptor antagonism using intact canine platelets, *J. Pharmacol. Meth.,* 20, 237, 1988.
15. **Tilley, J. W., Burghardt, B., Burghardt, C., Mowles, T. F., Leinweber, F.-J., Klevans, L., Young, R., Hirkaler, G., Fahrenholtz, K., Zawoiski, S., and Todaro, L.,** Pyrido[2,1-b]quinazolinecarboxamide derivatives as platelet activating factor antagonists, *J. Med. Chem.,* 31, 466, 1988.
16. **Tilley, J. W., Levitan, P., Welton, A. F., and Crowley, H. J.,** Antagonists of slow reacting substance of anaphylaxis. I. Pyrido[2,1-b]quinazolinecarboxylic acid derivatives, *J. Med. Chem.,* 26, 1638, 1983.
17. **Tilley, J. W., Coffen, D. L., Schear, B. H., and Lind, J.,** A palladium catalyzed carbonyl insertion route to pyrido[2,1-b]quinazoline derivatives, *J. Org. Chem.,* 52, 2469, 1987.
18. **Tilley, J. W., Levitan, P., Lind, J., Welton, A. F., Crowley, H. J., Tobias, L. D., and O'Donnell, M.,** N-(Heterocyclic alkyl)pyrido[2,1-b]quinazoline-8-carboxamides as orally active antiallergy agents, *J. Med. Chem.,* 30, 185, 1987.
19. **Strojny, N., Puglisi, C. V., and de Silva, J. A. F.,** Determination of the antiallergenic agent, N-[4-(1H-imidazol-1-yl)butyl]-2-(1-methylethyl)-11-oxo-11H-pyrido[2,1-b]quinazoline-8-carboxamide, in plasma by reversed phase high-performance liquid chromatographic analysis using fluorometric detection, *J. Chromatogr.,* 336, 301, 1984.
20. **Tilley, J. W., Clader, J. W., Zawoiski, S., Wirkus, M., LeMahieu, R. A., O'Donnell, M., Crowley, H., and Welton, A. F.,** Biphenylcarboxamide derivatives as antagonists of platelet activating factor, *J. Med. Chem.,* 32, 1814, 1989.
21. **Guthrie, R. W., Kaplan, G., Mennona, F., Tilley, J. W., Kierstead, R. W., Mullin, J., Zawoiski, S., LeMahieu, R. A., O'Donnell, M., Crowley, H., Yaremko, B., and Welton, A. F.,** Pentadienyl carboxamide derivatives as antagonists of platelet activating factor, *J. Med. Chem.,* 32, 1820, 1989.

22. **Casals-Stenzel, J., Muacevic, G., and Weber, K.-H.,** Pharmacological actions of WEB 2086, a new specific antagonist of platelet activating factor, *J. Pharmacol. Exp.,* 241, 974, 1987.

23. **Vargaftig, B. B., Lefort, J., Chignard, M., and Benveniste, J.,** Platelet-activating factor induces a platelet-dependent bronchoconstriction unrelated to the formation of prostaglandin derivatives, *Eur. J. Pharmacol.,* 65, 185, 1980.

24. **Halonen, M., Palmer, J. D., Lohman, I. C., McManus, L. M., and Pinckard, R. N.,** Respiratory and circulatory alterations induced by acetyl glyceryl ether phosphorylcholine, a mediator of IgE anaphylaxis in the rabbit, *Am. Rev. Respir. Dis.,* 122, 915, 1980.

25. **Denjean, A., Arnoux, B., Masse, R., Lockhart, A., and Benveniste, J.,** Acute effects of intratracheal administration of platelet-activating factor in baboons, *J. Appl Physiol. Respir. Environ. Exercise Physiol.,* 55, 799, 1983.

26. **Cuss, F. M., Dixon, C. M. S., and Barnes, P. J.,** Effects of inahled platelet activating factor on pulmonary function and bronchial responsiveness in man, *Lancet,* 2, 189, 1986.

27. **Rubin, A. E., Smith, L. J., and Patterson, R.,** The bronchoconstrictor properties of platelet-activating factor in humans, *Am. Rev. Respir. Dis.,* 136, 1145, 1987.

28. **Mitchell, H. W. and Denborough, M. A.,** The metabolism of arachidonic acid in isolated tracheal and lung strip preparations of guinea pigs, *Lung,* 158, 121, 1980.

29. **Brigham, K. L., Bowers, R. E., and Haynes, J.,** Increased sheep lung vascular permeability caused by *Escherichia coli* endotoxin, *Circ. Res.,* 45, 292, 1979.

30. **Ogletree, M. L. and Brigham, K. L.,** Effects of cyclooxygenase inhibitors on pulmonary vascular responses to endotoxin in unanesthetized sheep, *Prostaglandins Leukotrienes Med.,* 8, 489, 1982.

31. **Snapper, J. R., Hutchinson, A. A., Ogletree, M. L., and Brigham, K. L.,** Effects of cyclooxygenase inhibitors on the alterations in lung mechanics caused by endotoxemia in the unanesthetized sheep, *J. Clin. Invest.,* 72, 63, 1983.

32. **Ahmed, T., Wasserman, M. A., Muccitelli, R., Tucker, S., Gazeroglu, H., and Marchette, B.,** Endotoxin-induced changes in pulmonary hemodynamics and respiratory mechanisms, *Am. Rev. Respir. Dis.,* 134, 1147, 1986.

33. **Inarrea, P., Gomez-Cambronero, J., Pascual, J., del Carmen Ponte, M., Hernando, L., and Sánchez-Crespo, M.,** Synthesis of PAF-acether and blood volume changes in gram-negative sepsis, *Immunopharmacology,* 9, 45, 1985.

34. **Terashita, Z., Imura, Y., Nishikawa, K., and Sumida, S.,** Is platelet activating factor (PAF) a mediator of endotoxin shock?, *Eur. J. Pharmacol.,* 109, 257, 1985.

35. **Toth, P.D. and Mikulaschek, A. W.,** Effects of a platelet-activating factor antagonist, CV-3988, on different shock models in the rat, *Circ. Shock,* 20, 193, 1986.

36. **Etienne, A., Hecquet, F., Soulard, C., Spinnewyn, B., Clostre, F., and Braquet, P.,** *In vivo* inhibition of plasma protein leakage and *Salmonella enteritis*-induced mortality in the rat by a specific PAF-acether antagonist: BN 52021, *Agents Actions,* 17, 368, 1985.

37. **Handley, D. A., Van Valen, R. G., Melden, M. K., Flury, S., Lee, M. L., and Saunders, R. N.,** Inhibition and reversal of endotoxin-aggregated IgG- and PAF-induced hypotension in the rat by SRI 63-072, a PAF receptor antagonist, *Immunopharmacology,* 12, 11, 1986.

38. **Casals-Stenzel, J., Muacevic, G., and Heuer, H.,** Modulation of the endotoxin shock and anaphylactic lung reaction by WEB 2086, a new potent antagonist of PAF, *2nd Int. Conf. on Platelet-Activating Factor and Structurally Related Alkyl Ether Lipids,* Gatlinburg, TN, October 26—29, 1986, 107.

Part III
Molecular Modeling

Chapter 12

STRUCTURE ACTIVITIES IN PAF ACETHER ANTAGONIST SERIES USING MOLECULAR LIPOPHILIC POTENTIAL STUDIES

J. P. Dubost, M. H. Langlois, E. Audry, P. Braquet, J. C. Colleter, F. Croizet, and Ph. Dallet

INTRODUCTION

It is now accepted that lipophilicity is a very important molecular property in the search of relationships between the chemical structure of a molecule and its biological activity.[10]

Log P, the partition coefficient, usually describes this property and is widely used for classical quantitative structure activity relationships (Q.S.A.R.). However, this "one dimensional" representation becomes insufficient when stereochemical features of molecules are analyzed in the context of intermolecular interactions with the receptor. So, to avoid this failure we have recently introduced the notion of Molecular Lipophilic Potential[1,2] which takes into consideration that lipophilicity is a property distributed all over the different parts of a molecule. Lipophilic and hydrophilic regions in the surrounding space of a molecule are revealed thanks to this concept.[3,6] It is easier to compare different drugs even if they do not have the same framework.

For this reason we have applied this new tool to a series of 16 PAF acether antagonists (Table 1) in order to better understand how these drugs interact with the PAF receptor.

THE MOLECULAR LIPOPHILICITY POTENTIAL (MLP)

If a molecule is considered as the sum of n independent fragments, the logarithmic partition coefficient value can be broken down into a sum of hydrophobic fragmental constants f_i:[9]

$$\log P = \sum_{i=1}^{n} f_i \tag{1}$$

f_i is the lipophilic contribution of a constituent fragment of a molecules to the total lipophilicity.

For us a fragment is a nonhydrogen atom connected with zero, one, two, or three hydrogen atoms. We have used f_i values published by Broto in the *European Journal of Medicinal Chemistry*.[4]

Let us consider a molecule S in an organic phase constituted of nonpolar or slightly polar molecules L. Molecules L are distributed at random when they are far from S. This arrangement must be modified as the distance is decreasing. A lipophilic fragment (f_i positive) will tend to attract the molecules L and a hydrophilic fragment (f_i negative) will tend to repulse molecules L.

We have defined at each point M in the space surrounding the molecule S, a parameter called Molecular Lipophilicity Potential (MLP) as:

$$MLP = \sum_{i=1}^{n} \frac{f_i}{1 + d_i} \tag{2}$$

d_i is the distance (Å) between the fragment i and the point M.

TABLE 1
Structures of PAF Acether Antagonists Studied

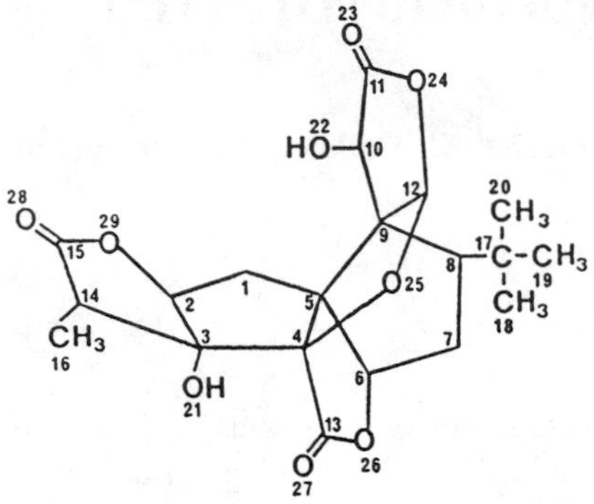

BN 52020
GINKGOLIDE A

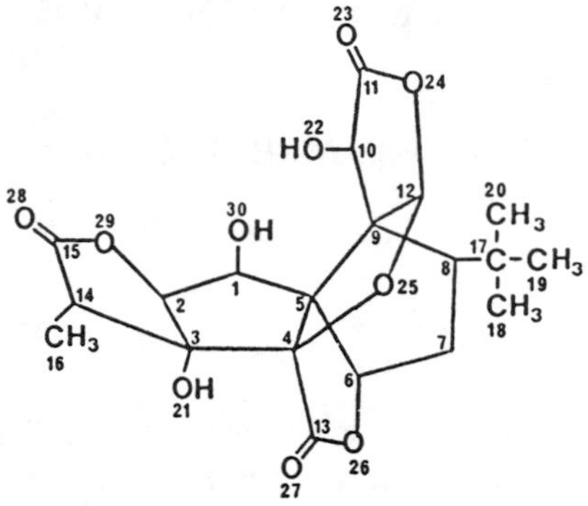

BN 52021
GINKGOLIDE B

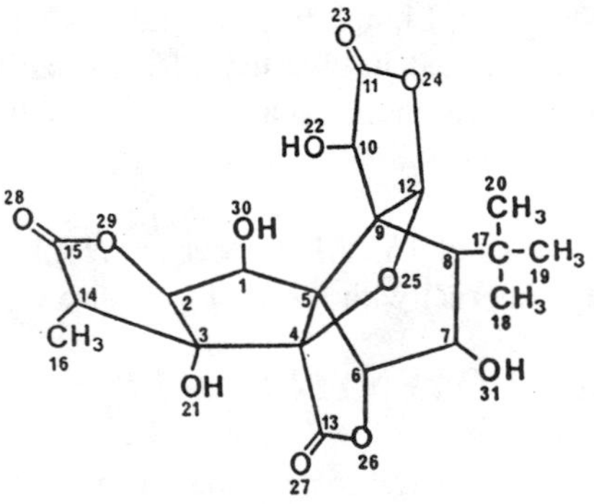

BN 52022
GINKGOLIDE C

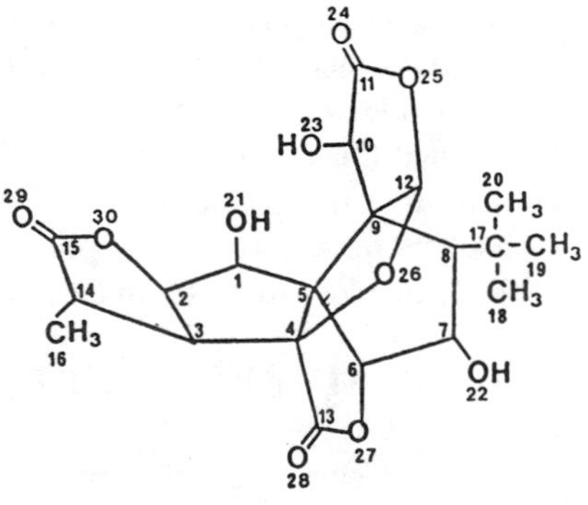

BN 52023
GINKGOLIDE M

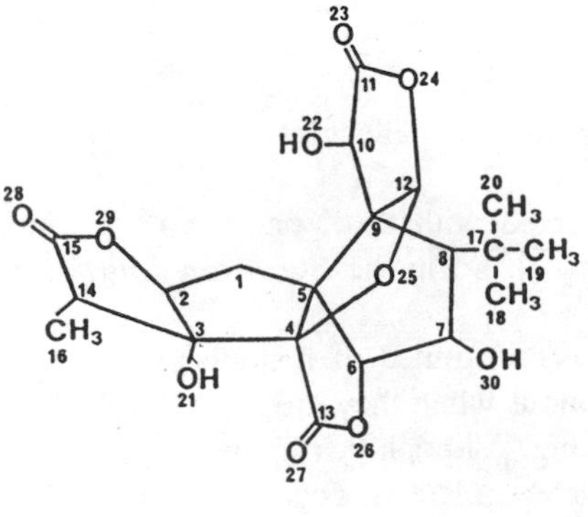

BN 52024
GINKGOLIDE J

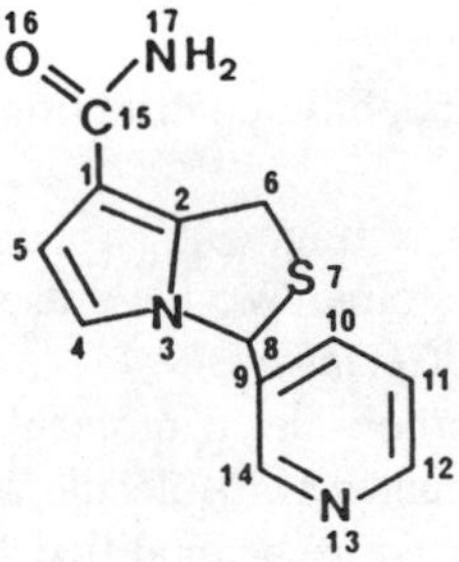

RP 48740

TABLE 1 (continued)
Structures of PAF Acether Antagonists Studied

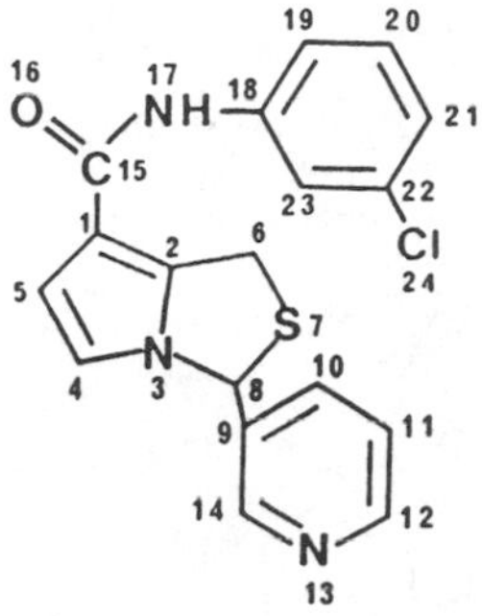

RP 52770

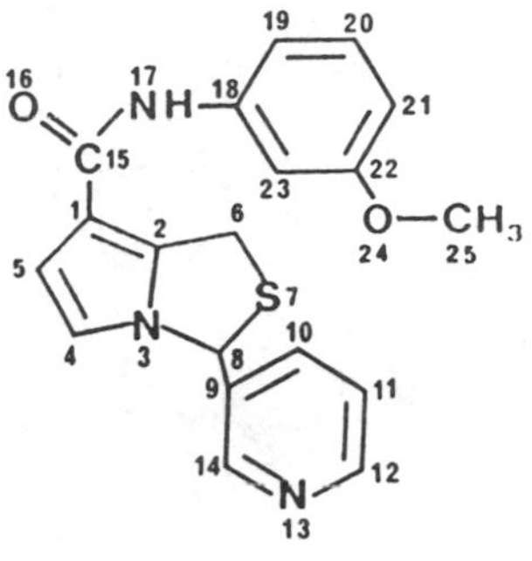

RP 52629

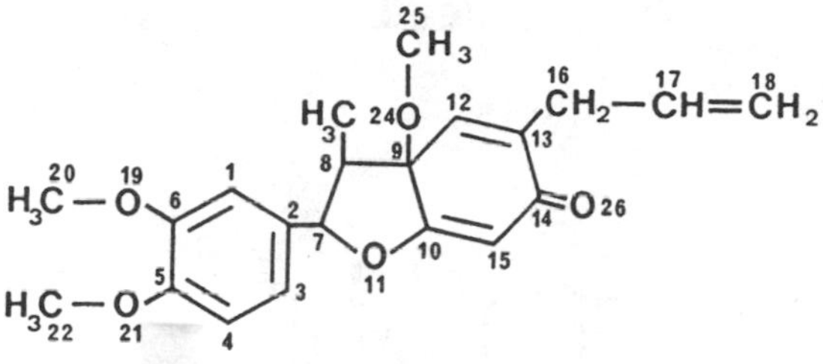

KADSURENONE

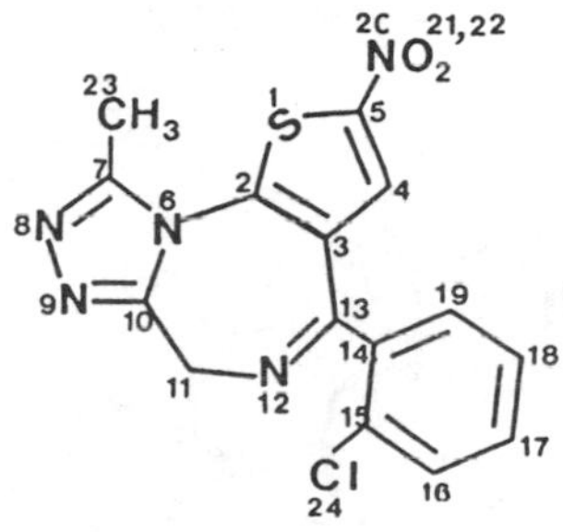

TBDZ A

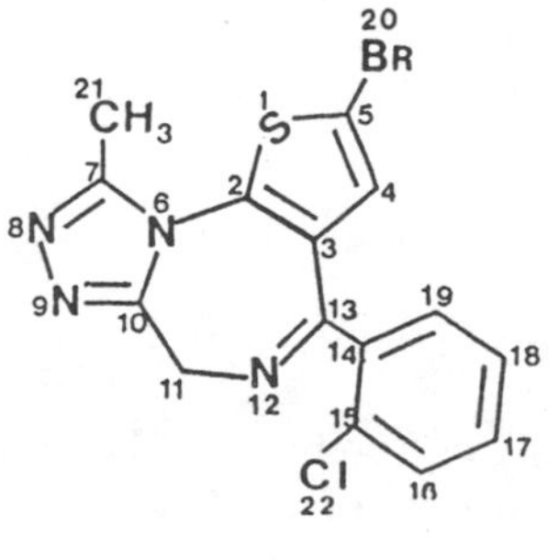

BROTIZOLAM

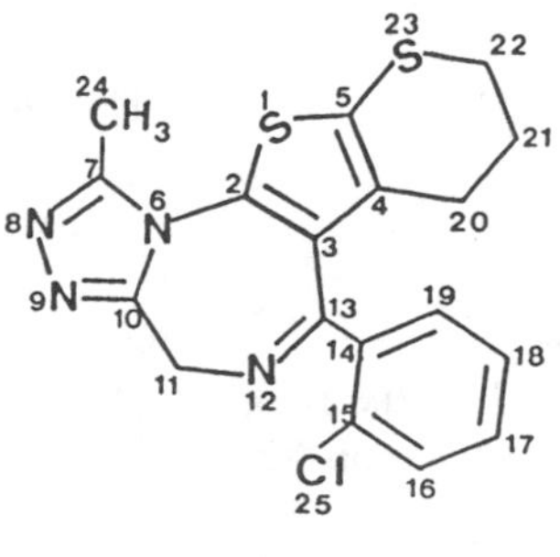

TBDZ B

TABLE 1 (continued)
Structures of PAF Acether Antagonists Studied

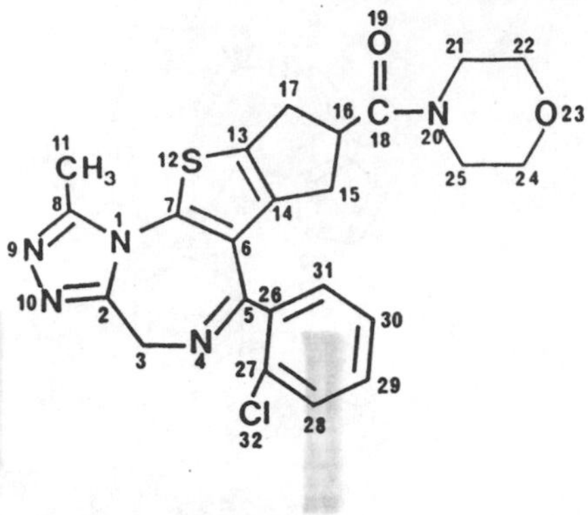

WEB 2170

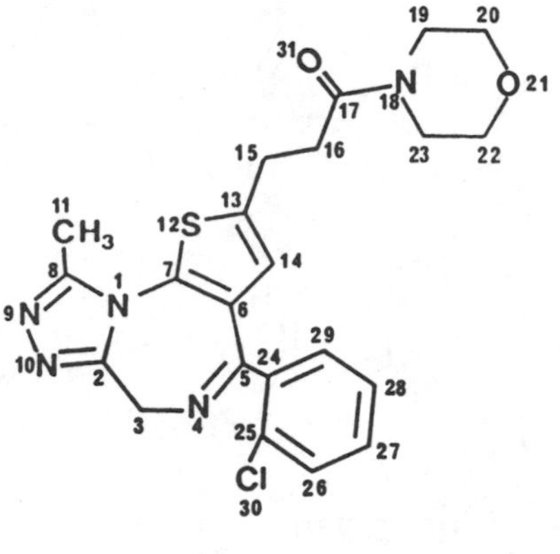

WEB 2086

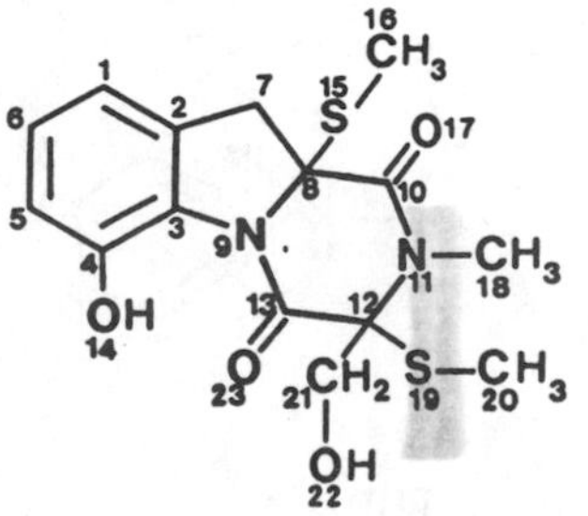

GLIOTOXIN A

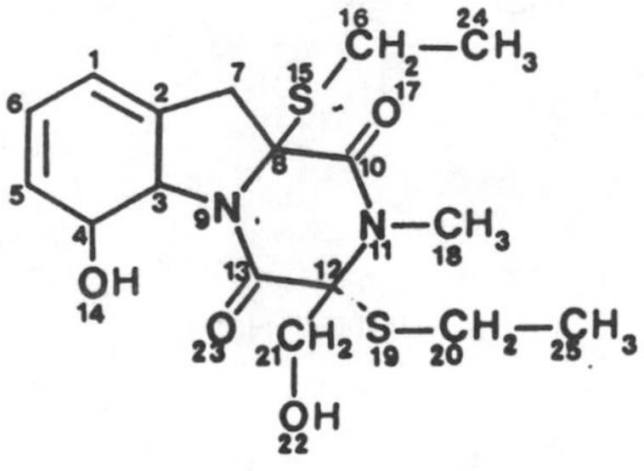

GLIOTOXIN B

If $n = 1$, then Equation 2 becomes:

$$MLP = \frac{f_i}{1 + d_i} \tag{3}$$

It is the lipophilicity potential generated by a fragment i on one point located at d_i. At d_i, MLP can be considered as the fraction of the maximum affinity of the fragment to a receptor.

Parallel to the definition of partition coefficient, MLP can be written:

$$MLP = \log \frac{P_1}{Q_1} \tag{4}$$

where P_1 is the probability for a molecule S to interact with the molecule L via a lipophilic interaction and Q_1 the contrary probability.

$$\text{as: } P_1 + Q_1 = 1 \tag{5}$$

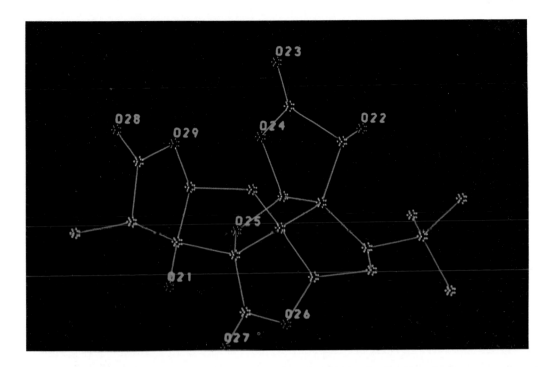

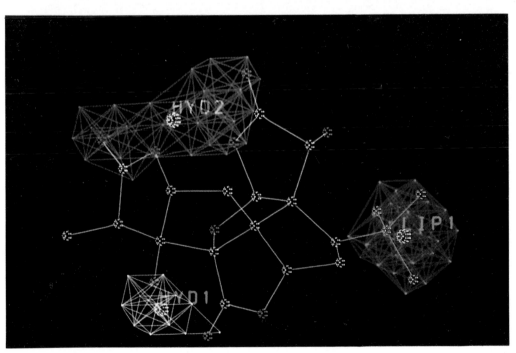

PLATE 1. Spatial conformation of BN 52020 (Ginkgolide A) determined by X-ray diffraction (8). (Top) Isolipophilicity curves. (Bottom) P_1 limits of each zone: LIP 1 — 0.8 to 0.9, HYD 1 — 0.2 to 0.3, HYD 2 — 0.3 to 0.4.

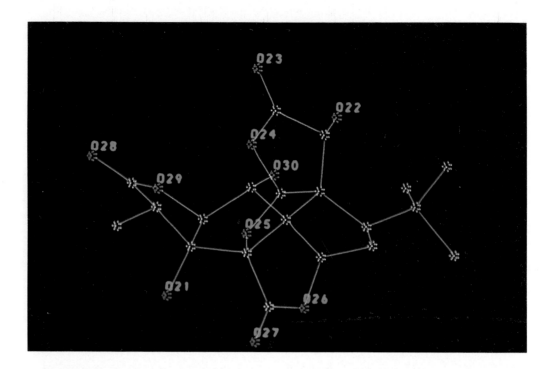

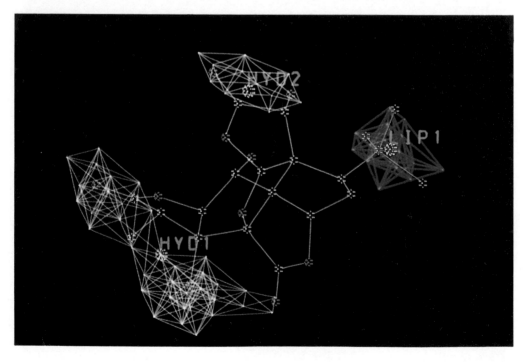

PLATE 2. Spatial conformation of BN 52021 (Ginkgolide B) determined by X-ray diffraction (7). (Top) Isolipophilicity curves. (Bottom) P_1 limits of each zone: LIP 1 — 0.8 to 0.9, HYD 1 — 0.2 to 0.3, HYD 2 — 0.2 to 0.3.

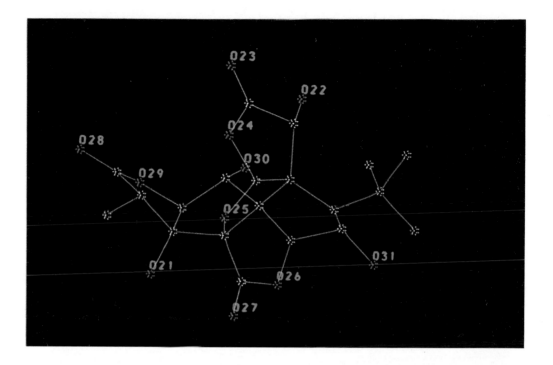

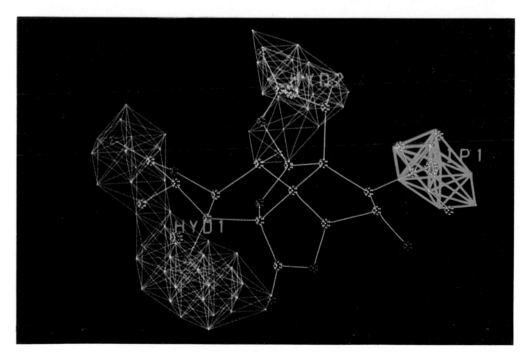

PLATE 3. Spatial conformation of BN 52022 (Ginkgolide C) determined by X-ray diffraction (8). (Top) Isolipophilicity curves. (Bottom) P_1 limits of each zone: LIP 1 — 0.7 to 0.8, HYD 1 — 0.2 to 0.3, HYD 2 — 0.2 to 0.3.

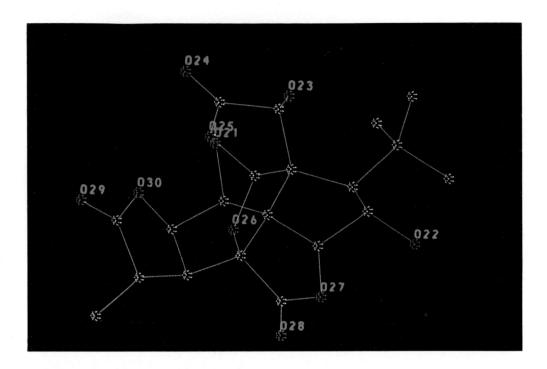

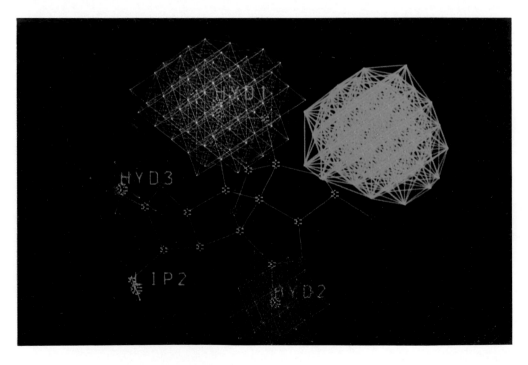

PLATE 4. Spatial conformation of BN 52023 (Ginkgolide M) determined by CHEMX molecular mechanism program. (Top) Isolipophilicity curves. (Bottom) P_1 limits of each zone: LIP 1-0.6 to 0.7, LIP 2 — 0.5 to 0.6, HYD 1 — 0.2 to 0.3, HYD 2 — 0.3 to 0.4, HYD 3 — 0.2 to 0.3.

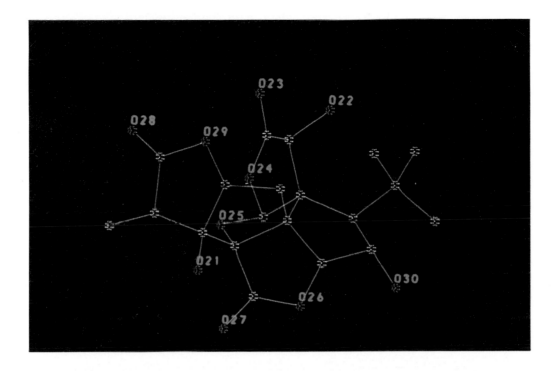

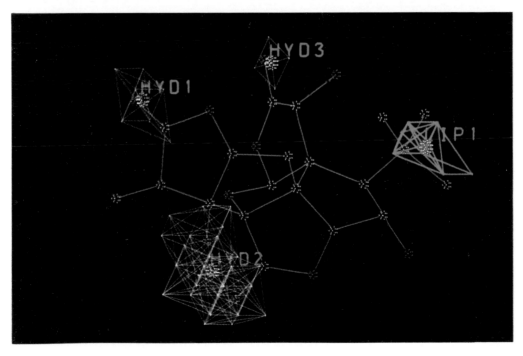

PLATE 5. Spatial conformation of BN 52024 (Ginkgolide J) determined by CHEMX molecular mechanism program. (Top) Isolipophilicity curves. (Bottom) P_1 limits of each zone: LIP 1 — 0.7 to 0.8, HYD 1 — 0.2 to 0.3, HYD 2 — 0.2 to 0.3, HYD 3 — 0.2 to 0.3.

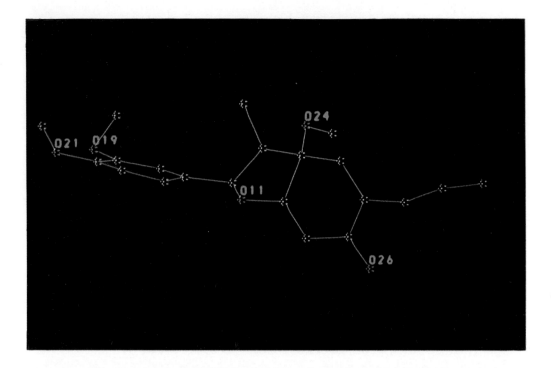

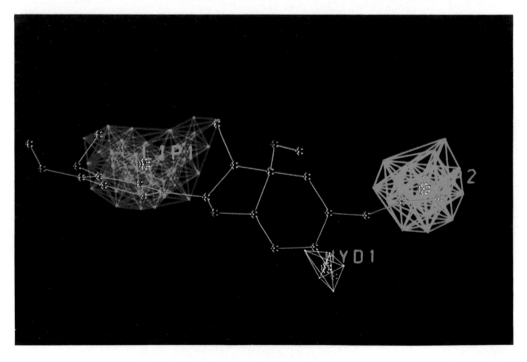

PLATE 6. Spatial conformation of kadsurenone determined by CHEMX molecular mechanism program. (Top) Isolipophilicity curves. (Bottom) P_1 limits of each zone: LIP 1 — 0.8 to 0.9, LIP 2 — 0.7 to 0.8, HYD 1 — 0.4 to 0.5.

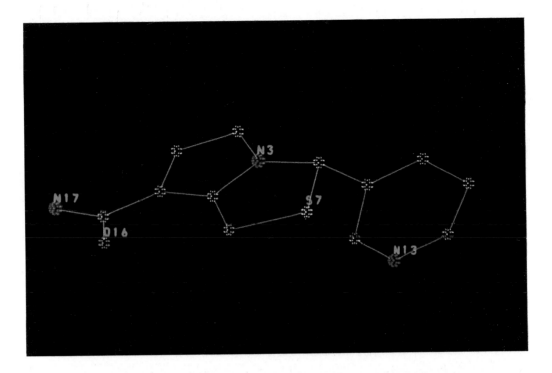

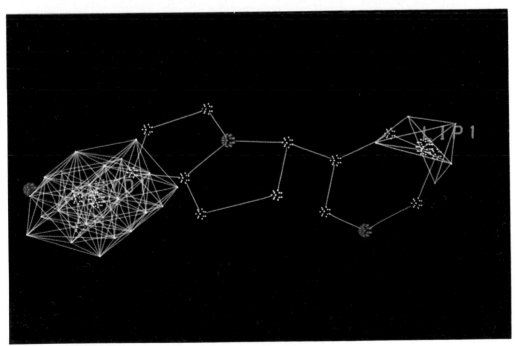

PLATE 7. Spatial conformation of RP 48740 determined by CHEMX molecular mechanism program. (Top) Isolipophilicity curves. (Bottom) P_1 limits of each zone: LIP 1 — 0.5 to 0.6, HYD 1 — 0.1 to 0.2.

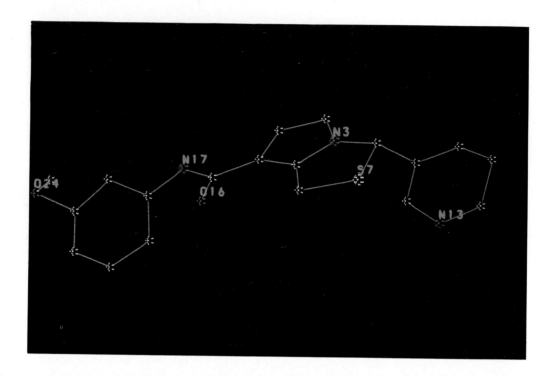

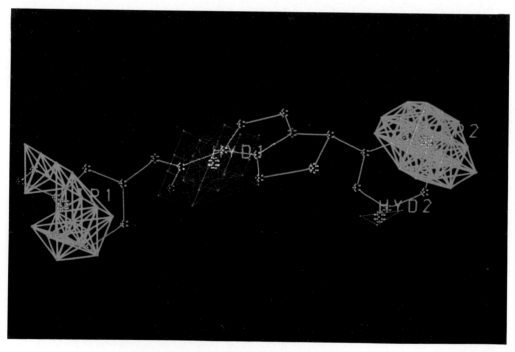

PLATE 8. Spatial conformation of RP 52629. (Top) Isolipophilicity curves. (Bottom) P_1 limits of each zone: LIP 1 — 0.7 to 0.8, LIP 2 — 0.6 to 0.7, HYD 1 — 0.3 to 0.4, HYD 2 — 0.1 to 0.2.

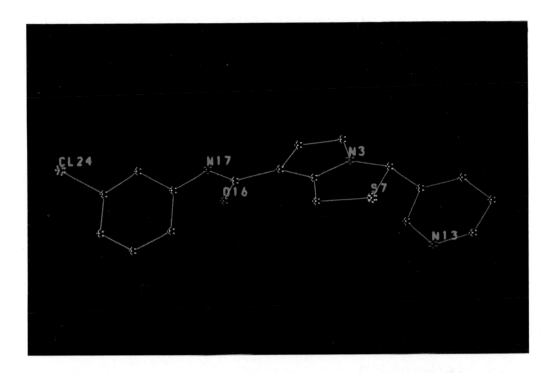

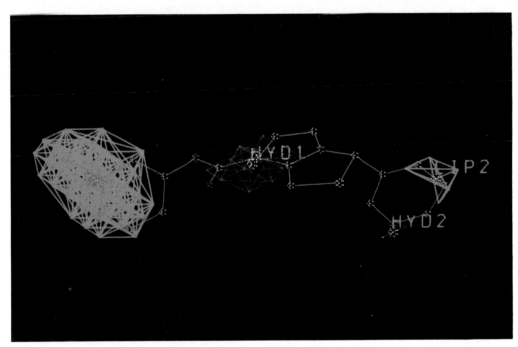

PLATE 9. Spatial conformation of RP 52770 determined by CHEMX molecular mechanism program. (Top) Isolipophilicity curves. (Bottom) P_1 limits of each zone: LIP 1 — 0.7 to 0.8, LIP 2 — 0.6 yo 0.7, HYD 1 — 0.3 to 0.4, HYD 2 — 0.4 to 0.5.

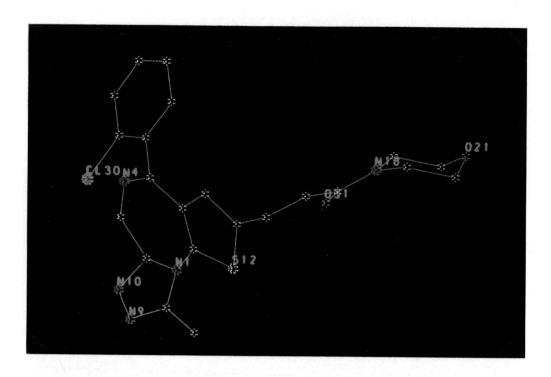

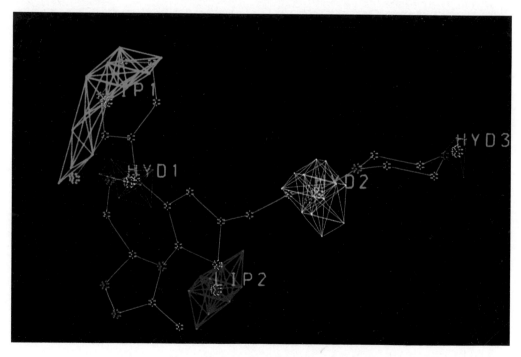

PLATE 10. Spatial conformation of WEB 2086 determined by CHEMX molecular mechanism program. (Top) Isolipophilicity curves. (Bottom) P_1 limits of each zone: LIP 1 — 0.7 to 0.8, LIP 2 — 0.8 to 0.9, HYD 1 — 0.3 to 0.4, HYD 2 — 0.4 to 0.5, HYD 3 — 0.3 to 0.4.

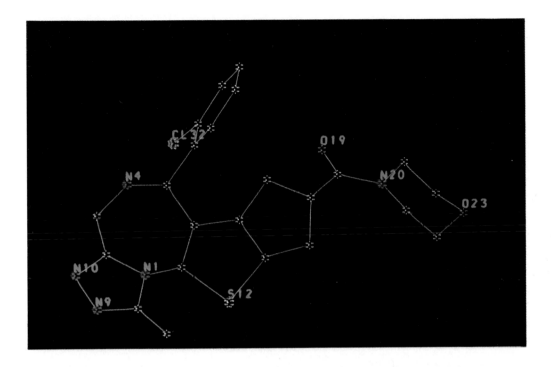

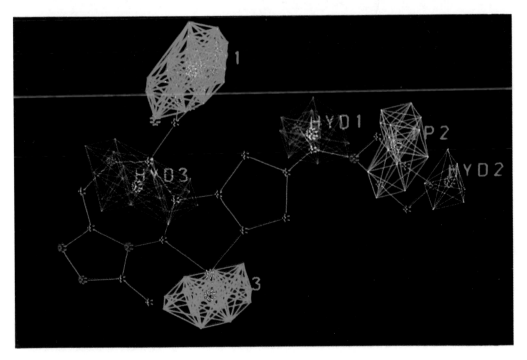

PLATE 11.   Spatial conformation of WEB 2170 determined by CHEMX molecular mechanism program. (Top) Isolipophilicity curves. (Bottom) P_1 limits of each zone: LIP 1 — 0.6 to 0.7, LIP 2 — 0.5 to 0.6, LIP 3 — 0.7 to 0.8, HYD 1 — 0.3 to 0.4, HYD 2 — 0.4 to 0.5, HYD 3 — 0.3 to 0.4.

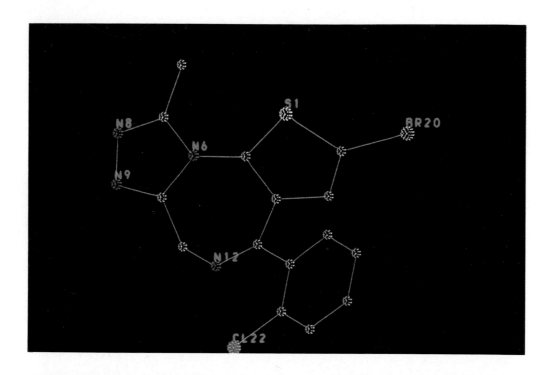

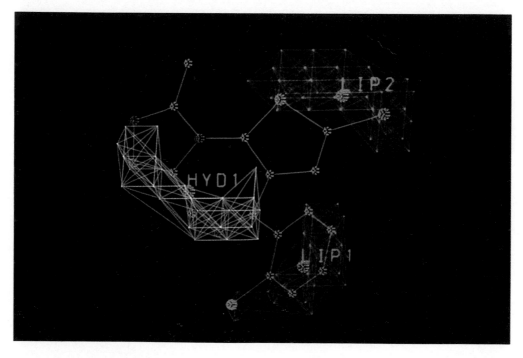

PLATE 12.   Spatial conformation of Brotizolan determined by CHEMX molecular mechanism program. (Top) Isolipophilicity curves. (Bottom) P_1 limits of each zone: LIP 1 — 0.8 to 0.9, LIP 2 — 0.8 to 0.9, HYD 1 — 0.4 to 0.5.

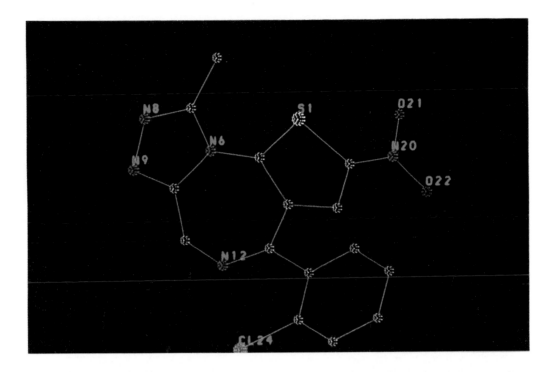

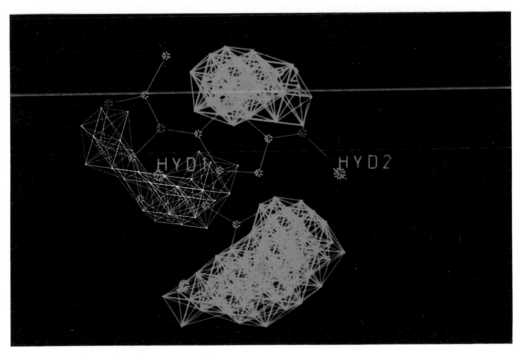

PLATE 13.   Spatial conformation of TBDZ A determined by CHEMX molecular mechanism program. (Top) Isolipophilicity curves. (Bottom) P_1 limits of each zone: LIP 1 — 0.7 to 0.8, LIP 2 — 0.7 to 0.8, HYD 1 — 0.4 to 0.5, HYD 2 — 0.4 to 0.5.

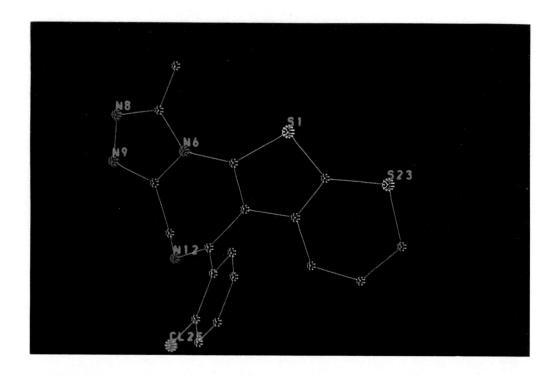

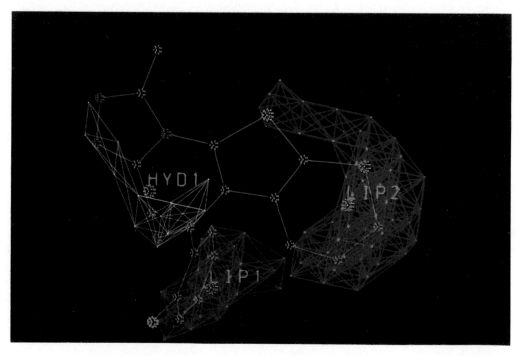

PLATE 14. Spatial conformation of TBDZ B determined by CHEMX molecular mechanism program. (Top) Isolipophilicity curves. (Bottom) P_1 limits of each zone: LIP 1 — 0.8 to 0.9, LIP 2 — 0.8 to 0.9, HYD 1 — 0.4 to 0.5.

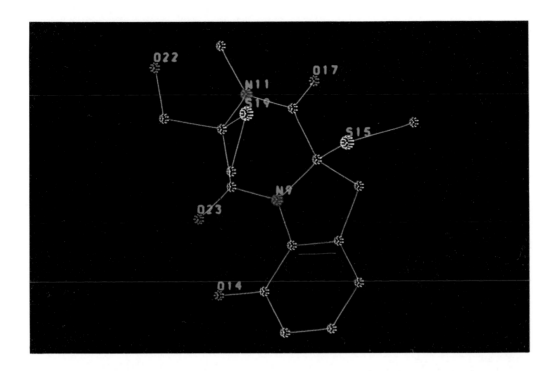

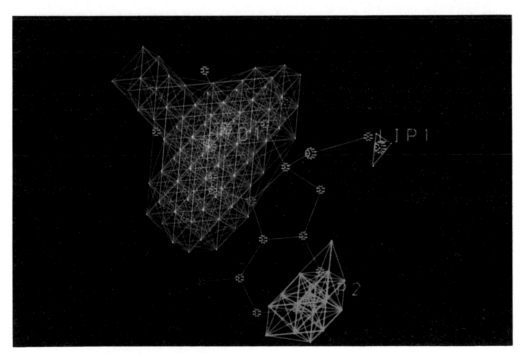

PLATE 15. Spatial conformation of Gliotoxin A determined by CHEMX molecular mechanism program. (Top) Isolipophilicity curves. (Bottom) P_1 limits of each zone: LIP 1 — 0.6 to 0.7, LIP 2 — 0.6 to 0.7, HYD 1 — 0.2 to 0.3.

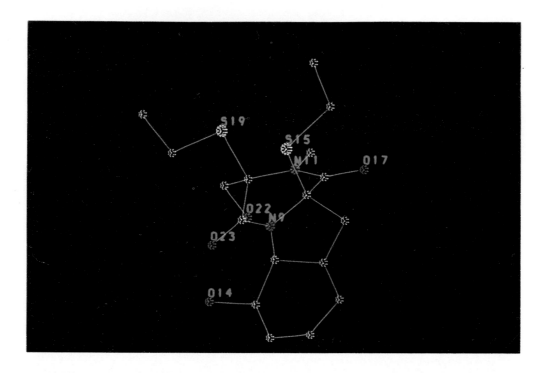

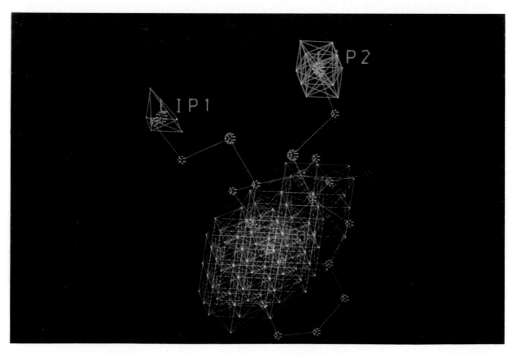

PLATE 16. Spatial conformation of Gliotoxin B determined by CHEMX molecular mechanism program. (Top) Isolipophilicity curves. (Bottom) P_l limits of each zone: LIP 1 — 0.5 to 0.6, LIP 2 — 0.5 to 0.6, HYD 1 — 0.1 to 0.2.

TABLE 2
P_1 Values Corresponding to MLP
Values

$$P_L = F \text{ (MLP)}$$

MLP			p_1		
1	< MLP <	∞	0.9	$\leq p_1 <$	1
0.6	$\leq$ MLP $\leq$	1	0.8	$\leq p_1 <$	0.9
0.4	$\leq$ MLP <	0.6	0.7	$\leq p_1 <$	0.8
0.2	$\leq$ MLP <	0.4	0.6	$\leq p_1 <$	0.7
0.1	$\leq$ MLP <	0.2	0.55	$\leq p_1 <$	0.6
−0.1	< MLP <	0.1	0.45	$< p_1 <$	0.55
−0.2	< MLP $\leq$	−0.1	0.4	$< p_1 \leq$	0.45
−0.4	< MLP $\leq$	−0.2	0.3	$< p_1 \leq$	0.4
−0.6	< MLP $\leq$	−0.4	0.2	$< p_1 \leq$	0.3
−1	< MLP $\leq$	−0.6	0.1	$< p_1 \leq$	0.2
−∞	< MLP $\leq$	−1	0	$< p_1 \leq$	0.1

$$P_1 = \frac{10^{MLP}}{1 + 10^{MLP}} \tag{6}$$

It is then possible to draw "equipotential" or isolipophilicity potential curves corresponding to probability areas varying from 0 to 1 (Table 2). Strong hydrophilic or lipophilic zones correspond to the hypothetical binding sites of a molecule.

Thus, the molecular geometrical representation of a drug can be simplified by using the MLP.

DETERMINATION OF SPATIAL CONFORMATION AND MOLECULAR LIPOPHILICITY POTENTIAL

The spatial conformations of drugs are those obtained either by radiocrystallography determination or by minimization of molecular energy using the molecular mechanism program of CHEMX.[5]

MLP determinations were made by using our own program.

RESULTS

For each molecule we give:

- its name
- its spatial conformation
- the 3D equipotential curves of strong hydrophilic or strong lipophilic zones and their center called, respectively, HYD n and LIP n where n will be the nth center of a hydrophilic or a lipophilic zone
- P_1 limits of each zone

DISCUSSION

If we consider the isolipophilicity curves of the different compounds, it is obvious there are always at least two zones for a molecule: a lipophilic one and a hydrophilic one. So we

TABLE 3
Distances (Å) between a Hydrophilic Center (Hyd) and a Lipophilic Center (Lip)

Molecule	Lip1 to Hyd1	Lip1 to Hyd2	Lip1 to Hyd3	Lip2 to Hyd1	Lip2 to Hyd2	Lip2 to Hyd3	Lip3 to Hyd1	Lip3 to Hyd2	Lip3 to Hyd3
BN 52020	6.9	6.7							
BN 52021	8.0	5.2							
BN 52022	7.9	5.5							
BN 52023	6.3	6.4	8.5	6.8	4.6	3.4			
BN 52024	8.0	7.4	4.7						
Kadsurenone	7.0			4.4					
RP 48740	7.5								
RP 52629	5.8	10.3		6.9	3.3				
RP 52770	6.3	11.2		6.7	2.9				
WEB 2086	4.0	7.7	11.2	4.8	6.0	9.1			
WEB 2170	4.6	9.2	4.3	3.3	2.5	9.4	6.4	8.8	4.4
Brotizolam	5.0			6.0					
TBDZ A	5.1	6.7		4.7	4.2				
TBDZ B	4.8			6.0					
Gliotoxin A	5.2			6.0					
Gliotoxin B	5.5			6.5					

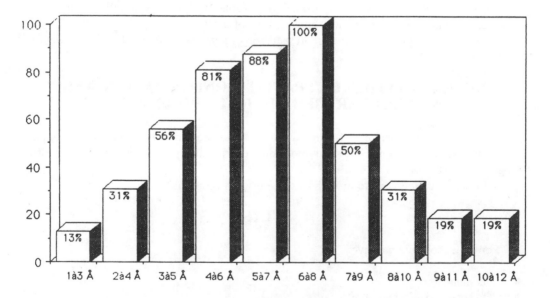

FIGURE 1.   Percentage of molecules having a distance D between a hydrophilic center and a lipophilic center such as $D = D_o \pm 1$ Å where D_o is an integer number between 2 and 11.

have calculated (see Table 3), for each molecule the distance D between the center of one of the lipophilic zones and the center of one of the hydrophilic zones. As shown in Figure 1, all molecules have at least one of the distances referred to as D such as:

$$D = 7 \pm 1 \text{ Å}$$

Depending on the molecular structure, the lipophilic zone envelopes:

- either an aliphatic group (tertiobutyl for BN 52020 to BN 52024, thioethyl for gliotoxin B)
- or an aromatic system (benzene ring in kadsurenone, WEB 2086, RP 52770, gliotoxin A, TBDZ A, pyridine ring in RP 52629, RP 48740, RP 52770)
- or a pseudo-aromatic system (thiophene in WEB 2170, WEB 2086, brotizolam, TBDZ B).

The hydrophilic zone is always near:

- either a carbonyl group (BN 52020 to BN 52024, gliotoxin A and B, RP 48740, RP 52629, RP 52770, WEB 2086, WEB 2170, kadsurenone)
- or a nitro group (TBDZ A)
- or a triazol ring (TBDZ B, brotizolam)

To conclude, we think that if molecules have to show an affinity for the receptor of the PAF acether, they must possess at least two areas of different lipophilicity separated by a distance of 6 to 8 Å.

The activity of these molecules may be modified by the relative importance of the lipophilic areas values.

REFERENCES

1. **Audry, E.**, *Th. Etat Es Sc. Pharm.*, Bordeaux, 1985.
2. **Audry, E., Dubost, J. P., Colleter, J. C., and Dallet, Ph.**, Une nouvelle approche des relations structure-activité le Potentiel de Lipophilie Moléculaire'', *Eur. J. Med. Chem. - Chim. Ther.*, 21, 71, 1986.
3. **Audry, E., Dubost, J. P., Dallet, Ph., Langlois, M. H., and Colleter, J. C.**, Le Potentiel de Lipophilie moléculaire: application à une série d'amines β-adrénolytiques, *Eur. J. Med. Chem. - Chim. Ther.*, 24, 155, 1989.
4. **Broto, P., Moreau, G., and Vandycke, C.**, Molecular structures perception, autocorrelation descriptor and SAR studies, *Eur. J. Med. Chem. - Chim. Ther.*, 19(1), 71, 1984.
5. CHEMX distributed by Chemical Design Ltd, Oxford, England.
6. **Dubost, J. P., Audry, E., Dallet, Ph., Montagut, M., and Carpy, A.**, Indirect molecular modelling approaches in the alpha adrenergic field, in *Q.S.A.R. in Drug Design and Toxicology*, Vol. 17, Elsevier, Amsterdam, 1987, 169.
7. **Dupont, L., Dideberg, L., Germain, G., and Braquet, P.**, Ginkgolide B (BN 52021) monohydrate a highly specific PAF/acether receptor antagonist isolated from *Ginkgo biloba* L., *Acta Crystallogr.*, C42, 1759, 1986.
8. **Dupont, L., Dideberg, L., and Braquet, P.**, Structure of Ginkgolide A (BN 52020) monohydrate and Gingkgolide C (BN 52022) ethanol-1-5-hydrate isolated from *Ginkgo biloba* L. *Acta Crystallogr.*, C43, 2377, 1987.
9. **Rekker, R. F.**, *The Hydrophobic Fragmental Constant*, Elsevier, Amsterdam, 1977.
10. **Van de Waterbeemd, H. and Testa, B.**, The parametrization of lipophilicity and other structural properties in drug design, in *Advances in Drug Research*, Vol. 16, Academic Press, New York, 1987, 87.

Index

INDEX

A

N-Acetylcarbamoyl derivative
  effects of distance between polar head moiety
    and, 106
  synthesis of, 102—105
Acetyltransferase, macrophage levels of, 10
Achiral analogs, 135, 149
ACTH, PAF effects on, 24
Actin, increased cytoskeletal levels of, 3
Acylcarbamoyl moiety, 120
N-Acylcarbamoyl derivatives, synthesis and structure-activity relationships of, 105—111
Adenylate cyclase, inhibition of, 3
Airway hypersensitivity
  in vitro studies on, 29—30
  in vivo studies of, 27—29
  PAF antagonists in, 27—30
Airway inflammation, PAF-associated, 181, 191
Airway miocrovascular leakage, prevention of, 162
Alkyl groups, 136
2-Alkylidene analogs, 136
Alkyl phospholipids, 97
Alkyl substutient, 239
Allergic conditions, PAF in pathology of, 47, see
  also Asthma
Allopurinol, and PAF-induced hypotension, 36
Allylphenol plus allylphenol derived neolignans,
  90—91
Alpha alkyl substituent, 239
Alpha-methyl group, effect of on hydrolysis rates,
  230—231
Alprazolam
  discovery of, 171
  displacement by, 4
  and PAF-induced chemoluminescence, 9—10
  in platelet aggregation, 5
  structure of, 51
Amidases, action of, 230
Amides, potency of in binding, 235—238
Aminoacylates
  biological results of
    in vitro studies, 120—128
    in vivo studies, 129—132
  chemistry of, 119
  synthetic scheme of, 121
Aminocarbamates
  biological results of
    in vitro studies, 120—128
    in vivo studies, 129—132
  chemistry of, 119
  synthetic scheme of, 122
Anaphylactic shock, see also Shock
  CV-3988 protective effect on, 105
  PAF-induced, 189—191
  passive cutaneous, 152

value of PAF antagonists in, 16
Angiotensin converting enzyme inhibitors, 21
Antigen-induced arthritis, 33
Anti-PAF action bioassay, 97
Arachidonic acid
  bronchoconstriction caused by, 252
  effect of PAF antagonists on
    metabolizing enzymes of, 251
  inhibition of ionophore-induced
    metabolism of in rat peritoneal macrophages,
    251
  products of metabolism of, 26
  promotion of release of, 3
  release of in thermal injury, 18
ARDS, 193, 197
Aromatic ring "a", 246, 256
Aromatic rings, effect of restriction of conformation
  of, 242
Arterial hypertension, PAF role in, 21—22
Arterial thrombosis, 131—132
Arthritis
  antigen-induced, 33
  PAF and antagonists in, 32—34
5-Aryl-2,3-dihydroimidazo[2,1a]isoquinoline, structure-activity relationships in, 221—227
Aryl-N-[4-(3-pyridinyl)butyl]carboxamides, structure
  of, 234
N-Aryl-3-(3-pyridyl)-1H,3H-pyrrolo[1,2-c]thiazole-
  7-carboxamides, 212
N-Aryl-pyrrolo[1,2-c]thiazole-7-carboxamides, optimization of, 208—209
Arylpropeneamides, structure-activity relationships
  of, 246—247
Asthma
  airway hypersensitivity in, 27
  complexity of, 256
  disease-related models of, 197
  eosinophils in, 12—14
  ovalbumin induced, 152—153
  PAF-induced, 47, 189—191
Astrocytes, PAF in metabolism of, 24
Atherogenesis, PAF role in, 21—22
Atherosclerosis, characteristics of, 43—44
Aza-glycerol, structural relationship of cyclic PAF
  analog to, 159

B

Bacteria, PMNL killing of, 9
BAPTA, inhibition of intracellular calcium and PAF
  release, 7
Benzodiazepine (BDZ), 171
Benzodiazepine (BDZ)-receptor antagonist, 171
Benzofuranoid C_6-C_3 dimers, 82

Z